Rapid Review of
Exotic Animal Medicine and Husbandry

Pet Mammals, Birds, Reptiles, Amphibians, and Fish

Karen L Rosenthal
MS DVM DiplAVBP
University of Pennsylvania, Philadelphia, Pennsylvania, USA

Neil A Forbes
BVetMed CBiol MIBiol RFP DipECAMS FRCVS
Great Western Referrals, Swindon, Wiltshire, UK

Fredric L Frye
BSc, DVM, MSc, CBiol, FIBiol, FRSM
Cloverdale, California, USA

Gregory A Lewbart
MS VMD DiplACZM
North Carolina State University, Raleigh, North Carolina, USA

T0272059

Manson Publishing/The Veterinary Press

Copyright © 2008 Manson Publishing Ltd
ISBN: 978-1-84076-055-2

A CIP catalogue record for this book is available from the British Library.

For full details of all Manson Publishing Ltd titles please write to:
Manson Publishing Ltd, 73 Corringham Road, London NW11 7DL, UK.
Tel: +44(0)20 8905 5150
Fax: +44(0)20 8201 9233
Email: manson@mansonpublishing.com
Website: www.mansonpublishing.com

Project manager: Paul Bennett
Copy editor: Peter Beynon
Design and layout: Cathy Martin, Presspack Computing Ltd
Colour reproduction: Tenon & Polert Colour Scanning Ltd, Hong Hong
Printed by: Grafos SA, Spain

Contents

Preface

Exotic animal medicine has evolved over the last two decades. Although gradual, the changes are profound. These changes are actually accelerated by the expectations of our clients, not necessarily by wide-ranging discoveries at our centers of learning. In fact, centers for research may lag behind the day-to-day cases we see in practice. As veterinarians, it is important for us to understand and recognize both the common and uncommon cases that enter our examination rooms. It is hoped that what follows in this book will help in this process.

Two decades ago veterinarians probably knew more about their avian patients than they did about their reptile or amphibian ones. And if veterinarians wanted to become familiar with the diseases of one particular group of exotic patients, they usually concentrated on the group where the most information could be found, which tended to be birds. Also, some veterinarians were content to be known as the 'doctor down the road' who could handle, take blood from, and treat your macaw or iguana. It was difficult to find concise, helpful information on just one group of exotic patients, but to find such information on more than one group was almost impossible. In fact, it was impossible. Veterinarians who treated birds were usually content knowing all they could about birds. Reptile patients were referred around the corner (if they were lucky), but it could be many miles around the corner if the nearest reptile colleague was not close by.

Over the last two decades the collective clinical experience in exotic animal medicine and surgery from colleagues throughout the world has led to a better understanding of health and disease in such patients. Numerous texts in a variety of formats have been published to bring this information to a greater audience, so veterinarians who have not had the opportunity to work with exotic animals can catch up with those who have. The self-assessment series of titles from which this book has evolved presented cases in a manner that imitated practice. There was a history, some examinations findings, and a patient with a lesion that could be illustrated. In many of these cases the reader was given the same options he or she would have in practice. What are the differentials? How can they be ruled out? How should the patient be treated? And the answers were just over the page, allowing for almost instantaneous learning.

This format was very well received. So well received in fact that demand dictated a book for each group of exotic animals seen in practice. Two decades ago, this was fine. However, this is no longer fine. The trend among organized veterinary exotic animal associations and journals is to consolidate rather than split. Many association meetings include more than one group of exotic animal presentations. Many colleagues do not see just avian or reptile patients, but wish to see all exotic patients. Clients would prefer to visit a veterinarian who can deal with all their exotic patients rather than visit someone who specializes in birds and someone else who specializes in reptiles. Sadly, our university system, in general, still lacks the resources to teach many of their veterinary students about exotic animal patients. For most newly graduated veterinarians, the ability to help these patients is a 'live and learn' process. This is not ideal for the patients and can be discouraging to fledgling veterinarians. This book was born in an effort to revive the successful format followed in the self-assessment series and to satisfy the appetite of all veterinarians who wish to learn more about exotic patients. We hope these pages will prove useful in the treatment of these wonderful patients.

Karen Rosenthal
Neil Forbes
Fred Frye
Greg Lewbart

Acknowledgement

In the course of writing and editing a book, there are numerous people, not apparent to the readership, without whom there would be no book. It could take another volume just to thank all of these people. But for this project there is one person in particular who needs to be acknowledged, and that is Peter Beynon. Without Peter's help, encouragement, and tireless editing, there would be mostly blank pages in this book. Peter, we cannot thank you enough for making this project a reality.

Abbreviations

ACE	angiotensin converting enzyme		KCl	potassium chloride
ACTH	adrenocorticotropic hormone		KHV	koi herpesvirus
AFA	ethyl alcohol, formalin, and acetic acid (solution)		KOH	potassium hydroxide
			LDH	lactic acid dehydrogenase
ALT (SGPT)	alanine aminotransferase		MIC	minimum inhibitory concentration
AP (SAP)	alkaline phosphatase		MMC	melanomacrophage center
AST (SGOT)	aspartate aminotransferase		MRI	magnetic resonance imaging
BUN	blood urea nitrogen		NaCl	sodium chloride
Ca	calcium		NSAID	nonsteroidal anitiinflammatory drug
CBC	complete blood count		OIE	World Organisation for Animal Health
CDV	canine distemper virus		OTC	over the counter
CHV1	cyprinid herpesvirus 1		PBFD	psittacine beak and feather disease
CNS	central nervous system		PCR	polymerase chain reaction
CPK (CK)	creatine phosphokinase		PCV	packed cell volume
CT	computed tomography		p/o	per os
DEFRA	Department for Environment, Food and Rural Affairs (UK)		PO_4	phosphate
			p.p.t.	parts per thousand
DMSA	dimercaptosuccinic acid		p.p.m.	parts per million
DNA	deoxyribonucleic acid		PTH	parathyroid hormone
DTM	dermatophyte test medium		PVC	polyvinyl chloride (piping)
ECG	electrocardiogram		RBC	red blood cell
EDTA	ethylenediamine tetra-acetic acid		RNA	ribonucleic acid
ELISA	enzyme-linked immunosorbent assay		s/c	subcutaneous/subcutaneously
GGT	gamma glutamyltransferase		SADV	sialodacryoadenitis virus
GI	gastrointestinal		SBI	swim bladder inflammation (virus)
HLLE	head and lateral line erosion		SCUD	septicemic cutaneous ulcerative disease
HPOA	hypertrophic pulmonary osteoarthropathy		SG	specific gravity
IFA	immunofluorescence assay		SVC	spring viremia of carp (virus)
i/c	intracoelomic		TP	total protein
i/m	intramuscular/intramuscularly		UV	ultraviolet
i/o	intraosseous/intraosseously		WBC	white blood cell
i/v	intravenous/intravenously			

Section 1
SMALL MAMMALS

Karen L Rosenthal

Classification of cases by species

Rabbits	1 to 40
Ferrets	41 to 56
Guinea pigs	57 to 66
Hamsters	67 to 73
Hedgehogs	74 to 81
Chinchillas	82 to 86
Rats	87 to 93
Mice	94 to 95
Squirrels	96 to 97
Gerbil	98

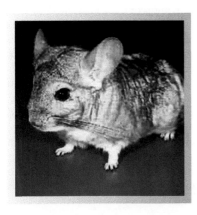
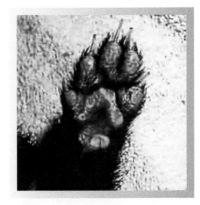
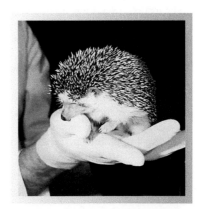

Introduction

Exotic animal medicine is, in my biased opinion, the most exciting area of veterinary medicine today. It is stimulating, it is dynamic, and it is demanding. The challenge can quickly turn to frustration if the knowledge that is needed to work with these animals is not immediately available. When we think of the more traditional areas of companion animal veterinary medicine, the information we require is usually right at our fingertips in the form of books, journals, review articles, or even calls to colleagues. The basic information for more traditional pets is taught to us at veterinary school and the diseases, diagnostics, and treatments become second nature while in practice. When asked by a new dog owner the lifespan of their pet, we do not need to consult a colleague halfway across the world to answer that question, but when a prospective new owner of a small mammal asks which of the common small mammal pets lives the longest, how many of us can rattle off the lifespan of chinchillas, ferrets, guinea pigs, or hedgehogs.

It is therefore apparent that even the basic knowledge of these exotic pets can be patchy at best. For many of us, the curriculum in veterinary school did not include the majority of these pets and what we learned was probably outdated and wrong. When asked a question in the examination room, often there is no knowledge base to fall back on, and no frame of reference. We need information. This is what this section hopes to accomplish, so that armed with the basics you will feel comfortable with these different pets and also have a source of information to enable you to go further and to diagnose and treat these great pets.

Exotic animal medicine has grown by leaps and bounds. In the 1970s and 1980s these were the bizarre animals brought in by eccentric owners. However, in the last two decades many of these species have become as popular in some areas of the world as dogs and cats. For example, in the UK by the second decade of this century, rabbits may surpass other pets to become the most popular house pet. Would anyone have imagined that in 1970? But then again, would any veterinarian treating horses and cattle in 1900 believe that people now pay money for their dogs and cats to be treated. Everything is relative.

Veterinarians want to do their best for all of their patients, and owners want the best care for their pets. The difficulty with exotic pets is that our knowledge changes so rapidly that it is difficult to keep up with the best diagnostic and treatment options. Sometimes, new diseases appear that are regional and it is not easy to find out this information. However, it is no longer acceptable to say that no one knows about rabbit dental disease or that it is impossible to treat adrenal gland disease in ferrets. It is no longer acceptable to categorize these animals as second-class pets. There will always be owners who won't pay for the care these pets need, but then there are always owners who won't pay for the care their dogs and cats need. Over the last two decades a 'tipping point' has been reached and there are now owners of exotic pets who want the same level of veterinary care for these pets as is provided for other companion animals. We can take this further and say that there are owners who want not only equal care to dogs and cats, but the same level as is given to people. Some owners do not think twice when explained the benefits of a CT scan; they do not ask how much but instead ask when it can be done. Owners have pushed veterinarians to give a very high level of care, which in turn has propelled our knowledge of how to diagnose and treat these pets as never before.

How has our knowledge of these animals increased? Some of it is through research. Research on the diseases of small mammals is mostly limited to their use as animal models or laboratory subjects. The information garnered from these studies is extrapolated to pets. Realistically, not many of these studies are relevant to the information we need to treat conditions seen in pet small mammals. Due to the lack of a large, profitable market, there is little research into drug treatments and nutrition of these pets. Some of the veterinary care of small mammals is extrapolated from the way we treat dogs and cats. This carries over well with carnivores such as ferrets, but can fall short when working with herbivores. The database of knowledge about herbivores and other small mammals, and much of the information contained within this book, has over the past three decades come mainly from anecdotal information.

Although the techniques used in small mammals are similar to those used in other pets, it is extremely important to understand the significance these methods make in their veterinary care. The four aspects of veterinary care that need to be emphasized are history gathering techniques, examination techniques, diagnostics, and special instrumentation. Many of the diseases in small mammal medicine concern poor husbandry techniques, so it is vital that the veterinarian who sees small mammals is well informed. Develop a fill-in form so that you never miss a question. By not asking the correct questions, you may totally miss the diagnosis. In small mammals, possibly the most important diagnostic test is the history form. Description of diet and housing are two of the most important aspects of history taking. Where has the pet been, which animals has it been exposed to, and where did the pet come from are some of the other important questions to ask. Examination techniques are very similar to those carried out in dogs and cats, but there are some aspects that are particularly important in small mammal examination. In rabbits it is always important to check the teeth for points, to auscultate the abdomen for gut sounds, and to examine the perineum for stool impactions. In ferrets it is always important to note changes to the normal hair coat. Diagnostic tests are also similar to those performed in dogs and cats, but the clinician needs to be aware of the size limitations and that many tests are not backed up with published studies. Also, it is important that the specialized instruments necessary to work with these animals are present in the veterinary practice (i.e. small needles and syringes, gram scales, and small surgical instruments). Finally, medications in dosage forms and volumes specifically designed for small mammals must also be available.

The advances in rabbit medicine are probably as significant as in any species over the last two decades. Although we may not have all the answers, we understand the pathophysiology of disease in these pets much better than we did even five years ago. One of the most vexing problems in rabbit medicine has been disease of the teeth and jaw abscesses. It is apparent now that in most rabbits these conditions are related. It is almost unheard of to have a jaw abscess without concomitant dental disease. In the past we admitted to not understanding the etiology of these jaw abscesses and explained them away as spontaneous infections of the bone. Not knowing the etiology, we would explain it as sepsis due to an infection in some far away part of the body. We would try treating for liver abscesses or pneumonia or pyelonephritis that we supposed existed, even though there was no supporting evidence. We now have a clearer picture of the etiology of jaw abscesses; elongated, overgrowing premolar and molar tooth roots causing damage to the maxilla and mandible and allowing the cesspool of bacteria in the mouth to invade the bone. No longer do we place the blame solely on *Pasteurella multocida* for these infections. In fact, *Pasteurella* organisms play only a role in jaw abscesses. Likewise, we understand the pathophysiology of dental disease much better today than we did ten years ago. We understand that incisor malocclusion may be secondary to cheek teeth disease. We cannot treat incisor disease successfully unless we also address the cheek tooth disease, the primary cause of the problem. Although we do not have all of the answers, our understanding permits us to diagnose the disease sooner, plan more effective treatments, and give a more realistic prognosis to the owners.

Another area of rabbit medicine in which great strides have been made in developing better veterinary care is proper nutrition. We have left behind the idea of a complete diet being fed *ad libitum*; 'any brand' rabbit pellets with some dried-out leafless alfalfa on the side. Although the entire story of proper rabbit nutrition has yet to be written, the dangers inherent in the diet we used to feed is becoming clearer to even the most stubborn adherent to a pelleted diet. It is more difficult to convince the owner that the convenience of a pelleted diet may be condemning their rabbit to a less than healthy lifestyle, but we have the information available now to at least allow the owner to understand why their rabbit has become sick on a pelleted only diet. It is likely that dental problems, at least partially, exist in rabbits due to the lack of proper fiber in the diet. This lack of fiber is directly related to the pelleted diet; specifically, the pelleted diet most owners find at the pet store. Although the connection between a pelleted diet and dental disease is supposed, it is very clear that the traditional, low-fiber, pellet only diet clearly contributes to poor cecal health. The lack of fiber, the high caloric content, and the high carbohydrate content of food can lead directly to a change in the normal cecal contents. The bacterial population changes, the entire milieu of the cecum changes, and gastrointestinal disease develops. Poorly formed stools, ileus, and eventually anorexia develop and the rabbit is brought to the hospital. The change in the bacterial population may predispose the rabbit to other bacterial infections.

Great strides have also been made in our understanding of some of the diseases that plague pet ferrets. The two most common diseases in older ferrets, insulinoma and adrenal gland disease, still perplex owners and veterinarians, but our understanding through the last decade has improved our care of these pets. We understand that surgery, not medical treatment, is the best overall treatment for insulinoma. We are better prepared to counsel owners on how to recognize signs of this disease in their pet ferrets. Our knowledge of adrenal gland disease has greatly increased over the last 15 years. We still may not understand the etiology, but we now have more treatment options and have a larger knowledge base with which to advise owners intelligently on the prognosis and choices they have for their pets with this disease. Other aspects of ferret medicine have also improved over the years. Gastrointestinal diseases have changed over the last decade, but we are in a better position to recommend treatment options. Vaccines are still used in ferrets and we understand better how to utilize them.

Guinea pigs and other small rodents are seen more frequently in veterinary practices today than they were even ten years ago. Since we have a larger database of knowledge, we are in a better position to advise the client on the treatment and prognosis of the diseases we see in these patients. We still run up against the problem of balancing the cost of testing against what the owner is prepared to pay. However, the basics of veterinary care are still important. How to take blood, what to feed, and how to handle these pets are skills that we are still learning, since we are not given this type of information in veterinary school. Ectoparasites continue to plague these small mammals, but they are easy and inexpensive to diagnose, the signs are usually obvious, treatments are easy to administer, and the pet can be cured. Of course, this whole process cannot start unless the veterinarian is armed with the knowledge that ectoparasites are common problems in small mammals.

Hedgehogs, both European and African, continue to be seen in large numbers by veterinarians. Skin disease is still a common complaint and both ectoparasites and fungal infections are diseases that are commonly treated. A basic knowledge of the care of hedgehogs is essential and knowledge of how to work with these shy animals is important.

The basics of small mammals transcend all species. It is important to understand anesthesia, venipuncture, handling, and diet of these increasingly common pets.

English and Latin names

Chinchilla	*Chinchilla langier*
Ferret	*Mustela putorius furo*
Gerbil (Mongolian)	*Meriones unguiculatus*
Guinea pig	*Cavia porcellus*
Hamster (Syrian)	*Mesocricetus auratus*
Hedgehog (European)	*Erinaceus europaeus*
Hedgehog (African)	*Atelerix albiventris*
Mouse	*Mus musculus*
Rabbit (cottontail)	*Sylvilagus nuttalii*
Rabbit (domestic)	*Oryctolagus cuniculus*
Rat	*Rattus norvegicus*
Squirrel	*Citellus tridecemlineatus*

Case 1: **Rabbit with GI ileus**

CLINICAL PRESENTATION. A two-year-old female rabbit is anorectic for three days. The rabbit is fed a diet consisting primarily of pellets, with hay and grain-based treats given on occasion. The owner reports that the rabbit refused to eat pellets for two days, but continued to eat hay, treats, and the newspaper bedding in the cage before becoming anorectic. The rabbit has produced scant, dry feces since the onset of anorexia. It has a small amount of palpable intestinal gas, but is otherwise normal in appearance and attitude

DIFFERENTIAL DIAGNOSES. GI obstructive disease does occur in rabbits. The most common causes include rubber, plastic, small masses of dried ingesta mixed with hair or carpet fibers, and stricture of the GI tract from postsurgical adhesions. These patients are acutely and severely depressed and exhibit abdominal discomfort. Radiography in these cases reveals significant dilation of the stomach.

INVESTIGATION. An abdominal radiograph is taken (**1**).

DIAGNOSIS. GI stasis.

ETIOLOGY. GI stasis is often the end result of GI hypomotility caused by a diet low in fiber and/or high in starch. When GI motility is slowed, the stomach and the cecum do not empty properly and the material they contain may become partially dehydrated. When the patient becomes anorectic, complete GI stasis occurs, resulting in further dehydration and impaction of the stomach and cecal contents. Often, radiographs reveal a 'halo' of air around the gastric contents. Frequently, this is what is occurring when rabbits are diagnosed with a gastric trichobezoar or 'wool block'. The term 'trichobezoar' is misleading because the problem is not exclusively an accumulation of hair. Nearly every rabbit has hair present in the gastric contents due to continual grooming. When the gastric contents become dehydrated, the hair, which represents only a portion of the stomach contents, is bound together in a matrix of compacted ingesta. This is different from a true trichobezoar, which is a tightly compacted mass composed of nearly 100% hair, as seen in cats or ferrets.

Rabbits usually crave high-fiber items, such as hay and paper, when they experience GI motility problems. Feces decrease in size and eventually cease altogether when the rabbit becomes anorectic. Early in the disease, these patients will have little or no abdominal discomfort and will appear bright and alert. Anorexia can eventually lead to hepatic lipidosis, which will result in further deterioration of the patient's condition. As the disease progresses, large quantities of painful gas build up through the entire GI tract.

MANAGEMENT. The single most common contributing factor in GI motility problems in the rabbit is low dietary fiber. The nondigestible fiber portion of the diet is essential to promote normal GI tract motility. In addition, a high-starch diet, ingestion of toxins, or inappropriate antibiotics can lead to changes in the cecal pH, resulting in dysbiosis, which in turn can cause cecal impaction and lowered GI motility.

Therapy is directed towards restoring normal GI tract motility and correcting underlying dietary problems. The stomach contents are rehydrated and GI motility stimulated through administration of a high moisture and fiber diet, parenteral fluids, and GI motility drugs. Grass hay and fresh leafy greens, such as dandelion greens, parsley, romaine lettuce, carrot top or kale, should be offered to the rabbit. Many rabbits will eat these high-fiber foods eagerly, avoiding the need for syringe feeding. If the rabbit refuses to eat on its own, appropriate assisted feedings can be given. The use of supplements that are high in fat or starch should be avoided. Also, the use of psyllium powder or other fiber products that draw water out of the colon should be avoided. Due to the nature of the physiology of the proximal colon, the use of these products may lead to cecal or colonic impaction. Typically, stools may not be produced for up to 72 hours after commencing assisted feeding. After replacing fluid deficits, lactated Ringer's solution (maintenance level of 75–100 mg/kg/day s/c, i/v, or i/o) is administered. For prevention, a diet of free-choice quality grass hay, fresh herbage and limited concentrate foods is recommended. High-starch treats must not be given.

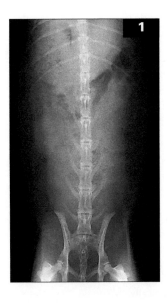

Case 2: **Rabbit syphilis**

CLINICAL PRESENTATION. A young doe in a herd of breeding rabbits has vesicles and ulcerated epidermis with a keratin rim on the vulva (**2**). There are no other clinical signs of disease in any of the other rabbits.

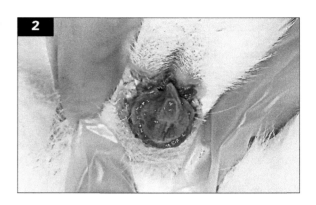

DIFFERENTIAL DIAGNOSES. Treponematosis (syphilis), bacterial dermatitis, contact dermatitis.

INVESTIGATION. Physical examination and response to treatment are typically diagnostic for rabbit syphilis. A definitive diagnosis is made by both cytology and histopathology. Material scraped from the lesions is examined under dark-field microscopy to demonstrate the spiral-shaped organisms. Diagnosis is also confirmed by a direct immunofluorescence test. Serologic assays, the indirect IFA, and a microhemagglutination test are used to detect subclinical carriers of the disease.

DIAGNOSIS. Rabbit syphilis caused by the spirochete *Treponema cuniculi*.

ETIOLOGY. Ulcerative lesions at the mucocutaneous junctions of the genitalia, anus, nose, eyelids, or lips are typical of this disease. Lesions on the face are a result of autoinfection from the rabbit grooming the infected genital area. The infection is transmitted by direct contact between breeding rabbits and from mother to young. Mild lesions may resolve spontaneously, but infected rabbits become carriers, with the spirochetes remaining latent in the lymph glands. Treponematosis is endemic and subclinical in many rabbitries. Other signs of this disease include abortions, metritis, and infertility.

PREVALENCE. This infection is more common in a breeding herd. It is less common in a single rabbit household.

MANAGEMENT. Two to three injections of benzathine penicillin G (42,000 iu/kg i/m) should be given given at seven-day intervals. This results in regression of the lesions and eliminates the infection. Although injectable penicillin is relatively safe, the rabbit should be fed a high-fiber diet to avoid potential cecal dysbiosis. Do not use beta-lactam antibiotics orally in the rabbit. To control the infection in a herd, it is necessary to treat the breeders. To eliminate treponematosis in a herd, only seronegative rabbits should be used for breeding.

PROGNOSIS. With proper treatment, this disease can be cured in most rabbits. It is always possible that the lesions may recede but a carrier state remains. Also, rabbits can become reinfected if exposed to diseased rabbits.

Case 3: **Rabbit mite infestation**

CLINICAL PRESENTATION. This rabbit (**3a**) has developed dandruff and is losing hair. On physical examination, reddened, hairless, scaly patches are noted over the head and back. The owner relates that the rabbit appears to be scratching the area of hair loss.

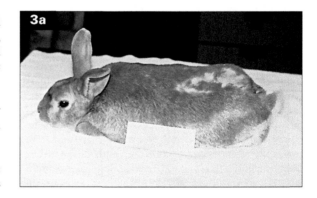

DIFFERENTIAL DIAGNOSES. Cheyletiellosis, other ectoparasites, dermatophytosis, barbering, bacterial dermatitis, contact dermatitis.

INVESTIGATION. On a superficial skin scrape, the organism shown in **3b** was recovered. The mite is identified by the large palpal claws on its anterior surface. It can often be seen grossly visible moving in the heavily scaled areas. It is also possible to use clear cellophane tape to collect the mites from the fur and skin. The tape is then examined microscopically.

ETIOLOGY. *Cheyletiella parasitivorax.* This organism is referred to as 'walking dandruff'.

PREVALENCE. This disease is seen occasionally in pet rabbits. It can easily spread from rabbit to rabbit.

MANAGEMENT. Ivermectin (0.20–1.0 mg/kg s/c q7d) is administered for 2–4 doses. Some workers also suggest dusting with carbaryl or permethrin powder at weekly intervals. Both of these medications can cause reactions in rabbits if they are exposed to them for an extended period of time; therefore, they are less safe than ivermectin. However, they can be used in the environment to kill any mites that may be outside the enclosure. Using lime/sulfur dips every two weeks for 2–3 treatments has also been suggested, but ivermectin appears to be very safe and effective. *C. parasitivorax* survives in the environment longer than most mites; therefore, the premises remain a source of infection and must also be treated. Flea elimination products, including desiccants that are safe for cats, work well, but

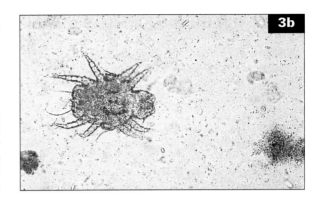

prolonged treatment may be necessary. These products must be used cautiously, especially in debilitated or obese rabbits, as deaths have been reported. On occasion, the mites affect humans and other animals.

PROGNOSIS. Excellent for a complete recovery.

Case 4: **Rabbit GI disease**

INTRODUCTION. Many pet rabbits are fed diets low in fiber. This low-fiber diet leads to numerous signs of disease such as anorexia, lethargy, and soft stools. In most cases, a thorough diet history will explain the signs of disease in these rabbits.

ETIOLOGY. The rabbit has evolved a unique GI anatomy and physiology in order to survive on high-fiber foods. Rabbits are herbivores and hindgut fermentors like horses (colon fermentor) and large ruminants. However, because of their small body size, rabbits are unable to store large volumes of coarse fiber for long periods of time, which would allow for bacterial and protozoal digestion. Rabbits have a system that eliminates fiber from the gut as rapidly as possible and employs its digestive process on the nonfiber portion of forage, which is directed into the cecum for fermentation. This system is driven by the presence of fiber in the diet.

The rabbit has the largest stomach and cecum of any monogastric mammal. The stomach of the rabbit is simple and acts as a storage vessel for the ingested feed. The rabbit has a well-developed cardiac sphincter, which is arranged in such a way that the rabbit cannot vomit. Suckling rabbits have a pH of 5–6.5 in their stomach.

The pH drops at the time of weaning. Adult rabbits have a remarkably low pH of between 1.5 and 2.2 in their stomach. The higher pH of young rabbits allows the normal microbial population of the gut to develop; however, it also predisposes young rabbits to develop pathogenic bacterial infections.

PREVALENCE. GI disease due to diets low in fiber is very common in pet rabbits.

MANAGEMENT. Rabbits should be fed diets that are appropriate for their unique GI anatomy and physiology. This should include grasses and hays. Even high-fiber pellets should be limited, as not only do rabbits need high fiber, but their GI systems need fiber length, not just fiber. Low-fiber pellets should be not be fed, even in limited amounts.

PROGNOSIS. Most rabbits respond well to a diet change, even if signs are present. In rabbits debilitated because of a poor diet, supportive care along with a diet change is usually successful. Therefore, the prognosis in most rabbits with signs related to a poor diet is very good.

Case 5: **Rabbit with an intraocular abscess**

CLINICAL PRESENTATION. This three-year-old spayed female rabbit has a progressively enlarging white area in its eye (**5**). Currently, there is a bulge in the cornea over the white area.

DIFFERENTIAL DIAGNOSES. Bacterial intraocular abscess, fungal intraocular abscess, neoplasia.

INVESTIGATION. The mass should be aspirated and cytology and culture performed. Skull radiographs and CT can determine the extent of destruction and if dental disease is part of the etiology. Ocular ultrasound will determine if a retrobulbar component is also involved.

DIAGNOSIS. This is an intraocular abscess.

ETIOLOGY. In the past, intraocular abscesses have been largely attributed to *Pasteurella multocida*. However, it is likely that there are multiple bacterial organisms responsible for this condition. Recent reports suggest that anaerobic bacteria are common in these abscesses. Also, extension of a dental abscess should always be considered.

PREVALENCE. These are common problems in rabbits. There is no particular signalment.

MANAGEMENT. Antibiotic treatment, both topical and systemic, can be used, but it may be unsuccessful in curing this infection. A more sure method of treatment cure is enucleation. Indications for enucleation include intraocular abscesses, trauma, and other end-stage ocular diseases. Surgery must be approached very cautiously, as the very large orbital venous sinus can cause significant, even fatal, hemorrhage if it is lacerated.

Two enucleation techniques in rabbits are described to avoid cutting the sinus:
- The first technique is a transconjunctival approach. The borders of the eyelids are removed and the palpebral conjunctiva dissected off the surface of the eyelids. Dissection is continued on to the bulbar conjunctiva along the globe, staying as close as possible to the surface of the globe to avoid damaging the venous sinus. Once all the periorbital structures are dissected free from the globe, a hemostatic clip is placed on the optic nerve and blood vessels and the globe removed.
- Alternatively, a transpalpebral approach can be used. Dissection is performed, staying as close to the wall of the bony orbit as possible in order to avoid damaging the venous sinus. All the structures are removed from within the bony orbit. If the sinus begins to bleed, hemostatic clips are placed blindly in order to control the hemorrhage. As a last approach, the globe is removed as quickly as possible, the bony orbit is packed with gel foam, and digital pressure is applied to control the hemorrhage. All conjunctival and glandular tissue is removed prior to closure. The eyelids are sutured closed once hemostasis is achieved. In most rabbits, 3-0 or 4-0 nylon works well.

PROGNOSIS. If this is an isolated abscess and enucleation is performed, it is unlikely that the infection will recur. However, if the condition is an extension of dental disease, enucleation will not by itself cure the primary problem. If medical treatment is attempted, the prognosis is variable.

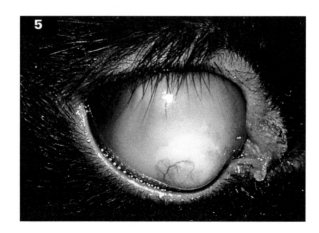

Case 6: **Rabbit with pinna necrosis due to thrombosis**

CLINICAL PRESENTATION. A three-year-old female rabbit is anorectic and has ileus. Initially, it is treated with intravenous chloramphenicol, an intravenous balanced electrolyte solution, and multiple syringe feedings. The patient does well until four days later, when it develops a dry, leather-like ear tip (6).

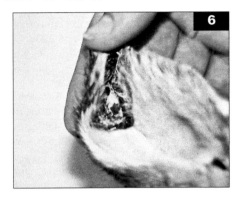

DIFFERENTIAL DIAGNOSES. Phlebitis with ischemic necrosis of the ear tip, trauma (especially in the long-eared breeds), disseminated intravascular coagulation, frostbite, fly or insect bites, and cold agglutinin disease.

INVESTIGATION. In this case, history is the most important diagnostic test. The fact that an ear catheter was placed and medication passed into that catheter makes ischemic necrosis the likely cause.

DIAGNOSIS. Phlebitis with ischemic necrosis of the ear tip resulting from the intravenous catheter.

ETIOLOGY. This is a common sequela resulting from the use of aural intravenous catheters, especially in the short-eared breeds. Administration of irritating intravenous medications makes this condition more likely to occur.

PREVALENCE. Common when catheters are placed in the pinna. This condition can also occur with aural venipuncture.

MANAGEMENT. The necrotic tissue is amputated surgically. The patient is given a broad-spectrum antibiotic for seven days. In addition, contact with flies or other insects must be prevented. Phlebitis with ischemic necrosis can be prevented by placing catheters in peripheral veins such as the cephalic and lateral saphenous veins.

PROGNOSIS. The prognosis for recovery is good with appropriate care.

Case 7: **The appearance of the normal fundus of rabbits and guinea pigs**

CLINICAL PRESENTATION. A rabbit and a guinea pig present for ocular examination. Both species have a unique appearance to the fundus. The fundus of a rabbit (7a) and a guinea pig (7b) are shown.

The fundus of the rabbit is normal. Lagomorphs possess a merangiotic retinal vascular pattern where vessels emanate from the optic nerve head and pass horizontally in association with the white medullary rays. The medullary rays represent myelinated nerve fibers. The optic nerve of the rabbit is far superior, which results in a blind spot coincident with a view of the ground. This is a place from where few rabbit predators approach. The optic disc has a deep physiologic cup that should not be misdiagnosed as indicative of glaucoma.

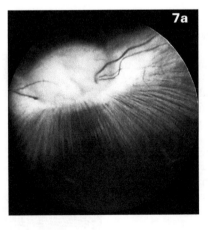
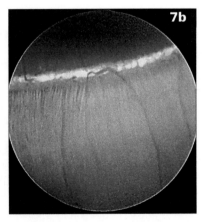

The fundus of the guinea pig is normal. Reportedly, the guinea pig has a paurangiotic retinal vascular pattern similar to that in the horse, but clinically it is considered to be anangiotic, as retinal vessels are never observed. The orange stripes in 7b represent choroidal vessels visualized through the avascular retina.

Case 8: **Rabbit handling and potential fractures and luxations**

INTRODUCTION. Rabbits have a fragile lumbar spine that can luxate or fracture easily if the animal is handled incorrectly. There are several described techniques for picking up a rabbit.

The hindquarters of the rabbit must always be supported when picking it up or transporting it. Rabbits should be removed from their containers on the floor to prevent potential 'escape' jumps from a high table. In addition, rabbits should be weighed on the floor to prevent similar accidents.

The three methods of picking up a rabbit are: (1) The loose skin over the back of the neck is grasped and the rabbit lifted up while placing the other hand under the hindquarters (**8**). (2) An open hand is placed under the thorax and, as the rabbit is lifted, the thorax is grasped and the other hand used to support the hindquarters. (3) The thorax is grasped as in (2) with one hand and the lower lumbar area firmly grasped with the other hand. This firm grip on the lumbar area will frequently cause a fractious rabbit to stop kicking and it protects the area of the spine that is often luxated or fractured. In each of these cases the rabbit is transported immediately to the examination table, where a mat or towel is placed to prevent the feet from slipping. Rabbits kicking out on a slippery surface can also damage their backs.

Vertebral fractures due to improper handling are not always cause for euthanasia. Radiographs can be used to determine the severity of any fracture(s). Luxations can be identified on radiographs and carry a better prognosis than fractures. Serial neurologic examinations are necessary to determine how well the rabbit is progressing.

ETIOLOGY. Fractures can be due to the pressure put on poorly calcified bones by the heavily muscled hindlimbs.

PREVALENCE. Common.

MANAGEMENT. Physical therapy on the hindlimbs is needed to prevent muscle atrophy. Constant attention to the bladder is necessary to prevent infection. Owners will need to manually express the bladder if the patient cannot. Urine scald is a common problem.

PROGNOSIS. Dependent on the severity of the fracture.

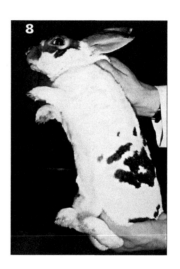

Case 9: **Housing recommendations for a pet rabbit**

INTRODUCTION. Improper husbandry can contribute to many clinical problems in the rabbit including pododermatitis, respiratory disease, and enteritis. Poor rabbit husbandry conditions are a common finding, and there are certain husbandry requirements that owners should be aware of.

Improper husbandry is usually due to the lack of correct information available for the rabbit owner. Rabbit owners may not contact the veterinarian until the pet is sick. It is important to obtain a detailed history in order to diagnose husbandry related disease.

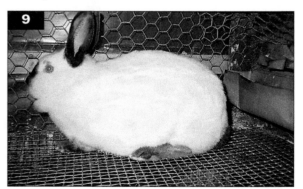

MANAGEMENT. The optimal temperature range for the rabbit is 16–21°C (60.0–69.8°F). Rabbits may be housed indoors or outdoors. If housed outdoors, the rabbit should be protected from extremes in temperature and from predators. An appropriate cage size should average about 0.30 m^2 per kilogram of body weight. The best cage material is galvanized wire or stainless steel. Wood cages are destroyed by chewing and are difficult to disinfect. Flooring that can be kept clean and dry must be provided. Wire mesh floors with 1 × 2.5 cm openings allow feces and urine to fall through to a drop pan (9). However, if the spacing of the wire is too wide, foot and toe injuries can occur. A cloth pad, newspaper, or a box filled with bedding in one area of the cage to give the pet a resting place off the wire should be provided. Solid floored cages can be used, but they are more difficult to keep clean. Bedding such as straw, hay, or pelleted products should be changed at least twice a week to prevent feces and urine accumulation. Dust must be kept to a minimum.

Rabbits tend to eliminate in one corner of the cage. They can be trained to use a litter box by placing the box containing an absorbent bedding in preferred areas. The rabbit should be allowed a minimum of 1–2 hours daily to exercise outside its cage in a supervised area. It is necessary to 'rabbit proof' areas to which the rabbit has access to prevent the destruction of electrical cords or furniture. Rabbits enjoy a variety of toys as a means of satisfying their need to chew and to combat boredom. Acceptable toys include untreated straw mats or baskets, cardboard boxes or tubes, paper bags, untreated wood scraps, hard plastic baby toys, hard rubber or metal balls containing bells, jar lids, and cardboard or plastic boxes filled with hay or straw used for digging.

Case 10: **Splay leg in a rabbit**

CLINICAL PRESENTATION. A seven-year-old intact female rabbit has bilateral hindlimb paresis and inappetence progressing over a two-week period. The rabbit maintains a splay-legged position, is weak on all four limbs, and is reluctant to stand. Spinal reflexes are normal in all four limbs. The ventrum and perineum are superficially ulcerated by constant contact with urine.

DIFFERENTIAL DIAGNOSES. Many different diseases can cause a rabbit to exhibit the appearance of 'splay leg'. These include metabolic diseases (i.e. renal failure and hepatic disease), neoplasia, ingested toxins, mucoid enteropathy, severe infections, cerebrovascular accident, trauma, encephalitis, vertebral spondylosis, spinal trauma, and neoplasia. The chronic staining of the perineum may be due to the fact that the rabbit cannot stand or groom itself, or it may be related to other illness. These other illnesses might include cystitis, cystic calculi, reproductive disease (e.g. pyometra, uterine neoplasia), renal disease, rabbit syphilis, obesity (perineal skin folds around the perineum trap urine), urinary incontinence, spinal disease, CNS disease, systemic disease resulting in generalized weakness, and disease causing painful movement (e.g. arthritis, pododermatitis).

INVESTIGATION. Hematology, plasma biochemistries, and urinalysis are performed and abdominal radiographs obtained. In this rabbit, CBC abnormalities included a nonregenerative anemia and hypoproteinemia. The plasma chemistry profile demonstrated an increased BUN and creatinine, with a normal total protein. A low specific gravity was the only abnormality on urinalysis, indicating a diagnosis of renal failure.

DIAGNOSIS. Splay leg.

ETIOLOGY. In this case the splay leg is due to renal disease. When rabbits are ill, they may develop a splay leg appearance in which they cannot stand or ambulate. It is important to perform a complete physical examination on all rabbits presenting with hindlimb paresis to differentiate neurologic disease from generalized weakness.

PREVALENCE. Not uncommon in older rabbits. In younger rabbits, splay leg can be due to genetic disease.

MANAGEMENT. In this case, supportive care, fluids, and nutrition are important for the metabolic health of this rabbit. Cleaning and topical treatment of dermatitis is also important.

PROGNOSIS. The prognosis for renal disease depends on the etiology. If due to degenerative disease, the prognosis is not good. The prognosis for 'splay leg' without a firm diagnosis is usually not good.

Case 11: **Managing pain in rabbits**

INTRODUCTION. Like all patients, rabbits benefit from postoperative pain relief. Signs of pain and distress in the rabbit are different to what one might expect in a dog or cat. Prey animals exhibit different reactions to predator species.

There are both behavioral and physiologic signs of pain in rabbits. Severe, acute pain or fright is accompanied by a characteristic high-pitched squeal. Generally, any change in temperament or behavior from normal may be an indication of pain or distress. Specific behavioral conditions include inability to sleep, decreased activity, sitting in a hunched position, unkempt coat condition, reluctance to move, timidity, depression, irritability, prolonged recumbency, lameness, and abdominal splinting.

Rabbits with abdominal pain may lie stretched out in the cage. A hunched posture and tooth grinding may also be seen in rabbits with abdominal discomfort. Two very important signs to watch for are decreased food and water intake. Physiologic findings that may indicate pain include hyperventilation, tachycardia, fluctuations in blood pressure, and hyperglycemia.

ETIOLOGY. The most common causes of pain in pet rabbits are abscesses, trauma, GI stasis, postsurgical discomfort, and dental disease.

PREVALENCE. Common.

MANAGEMENT. Although not approved for use in rabbits, a number of drugs have been reported efficacious or suggested for pain treatment in rabbits. These include opioid agonists, opioid agonist-antagonists, and NSAIDs. All have potential side-effects. Safe use requires an understanding of their pharmacologic properties.

The opioid agonist morphine (2–5 mg/kg s/c, i/m) produces good analgesia of 2–4 hours duration. Side-effects include possible ileus and respiratory depression.

Opioid agonist-antagonists (less side-effects than agonists) suggested for use in rabbits include buprenorphine (0.03–0.05 mg/kg s/c, i/m), butorphanol (0.1–0.5 mg/kg s/c, i/m) and nalbuphine (1–2 mg/kg i/m, i/v).

NSAIDs such as flunixin meglumine (0.3–1.0 mg/kg s/c, i/m), may be useful for treating mild to moderate musculoskeletal pain or pain due to inflammation. Meloxicam appears to offer pain relief in rabbits given at a dose range of 0.1–0.5 mg/kg p/o q12–24h. Meloxicam has replaced flunixin meglumine as the NSAID of choice in rabbits. Recently, the synthetic opioid-like drug tramadol has been used in rabbits. The reported dose range is 1–5 mg/kg q12h p/o.

PROGNOSIS. In general, if pain is controlled in rabbits, the prognosis for recovery from the cause of the pain is improved.

Case 12: **Rabbit anesthesia protocols**

INTRODUCTION. Injectable anesthetics are used commonly to sedate rabbits for examination, for intravenous catheter placement, as premedicants, or as induction agents before inhalant anesthesia.

MANAGEMENT. The rabbit must be handled and restrained carefully to prevent injury to its delicate spine and limbs. One protocol is to use tranquilizers such as acepromazine (0.1–1.0 mg/kg i/m) in combination with ketamine (20 mg/kg i/m) to improve the quality of anesthesia produced. Diazepam or midazolam (1–2 mg/kg i/m) can be given to provide sedation and muscle relaxation. When diazepam or midazolam (0.5–1.0 mg/kg i/m, i/v) is used with ketamine (10–20 mg/kg i/m) to improve the quality of anesthesia, the effect can be enhanced by giving the diazepam or midazolam i/v approximately 10–20 minutes after the i/m ketamine. Alternatively, the sedative analgesic xylazine (2–5 mg/kg i/m, s/c) can be given with ketamine (20–35 mg/kg i/m). Xylazine must only be used in healthy animals. Its use is associated with muscle relaxation and peripheral vasoconstriction, and decreases in the heart rate, arterial blood pressure, and respiratory rate. Recent trials in rabbit sedation/anesthesia protocols include the use of a combination of medetomidine (0.100–0.250 mg/kg) and ketamine (10–15 mg/kg), given i/m.

It is best to use inhalant anesthesia for surgical procedures. The two most commonly used inhalant agents are isoflurane and sevoflurane. Some workers continue to use injectable medication for shorter surgical procedures. Ketamine alone produces sedation and chemical restraint, but does not provide enough muscle relaxation and analgesia for most surgical procedures. Ketamine (20–35 mg/kg i/m) in combination with xylazine (2–5 mg/kg i/m) provides a variable plane of anesthesia and may require supplemental inhalant anesthesia for surgery. Decreases in blood pressure, respiratory rate, heart rate, and body temperature are associated with ketamine and xylazine combinations. Local irritation is reported following i/m administration of ketamine/xylazine. To avoid this, the total dose should be divided and administered at several sites. Supplemental medication for analgesia will still be necessary. A combination of ketamine (20–40 mg/kg i/m) and diazepam (5–10 mg/kg i/m) provides a variable plane of anesthesia, which can be supplemented as needed with an inhalant anesthetic. This high-dose combination is not recommended; the lower dose followed by isoflurane anesthesia is preferred.

Barbiturates have potent respiratory depressant effects in rabbits. Severe laryngospasm can also be a problem at light levels of barbiturate anesthesia. Barbiturates have a very narrow margin of safety. Tiletamine/zolazepam can cause renal toxicity in rabbits, with the tiletamine implicated as the causative factor in a dose-dependent manner.

Atropine is not routinely used as a premedication in rabbits. Some rabbits have atropinesterase and, therefore, metabolize atropine rapidly. Glycopyrolate is a more useful anticholinergic agent in rabbits.

Case 13: **Rabbit urine colored due to porphyrin pigments**

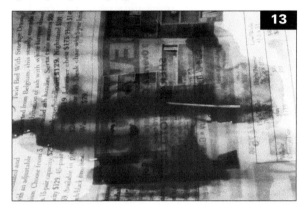

CLINICAL PRESENTATION. A six-month-old intact pet female rabbit is exhibiting increased frequency of urination. She eliminates small amounts of urine in several selected areas of the room where she is housed. The urine is reddish in color (**13**).

DIFFERENTIAL DIAGNOSES. Discolored urine with a 'reddish' tinge can be caused by blood from the urinary or female reproductive tract or from dietary pigments that result in porphyrinuria. Hematuria occurs with urinary tract infection, trauma, neoplasia, urolithiasis, bladder polyps, or reproductive disease (e.g. uterine aneurysm, adenocarcinoma, or pyometra). Blood from the uterus pools in the vagina and is expelled when the rabbit urinates. Uterine bleeding from an adenocarcinoma is sporadic and often appears as clots of blood within the voided urine. A differential diagnosis for increased urination due to medical conditions could be a urinary tract infection.

INVESTIGATION. It is imperative to perform a complete urinalysis to rule out blood as the cause of the red appearance as opposed to porphyrin pigments. Porphyrin pigments potentially can change the colors on a urine dipstick, so a complete urinalysis is recommended. A CBC and biochemistry panel is helpful to determine the health status of the patient. For example, if there is blood in the urine, anemia is expected. All diagnostics should be normal if urine changes are due to porphyrin.

DIAGNOSIS. In this case the red color of the urine is due to porphyrin pigments.

ETIOLOGY. Rabbits normally eliminate porphyrin pigments in the urine. These pigments can color the urine dark yellow to a deep red-orange. The factors that cause porphyrin production are unknown. Some foods can cause urine color changes. The frequency of urination in this sexually mature animal is consistent with territorial marking.

PREVALENCE. Porphyrin pigments causing colored urine is common in pet rabbits. It does not appear to be associated with any particular signalment.

MANAGEMENT. No treatment is necessary if porphyrin pigments are in the urine. Diet changes are not required. Territorial marking is difficult to treat the longer it occurs. An ovariohysterectomy will usually curtail marking behavior. In some cases of territorial marking, additional behavior modification may be necessary.

PROGNOSIS. The prognosis for rabbits with porphyrin pigments is excellent, as it is not due to a medical condition. Territorial marking will continue unless the circumstances that have caused it are removed.

Case 14: **Rabbit with corneal membranous occlusion**

CLINICAL PRESENTATION. The right eye of a four-month-old female rabbit that developed a progressive growth over the cornea in the last two weeks is shown (**14**). The rabbit appears otherwise healthy and the left eye is normal.

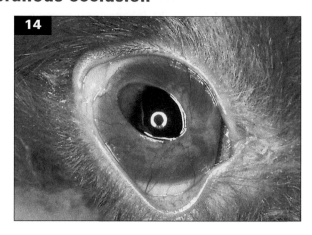

DIFFERENTIAL DIAGNOSES. There are no other conditions that cause this appearance in rabbits.

INVESTIGATION. No evidence of inflammation is present in this eye and microbiologic cultures are negative for *Mycoplasma* species and *Chlamydia* species. The Schirmer tear test is also normal at 8 mm/minute (the normal mean + SD Schirmer tear test for the rabbit is 5 +/- 3 mm/minute), suggesting a tear film disorder is not involved. Deeper intraocular structures are normal. A slit lamp examination is normal.

DIAGNOSIS. This condition is called corneal membranous occlusion or centripetal conjunctival migration, or pseudopterygium.

ETIOLOGY. The disorder is usually progressive, may be unilateral or bilateral, and, in extreme cases, results in blindness due to occlusion of the pupil. The cause of this condition is unknown, but it may represent a congenital symblepharon; however, it is also known to occur in adult rabbits. The architecture of the membrane may be quite complex and it is usually lined with conjunctival epithelium on both surfaces. Frequently, the membrane adheres only to the limbus and not the cornea. Rarely, loose to moderately firm, focal adhesions to the peripheral cornea occur.

PREVALENCE. Corneal membranous occlusion is infrequently seen in pet rabbits.

MANAGEMENT. The membrane is excised. Some rabbits require a superficial keratectomy if there are focal adhesions to the cornea. A small, perilimbal ring of conjunctival epithelium is preserved, as this is where the progenitor cells of the cornea are located. Unfortunately, recurrence following excision is common. In an attempt to prevent regrowth, the cut edge of the bulbar conjunctiva can be anchored to the episclera at least 2 mm away from the limbus with a few, fine absorbable sutures. A topical ocular NSAID is administered 3–4 times daily for 10 days postoperatively to reduce the possibility of membrane regrowth. A broad-spectrum topical ophthalmic antibiotic is applied 3–4 times daily until the corneal defect has healed.

PROGNOSIS. Some rabbits respond to surgery, and in some rabbits the corneal membrane continues to regrow.

Case 15: **Rabbit ovariohysterectomy protocols**

INTRODUCTION. Ovariohysterectomy is recommended in nonbreeding rabbits. Ovariohysterectomy is a preventive health measure. Rabbits that undergo this procedure are less likely to exhibit unacceptable sexually related behavior such as territoriality and urine marking. Ovariohysterectomy prevents the most common cancer in rabbits, adenocarcinoma. Uterine adenocarcinoma is found in 30–80% of intact does over three years of age.

MANAGEMENT. Rabbit skin and tissue is very delicate. Bruising and postoperative complications can be prevented by observing careful handling. The mesovarium, mesosalpinx, and mesometrium are often very fatty and friable in mature rabbits and tear easily if too much tension is applied. Clamps must not be used

on these tissues. The rabbit has a duplex uterus with two uterine horns and no uterine body (**15**). The vagina extends cranially, ending at the double cervix. The vagina must be identified properly and not mistaken for a (nonexistent) uterine body.

In young rabbits a small (2–4 cm) ventral midline incision is made, centered between the umbilicus and the rim of the pelvis. A larger incision is created if needed in older animals with more developed reproductive organs or uterine pathology in order to fully exteriorize the ovaries and uterus. The bladder is emptied prior to surgery, and the voluminous bowel must be avoided when making the abdominal incision. The duplex uterus can be identified dorsal to the bladder in the caudal abdomen and elevated without the use of a spay hook.

One ovary is isolated and the branching ovarian vessels double ligated with synthetic absorbable suture. The associated uterine tube and infundibulum are identified and included with the tissues to be removed. The mesometrium contains many vessels distributed in a fan-like pattern. These are difficult to identify in fat animals, but they are tied by ligatures placed in the mesometrium. The large uterine vessels close to the cervix on each side are identified and double ligated. Each uterine horn is clamped, ligated, and removed as close to the cervix as possible. Alternatively, the vagina just caudal to the double cervix is clamped and ligated to ensure that all uterine tissue is removed. This is a more secure way of being certain that no tissue is left to produce uterine adenocarcinoma. The vaginal stump is oversewn to prevent leakage of urine into the abdomen. The abdominal wall is closed with synthetic absorbable suture. The skin is closed with synthetic absorbable suture in a buried continuous intradermal pattern or with skin staples.

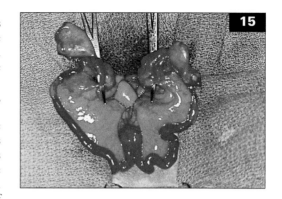

Case 16: **Rabbit reproductive biology**

INTRODUCTION. Rabbits become sexually mature from three and a half to nine months of age. The smaller the breed, the earlier the onset of sexual maturity. Young rabbits should be separated into same sex groups by 10–12 weeks of age in order to avoid breeding and unwanted litters. Five-week-old rabbits are shown (**16a**). The owner wants to know at what age can the kits be sexed, and how is this done.

MANAGEMENT. The kits are best sexed at birth or at weaning (5–8 weeks of age). In the interim, it is difficult to exteriorize the genitalia. The perineum is stretched to expose the anogenital structures. The male has a conical to cylindrical-shaped penis, with a rounded to oval urethral opening. The female has a vulva that protrudes slightly, with a slit-like opening (**16b**). In sexually mature males the scrotal sacs may be seen lateral to the perineum. Male rabbits can retract the testicles into the inguinal canal, making sex determination more difficult.

The gestation period of the rabbit is 29–35 days and litter size ranges from 4–12. Fetuses can be palpated in the uterus as early as ten days post breeding. At this stage they can be felt as masses approximately 1–1.5 cm in diameter located in the caudal ventral abdomen. At 18 days post breeding, the fetuses are approximately 2.5–3 cm in length. Palpation must be gentle to avoid damage to the fetuses. If necessary, radiography or ultrasonography can be used after 21 days to determine if the rabbit is pregnant.

Care must be taken when breeding rabbits to protect them from trauma. Does are territorial and may kill a new rabbit introduced into the cage. For this reason, it is important to bring the doe to the buck's cage for breeding. If the doe does not accept the buck within a few minutes and fighting occurs, they must be separated. They can be introduced again at 12–24 hour intervals until one to two successful matings have occurred.

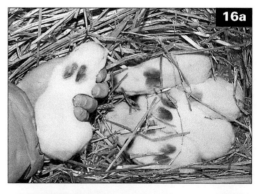

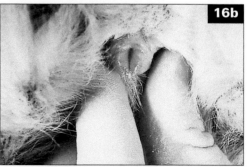

Case 17: **Dyspnea in a rabbit due to chronic pulmonary changes**

CLINICAL PRESENTATION. An adult rabbit presents with a history of dyspnea after a mild amount of exercise. Thoracic disease is common in pet rabbits.

DIFFERENTIAL DIAGNOSES. The major differential is emphysema, likely caused by chronic interstitial fibrosis due to previous pneumonia. Other differentials include acute pneumonia, thoracic neoplasia, and heart disease.

INVESTIGATION. Lateral (**17a**) and ventrodorsal (**17b**) radiographs of the thorax are obtained. In a normal rabbit the thymus is proximal and ventral to the heart and extends to the thoracic inlet. The esophagus, aorta, pulmonary vessels, and lymph nodes lie in the mediastinal space dorsal to the heart. The heart is located between the 4th and 6th pair of ribs and lies to the left of the midline. The lungs are divided into cranial, middle, and caudal lobes. The left cranial lobe is much smaller than the right cranial lobe. The right caudal lobe is subdivided into lateral and medial lobes. These radiographs show an interstitial pattern. Hyperinflated lungs are seen on the lateral view but not on the ventrodorsal view. The radiopaque area noted on the ventrodorsal view is the diaphragm, which is overlapped by a hyperinflated lung.

A CBC and plasma biochemistry panel should be performed to determine the metabolic status of the patient.

DIAGNOSIS. The pathological diagnosis is emphysema with chronic interstitial fibrosis. The condition was caused by a previous episode of aspiration pneumonia.

ETIOLOGY. It is likely that *Pasteurella multocida* has been overemphasized as a cause of pneumonia and other gram-negative bacteria should be considered. Also, anaerobic bacteria can cause disease.

PREVALENCE. Pneumonia, both clinical and subclinical, appears to be common in pet rabbits.

MANAGEMENT. Even though this condition is not due to an active infection, antibiotics are administered to prevent a secondary infection. The primary method of management is to decrease stress and limit activity. Also, it is important to keep the rabbit trim and on a good diet. The diet should be a high-fiber diet with free-choice hay and greens.

PROGNOSIS. This condition cannot be cured, but dietary management and stress management may give affected rabbits a good quality of life.

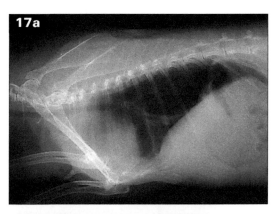

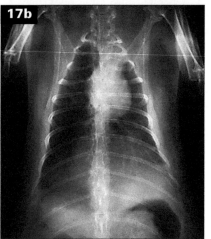

Case 18: **Rabbit intubation technique**

INTRODUCTION. To improve airway access, it is important to be able to intubate rabbits. At least three techniques are used for rabbit endotracheal intubation: direct visualization, stylet-assisted, and blind. For each method, the rabbit is positioned in sternal recumbency with the neck extended. The tongue is pulled through the diastema on one side so that it will not be cut or bruised by the teeth or laryngoscope blade (**18a**).

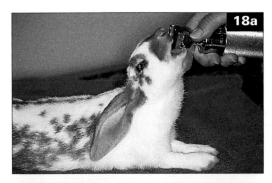

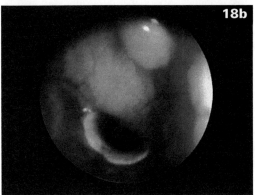

TECHNIQUE. The direct visualization technique is suitable for use in larger rabbits. The lighted laryngoscope blade is introduced at the diastema and gently advanced over the base of the tongue until the larynx is brought into view (**18b**). If laryngospasm is a problem, the larynx can be swabbed with a cotton-tipped applicator that has been soaked with a topical anesthetic (e.g. a small amount of 1% lidocaine [approximately 0.25 ml]). Benzocaine containing spray has been associated with methemoglobinemia in rabbits and rats. Premedication with terbutaline may also decrease the incidence of laryngospasms and bronchospasms. The endotracheal tube is passed gently into the larynx and the laryngoscope removed. A semi-rigid atraumatic stylet is used to direct the tube for accurate placement.

The stylet-assisted technique is used in smaller rabbits because there is not enough room for simultaneous placement of the laryngoscope blade and the endotracheal tube. In these animals a flat laryngoscope blade (Miller) is easiest to introduce into the mouth to visualize the larynx. A 3.5 or 5.0 Fr urinary catheter is passed into the larynx, the laryngoscope is removed, and the endotracheal tube is advanced over the catheter into the airway. The catheter is removed quickly to prevent airway obstruction. With both the direct visualization and stylet-assisted techniques, an endoscope is a helpful tool with which to visualize the larynx and place the endotracheal tube.

For the blind endotracheal intubation technique, the animal is positioned with the neck extended as described above. The endotracheal tube is passed along the dorsal midline of the tongue toward the larynx, at the same time listening for breath sounds and watching for condensation in the tube. The tube is slipped into the larynx as the glottis opens during inspiration. Loss of breath sounds, loss of condensation and/or the presence of audible swallowing indicate that the tube is in the esophagus. The rabbit may respond to proper tube placement by moving or coughing. Correct placement is confirmed with the laryngoscope by auscultation of the chest during lung inflation, or by testing for air passage through the tube.

Case 19: **Rabbit with dysuria due to urinary tract calculi**

CLINICAL PRESENTATION. An owner reports dysuria in a rabbit for the last three days.

DIFFERENTIAL DIAGNOSES. Urinary tract calculi, bladder sludge, and infectious cystitis.

INVESTIGATION. Radiographs are taken and radiopaque material is seen in the bladder (**19a, b**). If calculi are in a ureter or kidney, these structures may need to be removed; therefore, a preoperative radiographic contrast study is one methodology used to check the function of the opposing kidney. Abdominal ultrasound can also be used to check the health of the urinary system. A CBC, plasma biochemical panel, and a urinalysis should all be performed to determine the metabolic status of the patient. Urine bacterial cultures are also performed.

DIAGNOSIS. Urinary tract calculi.

ETIOLOGY. Urinary tract calculi of varying sizes and abnormally large amounts of calcium carbonate (commonly referred to as 'sludge') are common in the rabbit. The rabbits have calciuria, with one or more of the following signs: anorexia, dysuria, stranguria, reluctance to move, a hunched posture, and perineal staining with calcium carbonate precipitate.

PREVALENCE. Common problem in pet rabbits.

MANAGEMENT. The urolithiasis is treated by flushing the urinary tract or performing a cystotomy. Since low-grade cystitis may be present, antibiotics are administered.

If bladder sludge is present, the first treatment can include diuresis with s/c fluids for 48 hours. If this is unsuccessful, the bladder can be flushed repeatedly with the rabbit anesthetized. The use of a mildly acidic solution may aid in this process. Gentle flushing is continued until the urine is clear. Analgesics are used post catheterization, as urethral spasm is common. These patients should be diuresed with parenteral fluids. Rabbits should be hospitalized until they are urinating normally. If bladder sludge cannot be removed by flushing, a cystotomy is necessary. The bladder mucosa is cultured and the calculi analyzed for mineral composition. Closure is routine. Analgesics are given post surgically.

Follow-up radiographs and urinalysis should be performed routinely to check for recurrence. If needed, water consumption can be increased by the addition of fruit-flavored drink additives (e.g. fruit juice, oral electrolyte solutions) to the water. There are suggestions that reducing dietary calcium decreases the amount of calcium excreted in the urine, but this has not been proven to be useful.

PROGNOSIS. Prevention of recurrence is hampered because the pathology of this disease is not yet fully understood; therefore, owners should be advised that this disease, even with appropriate management changes, may recur.

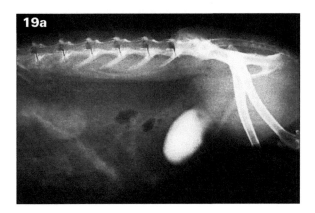

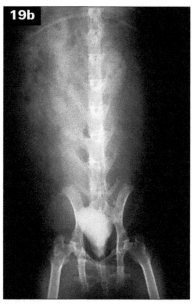

Case 20: **New Zealand White rabbit with glaucoma**

CLINICAL PRESENTATION. A six-month-old New Zealand White rabbit appears to be blind in both eyes. A white ring is visible at the limbus (**20**). The rabbit is one of a litter of four purchased from a laboratory colony to be a pet. The rabbit had apparently normal vision until recently.

DIFFERENTIAL DIAGNOSES. The white ring likely represents the affects of glaucoma. As the rabbit is a New Zealand white, the most likely cause is genetic, but other causes include infection, neoplasia, and granuloma.

INVESTIGATION. A complete ocular examination should be performed on both eyes. Intraocular pressures should be measured and an examination of the angle performed.

DIAGNOSIS. The white ring is due to early corneal edema resulting from raised intraocular pressure from glaucoma.

ETIOLOGY. This is an inherited condition in this breed. The bu gene causing buphthalmos is quite widespread in the laboratory population of New Zealand White rabbits. The gene is recessively inherited.

PREVALENCE. Litters produced by parents with normal vision but carrying the bu gene will have an average of one in four of the offspring develop the condition. Animals homozygous for bu are not always affected because the gene is only partially penetrant. Since the genetics of the parents is unknown, it is difficult to predict if the other three rabbits will develop this problem. Other causes of glaucoma are observed in rabbits, but the incidence rate appears to be the same as in dogs and cats.

MANAGEMENT. Glaucoma in rabbits does not appear to cause the same painful ocular sequelae that occur in the dog or cat. Usually, by the time the owner has noticed changes in the eye, the animal is already blind. The affected eyes do not become severely buphthalmic; therefore, secondary trauma due to an exposed bulging eye is uncommon. Surgery to relieve intraocular pressure can be performed early in the disease in an attempt to prevent blindness, but late in the disease it is of questionable value. Other causes of glaucoma can be treated as they are in dogs and cats.

PROGNOSIS. The bu gene also carries with it some semilethal effects such as low litter size (note that only four animals were born in this litter), high infant mortality, and occasionally sudden death. Owners should be advised not use these animals for breeding. Since most rabbits do not exhibit overt signs of pain with glaucoma, owners recognize the signs too late to save vision. Eventually, the eyes becomes quiet and the rabbit appears unaffected by the loss of vision.

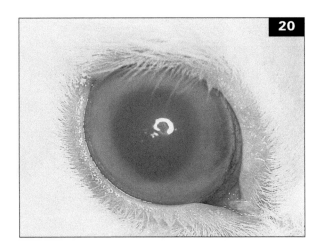

Case 21: **Hypermature cataracts in New Zealand White rabbit**

CLINICAL PRESENTATION. A New Zealand White rabbit has chronically red eyes. According to the owner, the left eye has dramatically changed appearance in the past 24 hours. It used to look like the right eye (**21a**), but it now appears as shown in **21b**.

DIFFERENTIAL DIAGNOSES. Uveitis and infection can appear grossly similar.

INVESTIGATION. A CBC, plasma biochemistry panel, and urinalysis are performed to rule out metabolic causes of cataract development. An ophthalmologic examination, including ocular pressure measurement, is needed to rule uveitis in or out. Examination of the lens and anterior chamber is necessary to make a definitive diagnosis.

DIAGNOSIS. Both eyes have hypermature cataracts.

ETIOLOGY. The red appearance is from lens-induced uveitis. The leakage of lens protein initiates an autoimmune response that results in chronic inflammation of the uveal tract. The anterior chamber of the left eye is full of blood. This is technically called hyphema. It is likely that the severe inflammation in the left eye resulted in frank intraocular hemorrhage. The vessels of the chronically inflamed iris are so fragile that even minor trauma results in bleeding.

PREVALENCE. Cataracts are not uncommon in pet rabbits. Causes can be infection or metabolic, genetic, or degenerative diseases. Secondary lens-induced uveitis is not an uncommon sequela to long-standing cataracts in rabbits. This can be seen in all breeds.

MANAGEMENT. The lens-induced uveitis is treated by controlling the inflammation using ophthalmic NSAIDs. In rabbits, steroids should be used with great caution and they are not recommended. Removal of the cataract to control the inflammation is not practical for most rabbits. Once the eye becomes inflamed from lens-induced uveitis, the likelihood of complications subsequent to cataract surgery increases dramatically. It is important to determine if a primary cause of the cataracts is present (e.g. diabetes mellitus). Ocular antibiotics are used if there is an infectious component to this disease.

PROGNOSIS. Antiinflammatory medication and decreased leakage of lens material may eventually control the uveitis. Cataracts may become hypermature and some sight may be restored.

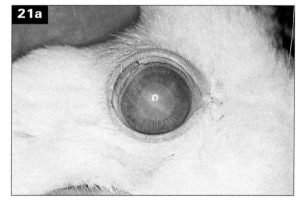

21a

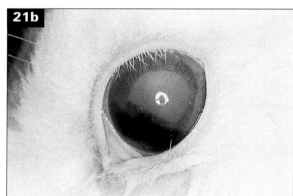

21b

Case 22: **Rabbit with loose stools due to a poor diet and subsequent GI hypomotility**

CLINICAL PRESENTATION. A two-year-old neutered male rabbit has these intermittent thick, pudding-like stools during the day (**22**). The soft stools are produced daily along with normal-sized dry droppings. The rabbit is fed a commercial rabbit pellet (16% fiber, 14% protein) free choice and is given a teaspoonful a day of rolled oats and one salt-free cracker.

DIFFERENTIAL DIAGNOSES. Poor diet leading to dysbiosis. Other causes of enteritis include bacterial, parasitic, and metabolic conditions.

INVESTIGATION. The most important diagnostic test is the diet history. Normal hematology and biochemistry results, along with a positive history, rules in dietary related disease. Fecal floats and cultures can be performed.

ETIOLOGY. Low-fiber diets (<18%) create cecal–colonic hypomotility. This predisposes the animal to abnormal cecal fermentation due to prolonged retention of digesta in the cecum. Low-fiber diets and those high in carbohydrates stimulate production of volatile fatty acids, resulting in pH alterations and ultimately changing the cecal microflora. This loss of intestinal homeostasis causes soft stools in the rabbit. The soft stools are actually liquid cecal contents, which should be formed cecotropes that the rabbit would normally ingest. Other signs include obesity and GI ileus (sometimes incorrectly identified as a 'gastric hairball'). Simple sugars and starches provide an environment in which pathogens such as *Escherichia coli* and *Clostridium* species proliferate. The addition of dietary glucose causes the production of iota toxin by *C. spiroforme*, the bacteria responsible for enterotoxemia in the rabbit. Diets high in fiber seem to have a protective effect against enteritis. The beneficial effect is associated with the indigestible fiber component, lignocellulose. Digestible fiber sources do not have this property. Fiber stimulates cecal–colonic motility. Other effects of fiber are indirect. High-fiber diets naturally have a lower carbohydrate concentration, which decreases the chance of carbohydrate overload enterotoxemia.

PREVALENCE. Low-fiber diets are common in pet rabbits. Obesity and GI stasis are common presentations to veterinarians.

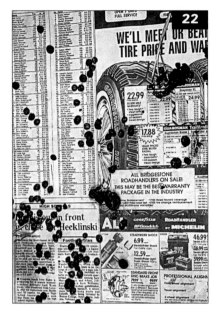

MANAGEMENT. Rabbits with soft stools are treated with supportive care and fed a diet high in fiber and hay. Adult pet rabbits should be offered a good quality grass hay (marsh, orchard, timothy, or Bermuda) *ad libitum*. The protein and calcium content of alfalfa is greater than that required by an adult rabbit. A good quality, high-fiber pellet (18–24% fiber) is fed in limited amounts to maintain normal body weight. Most adult nonbreeding rabbits can be maintained on unlimited grass hay and fresh herbage without pellets in their diet. Fresh herbage is offered at a rate of a minimum of one cupful/kg body weight daily. Foods high in starch (such as grain) or refined sugar must not be fed.

PROGNOSIS. Excellent if the rabbit is not very debilitated. Fluids and assisted feeds are key to improvement.

Case 23: **The consequences of rabbit mishandling**

CLINICAL PRESENTATION. A three-year-old rabbit is acutely paralyzed in its hindlimbs. The paralysis occurred after the rabbit was handled by several small children. The patient is alert and responsive, with normal mentation and normal appetite. The forelimbs have no neurologic abnormalities; the hindlimbs are bilaterally hyporeflexive and show no evidence of voluntary motion.

DIFFERENTIAL DIAGNOSES. The most likely cause is a traumatic vertebral fracture. Less likely, but necessary to consider, is a herniated disc. Another consideration would be acute aggravation of chronic pain associated with spondylosis with associated osteophytes, arthritis, discospondylitis, and metabolic disease. All of these differentials are possible, but with acute paralysis the etiology is almost always trauma leading to vertebral fracture.

INVESTIGATION. A CBC, biochemistry panel, and urinalysis should be performed to rule out metabolic disease. Radiographs will rule out bony disease. In this rabbit the lateral radiograph reveals a comminuted fracture visible in the fourth lumbar vertebrae, resulting in misalignment of the vertebral column caudal to the fracture (**23**).

DIAGNOSIS. The most likely diagnosis in a rabbit that is acutely paralyzed in the hindlimbs is a vertebral fracture, most likely in the lumbar vertebra.

ETIOLOGY. Rabbits have extremely powerful hindlimbs and a poorly calcified vertebral column. If adequate control of the hindlimbs is not maintained during restraint, vertebral fractures or luxations can occur if the rabbit kicks and hyperextends the spine.

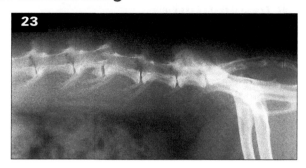

PREVALENCE. Vertebral fractures are common in rabbits that are improperly handled.

MANAGEMENT. Some rabbits can exhibit improvement weeks to months later with supportive care including cage rest and antiinflammatory drugs. Each case should be evaluated individually. All potential rabbit handlers should be taught the correct way to carry a rabbit. The hindlimbs should never be allowed to fully extend and kick. Various holds and carrying techniques can be used to prevent the limbs from fully extending.

PROGNOSIS. The prognosis depends on the severity of the fracture and the level of supportive care. In this case the prognosis is poor, as the alignment of the vertebral column is not maintained. The prognosis is poor in cases where the spinal cord is severely damaged or severed. In cases where there is only severe bruising and inflammation of the cord, and if proper supportive care is maintained, the prognosis for a good quality of life improves. Routinely euthanizing all rabbits with spinal fractures is not recommended.

Case 24: **Methods of assisted feeding in rabbits**

INTRODUCTION. Anorexia is a common sign of disease in the pet rabbit. Anorectic rabbits can develop hepatic lipidosis relatively quickly. It is extremely important to support rabbits nutritionally during illness otherwise they can succumb to the effects of hepatic lipidosis.

MANAGEMENT. Anorexia is treated over the short term with syringe feedings. Various products can be used in the syringe. Commercial products are available, as are homemade mixtures. One recipe calls for ground rabbit pellets or alfalfa powder (obtained through health food stores) mixed with puréed fresh vegetables, canned pumpkin, or strained human vegetable baby food. An oral electrolyte solution is added to thin the mixture and

approximately 10–15 ml/kg p/o q8–12h is fed. Dry commercial products can be made up as directed or mixed with a human caloric liquid food supplement.

If prolonged forced alimentation is expected, or if the patient is difficult to handle, a 5–8 Fr nasoesophageal feeding tube is placed. Good restraint is needed in the conscious rabbit and a small amount of lidocaine gel on the tip of the tube and a drop of lidocaine on the nasal mucosa will decrease any discomfort on placement. The catheter is secured to the skin over the dorsum of the nose and the cranium either with surgical glue or sutures. An Elizabethan collar is used only if necessary (which is rare). Before administering food, the rabbit's thorax is radiographed to ensure the tube is properly placed. Rabbits may not cough or otherwise indicate improper tube placement in the trachea when sterile saline is introduced. A high-calorie, nondairy human or equine liquid food supplement is given for the short term, or the previously mentioned syringe feeding mixture for the long term. The food is passed through a fine strainer to avoid clogging the nasoesophageal tube. The nasoesophageal tube is flushed with saline before and after feedings to maintain a clear line. Even while the nasoesophageal tube is in place, the patient should be offered fresh hay (grass is preferred) and a variety of fresh greens daily (romaine lettuce, parsley, carrot tops, and dandelion greens are often enjoyed). Once eating has resumed with normal stool production, tube feeding can be discontinued.

PROGNOSIS. The prognosis of the primary etiology is enhanced with adequate nutritional support.

Case 25: **Rabbit castration methods**

INTRODUCTION. Rabbits have large inguinal rings and canals that allow the testicles to move freely into and out of the abdominal cavity. However, inguinal herniation of abdominal viscera is rare. The epididymal fat pad prevents herniation of intestines through the rabbits' inguinal canal (**25**). The epididymal fat pad within the abdomen extends down into the inguinal canal when the testicle is in the scrotum. This large fat deposit prevents viscera from passing through the inguinal canal.

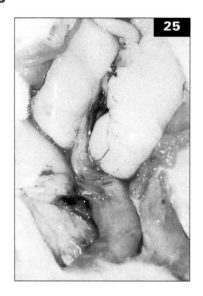

MANAGEMENT. With the rabbit in dorsal recumbency, the fur around the cranial aspect of the scrotum and penis as well as along the inner thighs is clipped and prepared for aseptic surgery. The first technique described is for a closed castration. A 1–1.5 cm incision is made through the scrotum longitudinally on each side of the midline about midway along the length of the scrotum. The tunic is grasped and the testicle removed from the scrotum with the tunic intact. The tunic adheres tightly to the end of the scrotum by the proper ligament of the testis. This ligament is broken down to allow exteriorization of the testicle. As rabbits age, this attachment becomes more fibrotic and it is more difficult to break down. Caudal traction is applied to the testicle and dry gauze used to strip the facial attachments, allowing the narrow portion of the cord to be exteriorized. Once the testicle has been adequately exteriorized, the base of the tunic containing the cord is ligated using a two- or three-clamp technique. The disadvantage of this technique is that if the suture is not tight enough, the spermatic vessels may slip out of the ligature.

A second technique involves performing an open castration and closing the inguinal ring. An incision is made as described above and the vaginal tunic incised to allow exteriorization of the testicle, spermatic cord, and vascular supply. The spermatic cord is double ligated and the testicle removed. The vascular pedicle craniad is traced and the inguinal canal identified. A single interrupted suture is placed across the inguinal canal, being careful not to compress the blood vessels passing through the canal.

A third technique involves an open castration, removing only the testicle and leaving the epididymal fat pad intact. The fat pad prevents herniation of intestine through the inguinal ring.

With all of these techniques, the scrotal incision may be left open to heal by second intention or sutured closed using either an intradermal pattern, tissue adhesive, or skin staples. 4-0 absorbable synthetic sutures are used.

Case 26: **Torticollis in rabbits**

CLINICAL PRESENTATION. A five-year-old male rabbit acutely develops a head tilt. The external ear canal appears normal; however, the tympanum is opaque and bulging slightly.

DIFFERENTIAL DIAGNOSES. Bacterial infection, protozoal infection, parasitic infection, trauma, neoplasia, toxin ingestion.

INVESTIGATION. With the rabbit under anesthesia, a spinal needle is inserted through the tympanum and an aspirate is removed for microbiologic culture. Skull radiographs are taken and otitis media of the right ear is evidenced by the increased radiographic opacity within the osseous bulla (**26a**). A CT scan (**26b**) or MRI gives a much more detailed description of the lesion, allowing a more accurate prognosis.

DIAGNOSIS. Otitis media of the right ear.

ETIOLOGY. The most common causes of head tilt are not known, as many rabbits do not go through the full diagnostic array of testing and few rabbits are examined histologically at death. It is assumed that gram-negative bacteria and anaerobes are common causes of this disease, possibly by extension from dental disease. Toxins have been suggested, but are likely to be uncommon causes. Infection with *Encephalitzoon cuniculi* is also commonly suggested, but evidence does not exist to prove this organism is a common cause of head tilt in rabbits. Degenerative disease, trauma, and neoplasia should be considered.

PREVALENCE. Common in any age rabbit, but usually seen in older rabbits.

MANAGEMENT. If the infection emanates from the ear canal, the infection is treated aggressively with a ventral bulla osteotomy. The bulla is palpated caudal and medial to the vertical ramus of the mandible. An incision is made, about 4–5 cm long, medial to the mandibular salivary gland between the angular process of the mandible and the wings of the atlas. The subcutaneous muscle is incised longitudinally along the same plane as the skin incision. The digastricus muscle is separated bluntly from the hyoglossal and styloglossal muscles, avoiding the hypoglossal nerve, which runs on the lateral aspect of the hyoglossal muscle. Blunt dissection is continued down (dorsally). The bulla is palpated as a round structure between the jugular process of the skull and the angular process of the mandible. Blunt dissection is continued until the surface of the bulla is reached. A self-retaining retractor is placed to maintain exposure. The periosteum of the bulla is incised with a scalpel and a periosteal elevator used to expose the bone of the osseous bulla. A small muscle courses along the ventral surface of the bulla from caudal to cranial. It has a tendinous attachment to the jugular process of the skull. The incision is made medial to this structure. The bone lateral to it is very hard and difficult to penetrate. Medial to this muscle, the bone is very thin and easily penetrated. The bulla is penetrated with a Steinmann pin and the opening enlarged with rongeurs. Samples are collected for histology and microbiologic culture. The bulla is irrigated and all the debris removed. The entire

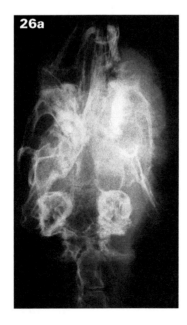

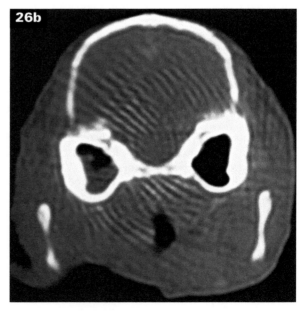

epithelial lining of the bulla is removed using a small curette. During curettage, care must be taken to avoid the dorsomedial aspect of the bulla cavity, which is the location of the ossicles and the promontory. Damage to these structures results in vestibular signs.

Once the bulla has been adequately debrided, an ingress-egress drain is placed. Placing antibiotic impregnated beads should also be considered. The muscles and subcutaneous tissues are closed loosely and the skin is closed routinely. A drain is used to irrigate the middle ear for 7–10 days. The rabbit is maintained on appropriate antibiotic therapy based on the results of the microbiologic culture and sensitivity. Radiographs are taken one month after treatment to assess the status of the disease.

PROGNOSIS. If surgery is performed, the infection may be cured. Straightening of the head and neck, though, is unlikely to occur. If medical treatment is attempted without surgery, it cannot be predicted how the patient will do.

Case 27: **Pregnancy toxemia in a pet rabbit**

CLINICAL PRESENTATION. This three-year-old intact female rabbit develops an acute onset of generalized weakness, depression, and incoordination (**27**). It is obese, maintains a splay-legged position, is weak on all four limbs, and is reluctant to move. Spinal reflexes are normal in all four limbs. The breath has an acetone odor and several masses are palpable within the uterus. The rabbit is housed with an intact male and has had two normal litters previously, the most recent occurring one year ago.

DIFFERENTIAL DIAGNOSES. Pregnancy toxemia, any metabolic disease (e.g. renal disease, hepatic disease), cardiac disease, systemic illness (e.g. septicemia), and dystocia.

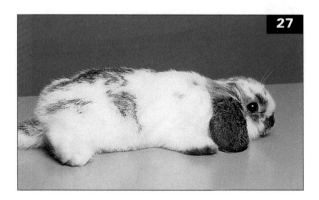

27

INVESTIGATION. The abdomen is radiographed to confirm pregnancy. Urinalysis will demonstrate ketonuria, proteinuria, and an acid pH. A CBC and plasma biochemistry panel are performed to rule out other diseases and determine the metabolic status of the patient.

DIAGNOSIS. Pregnancy toxemia.

ETIOLOGY. Although the cause of pregnancy toxemia in rabbits is unknown, hepatic lipidosis is usually observed at necropsy, and the syndrome is seen most commonly in does that are obese and/or have fasted. Affected rabbits become ketotic and are systemically weak. As in this case, the does develop generalized muscle weakness leading to the splay leg appearance, anorexia, tachypnea, and an acetone odor to the breath due to ketoacidosis.

PREVALENCE. Pregnancy toxemia usually occurs in the last week of gestation, although it is sometimes seen immediately post partum. It is most common in obese does (i.e. does that are on a poor plane of nutrition).

MANAGEMENT. Supportive therapy must be provided, including i/v or i/o fluids and injectable antibiotics. Assisted feedings are provided; an esophageal feeding tube is placed if necessary. If the doe does not respond to therapy and death is imminent, a cesarean section should be performed if the owner wants to attempt to save the litter. The owner is advised that raising orphan rabbits is often unrewarding. Does used for breeding should not be allowed to become obese. Nutrition should be closely watched, especially as gestation proceeds. Anorexia should be avoided in these rabbits. Rabbits should not be bred when they are obese; they should be calorie restricted and exercised before the breeding season.

PROGNOSIS. Guarded to grave.

Case 28: Myxomatosis lesions in a rabbit

CLINICAL PRESENTATION. Two adult rabbits were housed in a hutch in the garden of a semi-rural area in the UK. The previous year, both the rabbits were vaccinated with an attenuated Shope fibroma virus vaccine in an attempt to prevent myxomatosis. Both rabbits were recently exposed to a field strain of myxoma virus, resulting in one rabbit's death. The surviving cage mate (**28**) developed lesions on its face 7–10 days after exposure, with no other clinical signs.

DIFFERENTIAL DIAGNOSES. Myxomatosis lesions, neoplasia, papilloma, abscess.

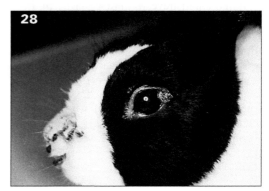

INVESTIGATION. The diagnosis can be confirmed on biopsy and histopathology of the lesion, or on virus isolation. It is important to submit intact epidermis.

DIAGNOSIS. These lesions are the result of myxomatosis caused by a pox virus.

ETIOLOGY. Myxomatosis is usually an acute infection with high morbidity and mortality, although less virulent strains of virus are recorded. In this case it is likely that the rabbit was either exposed to a nonfatal infection in the previous season, or was vaccinated successfully with Shope fibroma virus (available in the UK). The degree of protective immunity produced by this vaccination in the UK is variable. The rabbit that died likely did not develop protection against myxomatosis despite previous vaccination. This virus, like other pox viruses, is spread by insects. Vaccination and limiting exposure to biting insects is the best way to prevent infection.

PREVALENCE. This disease is present in the UK and areas of Europe. It is not seen in most areas of the US.

MANAGEMENT. Prophylactic treatment with an antibiotic such as enrofloxacin (15–20 mg/kg p/o q24h) should be considered. No specific treatment is available for the viral infection, which is self-limiting.

PROGNOSIS. The prognosis for this rabbit is good, as long as secondary bacterial respiratory disease is avoided.

Case 29: Young rabbits with nonspecific signs of disease associated with overgrowth of fecal coccidial organisms

CLINICAL PRESENTATION. Several young rabbits in a rabbitry develop anorexia and diarrhea. Some die due to loss of and lack of intake of fluids and nutrients.

DIFFERENTIAL DIAGNOSES. Coccidiosis, GI bacterial overgrowth, inappropriate use of antibiotics, viral infection, or GI toxemia.

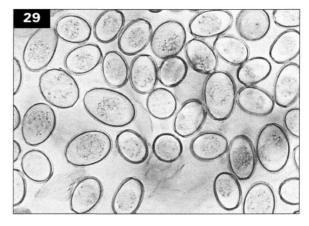

INVESTIGATION. A fecal flotation is performed and *Eimeria stiedae* organisms are recovered (**29**). Some of these ellipsoidal organisms measure 28–40 × 16–25 mm and have a micropyle (cap/operculum). Many other *Eimeria* species organisms are seen on the slide, including ones without micropyles. *E. stiedae* organisms can also be found in bile samples and on histologic examination of the liver.

DIAGNOSIS. Coccidiosis.

ETIOLOGY. *E. stiedae* is an extremely pathogenic protozoan parasite that lives in the bile duct epithelium of the rabbit. In severe infections this parasite produces hepatic dysfunction and may cause death. Rabbits are infected by ingesting infective oocysts from the environment (e.g. in the food, water, or bedding).

Oocysts hatch and release sporozoites that penetrate the intestinal mucosa and travel via the mesenteric lymph nodes and hepatic portal system to the liver. Here they enter epithelial cells of the bile ducts and liver parenchymal cells. They multiply asexually (schizogony), rupture the cells, and each newly released organism invades a new cell and multiplies asexually again. Eventually, asexual multiplication ceases and they undergo sexual reproduction in the cells and produce oocysts that are passed unsporulated through the bile ducts into the intestine. The oocysts pass out with the feces and must sporulate to the infective stage in the environment. This takes at least two days; therefore, reinfection cannot take place through the eating of cecotropes. Disease and illness occur during the asexual multiplication stages and the host may die before oocysts are shed in the feces. The prepatent period is 18 days. Unfortunately, it is difficult to distinguish *E. stiedae* from other *Eimeria* species that infect the intestinal tract of rabbits. These intestinal coccidia may produce diarrhea, particularly in the young, because they multiply in the intestinal epithelium before producing oocysts that are passed in the feces.

PREVALENCE. Coccidial organisms are the most common parasite of the rabbit GI tract. *Eimeria stiedae* is common in rabbitries with poor husbandry.

MANAGEMENT. In rabbitries, infection is prevented by the prophylactic use of coccidiostats.

PROGNOSIS. Mild infections may decrease weight gain and growth. Serious infections will kill rabbits.

Case 30: Facial dermatitis in a rabbit due to an obstructed nasolacrimal duct

CLINICAL PRESENTATION. A pet rabbit has a unilateral facial dermatitis (30). The lesion has become progressively larger over the past two weeks. The rabbit is otherwise normal and does not appear to be in any discomfort.

DIFFERENTIAL DIAGNOSES. Nasolacrimal blockage from infection or overgrown cheek teeth roots, conjunctivitis, or abscess.

INVESTIGATION. Only the lower nasolacrimal cannaliculus and punctum is present in rabbits. Lacrimal duct cannulation can be achieved without general anesthesia, using local ophthalmic anesthetic drops to desensitize the eye. To visualize the punctum, the lower lid can be pulled down and rolled outward or the lid edge can be grasped and gently pulled laterally. Cannulation can be challenging in the presence of a persistent discharge and severe inflammation of the peripunctal area, as the opening becomes scarred and smaller in diameter. Pressure can be applied below the punctum to cause the lips of the punctum to 'pout', thus allowing better access to the duct.

DIAGNOSIS. Facial dermatitis due to tear overflow or epiphora caused by an obstructed nasolacrimal duct.

ETIOLOGY. The nasolacrimal duct of the rabbit is unusual in that it has two sharp bends along its course. A build-up of purulent material at these duct deviations leads to obstruction. In addition, the ducts pass close to the root apices of the cheek teeth and incisor teeth and may become obstructed if there is tooth root disease.

PREVALENCE. This is a common problem in pet rabbits, independent of signalment.

MANAGEMENT. The best chance for a complete cure lies in aggressive therapy early in the course of the disease. Skull radiographs should be obtained to evaluate for dental disease. The duct is cleared by cannulation and irrigation with a sterile saline solution. A few drops of the flushed secretions exiting the nares are collected by free catch onto a culturette for bacterial culture and sensitivity. Appropriate antibiotics are used both topically and systemically for several weeks. The rabbit is rechecked and the tear ducts flushed with an antiseptic or antibiotic solution at 7–10 day intervals or sooner until the condition resolves.

PROGNOSIS. A guarded prognosis should be given for a complete cure if blockage is due to dental disease. Also, a guarded prognosis is given if this is long-standing and fibrosis has occurred in the duct itself. Prognosis is improved if treatment is instituted early in disease.

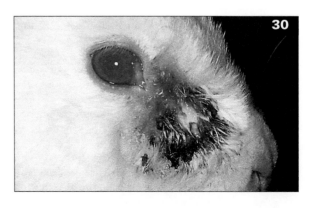

Case 31: **Rabbit with abnormal dentition**

CLINICAL PRESENTATION. A five-year-old pet rabbit is losing weight and having difficulty with prehension and chewing. Signs were first noticed several months ago and the rabbit's condition has been deteriorating. The rabbit is emaciated and has an abnormality of the incisor dentition (**31**). The ventral border of the mandible is smooth.

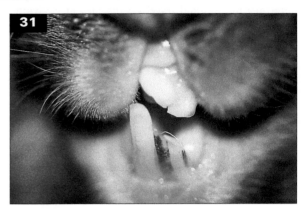

DIFFERENTIAL DIAGNOSES. Obliquely worn incisor teeth may be due to trauma, abnormal growth of the cheek teeth roots, tooth root abscess, or genetic disease.

INVESTIGATION. An oral examination, both awake and sedated, is necessary to determine the extent of disease in the mouth. A more detailed view of the problem is made with skull radiographs and/or a skull CT scan. Treatment success and prognosis is better evaluated with imaging views.

DIAGNOSIS. Obliquely worn incisor teeth.

ETIOLOGY. The most likely cause of this degree of oblique wear is uneven tooth regrowth following trauma. The owner later relates that the rabbit was dropped approximately one year previously, fracturing both upper first incisor and left lower incisor teeth above the gingiva. The right lower incisor was not trimmed until the fractured teeth had regrown, resulting in abnormal occlusion. The right upper first incisor was also growing back at an abnormal angle, thus exacerbating the situation. In cases showing a mild degree of oblique incisor wear, an abnormal chewing action, such as that caused by a unilateral cheek tooth problem, should be suspected.

PREVALENCE. Dental disease is common in pet rabbits. The most common etiology is presumed to be a poor diet or genetics or a combination of both. Trauma is a less likely cause.

MANAGEMENT. Once the trauma has occurred, the goal of treatment is to prevent oblique wear of the incisors. Therefore, the incisors should be trimmed, preferably using a dental burr, every 2–4 weeks to allow proper tooth alignment as they regrow. In addition, a complete physical examination, including visualization of the molars, is performed with each visit. Alternatively, the incisors can be removed.

PROGNOSIS. In cases where the incisors fail to grow back into occlusion and constant trimming is necessary, extraction is not only a viable option, but carries a good prognosis for a complete recovery.

Case 32: **Rabbit with incisor malocclusion**

CLINICAL PRESENTATION. Genetic malocclusion as well as trauma should be considered in the rabbit described in *Case 31*. This would be true particularly if it was a 15-month-old dwarf breed rabbit.

DIFFERENTIAL DIAGNOSES. Hereditary malocclusion, trauma.

INVESTIGATION. A thorough oral examination is carried out under sedation or anesthesia to check for other dental abnormalities. Skull radiographs, dental radiographs, and/or CT scan images can determine the extent of disease. This should be done before any treatment is instituted, as it provides the best chance of detecting both intraoral cheek tooth problems and tooth root disease. In this particular case the maxillary and mandibular incisor tooth roots are abnormal following

the earlier trauma. The intraoral overgrowth of the first mandibular premolar teeth shows as a clearly stepped occlusal line on the lateral radiograph (**32**). Grossly deformed mandibular cheek tooth roots are also visible.

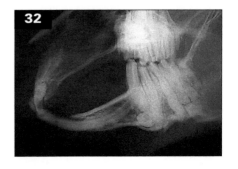

DIAGNOSIS. Hereditary incisor malocclusion.

ETIOLOGY. Dwarf breed rabbits are particularly prone to hereditary malocclusions including relative mandibular prognathism. These usually become apparent by 12 months of age, causing serious dysfunction by the time the animal is 18 months old. Tooth overgrowth occurs, impeding mastication, which ultimately leads to starvation if not treated. Unfortunately, affected individuals may have already produced several litters by the time a problem is recognized.

PREVALENCE. Unknown.

MANAGEMENT. Secondary cheek tooth malocclusion is common after a prolonged period of incisor dysfunction. The reverse is also true. Once a significant degree of secondary malocclusion develops, repeated dental procedures are needed for maintenance. Rabbits that show evidence of hereditary malocclusion must not be bred from. To minimize the effects of incisor malocclusion and resulting cheek tooth disease, it is imperative that owners feed a diet high in fiber, with a limited amount of pellets or no pellets at all.

PROGNOSIS. Palpable irregularities of the ventral mandible are common in cases of cheek tooth malocclusion in rabbits due to a high incidence of root elongation, and they are an indicator of a poor long-term prognosis.

Case 33: **Normal rabbit GI anatomy and physiology**

DISSCUSSION. A diagram of the rabbit GI tract is shown (**33**). Each of the labeled structures plays an important role in the digestive processes in the rabbit GI tract. Since much disease is associated with the digestive process, it is important to understand each of these structures and their function:
1. Cardia of the stomach. This area has a well-developed sphincter that prevents vomiting. The fundus is exocrine and secretes acid, intrinsic factor, and pepsinogen. The pH of the stomach of adult rabbits is usually <2.
2. Pancreas. The pancreas is diffuse in the mesentery of the small intestine. Multiple ducts empty into the terminal duodenum separately from the bile duct.
3. Sacculus rotundus or cecal tonsil. This is the terminal part of the ileum and contains many lymph follicles.
4. Cecum. The cecum comprises 40% of the GI tract of the rabbit. It is the organ where the major bacterial fermentation of cellulose occurs.
5. Proximal colon. This is the first limb of the colon, having rows of sacculations or haustrae that control movement of ingesta out of or back into the cecum.
6. Fusus coli. This is a heavily innervated structure that regulates the passage of material into the descending colon. Retrograde peristalsis transports ingesta with less fiber back to the cecum, where cecotropes containing vitamins, minerals, and amino acids are formed. Cecotropes are eliminated once or twice a day and ingested directly from the anus.

A healthy cecum in rabbits is essential for the digestive process to proceed normally. The rabbit has the largest cecum of any monogastric mammal. The cecum is a large blind sac. It contains about ten times the volume of the stomach and 40% of the total volume of the GI tract. The serous membranes of the cecum are extremely thin and delicate compared with those of other sections of the bowel, and they may tear easily when handled or sutured. The cecum provides an anaerobic environment suitable for the fermentation of ingesta by a highly complex population of microorganisms.

The result of fermentation in the cecum is called soft feces, night feces, or cecotropes. Cecotropes, which are rich in nutrients such as fatty acids, amino acids, and vitamins, are excreted separately from feces, which are nutrient poor. By consuming cecotropes, rabbits ingest nutrients that would otherwise be lost. They are eaten directly from the rectum. The arrival of cecotropes at the anus triggers a neural response, which results in licking the anal area and consumption of the cecotropes. Cecotropes are easily distinguished from feces. They are covered with a thin layer of mucus, are soft and moist, and tend to stick together and have a strong odor. Feces are hard, dry pellets.

Cecotrope intake depends on the protein and fiber concentration of the diet. Cecotrophy is greater if the ration contains less protein and/or more fiber. Rabbits consume the total quantity of the produced cecotropes if the diet is energy deficient.

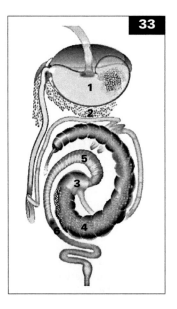

Case 34: **Treatment of rabbit cheek teeth spikes (points)**

CLINICAL PRESENTATION. The buccal surfaces of the maxillary (**34a**) and lingual surfaces of the mandibular cheek teeth (**34b**) of a rabbit that has not eaten well for two weeks are shown. These represent overgrown enamel spikes (points).

DIFFERENTIAL DIAGNOSES. Overgrown enamel spikes, dental related abscess.

INVESTIGATION. An oral examination, best done with the rabbit sedated, will find the spikes on the teeth of this rabbit.

ETIOLOGY. Overgrown enamel spikes are the result of either a diet low in fiber and/or genetic diseases.

PREVALENCE. Very common in pet rabbits.

MANAGEMENT. Some workers recommend trimming or filing off sharp enamel spikes and restoring a normal occlusal surface. This is more easily said than done, particularly as the occlusal plane is not horizontal in rabbits. In many cases there is an excessive curvature of the tooth roots, leading to apparent tipping of the affected teeth out of alignment in the dental arcade. These teeth are subject to abnormal occlusal forces, which may tip them further out of alignment. In early cases an attempt at treatment is usually worthwhile provided that no complicating factors are found during preoperative assessment. A low-speed drill is used to remove the spikes. They should not be filed as that can damage the teeth. Affected rabbits should be examined every 2–3 months, because recurrence of enamel spikes is common.

In extreme cases, progressive damage to the tongue may lead to extensive scarring. Because it is only the mucosal surface that is sensitive, its destruction and scarring can allow the pain to subside until a new area becomes involved. In addition to removing the offending enamel spikes, supportive therapy, including analgesia, must be provided to get the animal through the acute stage of the disease. Re-examine the patient at regular intervals, because some rabbits require lifelong treatment of recurring enamel spikes. Hay and fresh herbage should be given to improve the diet. Such a diet requires thorough chewing and provides a natural level of tooth wear. Pellets and grain should only be provided for individuals with an exceptionally high energy demand (e.g. breeding does, debilitated animals, and some fast growing youngsters).

PROGNOSIS. The prognosis is poor for a return to normal.

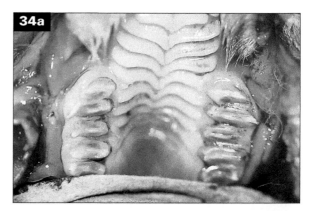

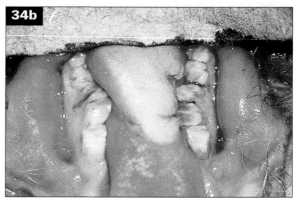

Case 35: **Techniques for rabbit venipuncture**

INTRODUCTION. It is common for pet rabbits to become ill and present with nonspecific signs of disease. It is therefore imperative to collect blood samples and interpret the results to aid the diagnosis of the disease process. Venipuncture is the most common procedure performed in rabbits. There are four common sites that can be used for venipuncture in the pet rabbit: the jugular vein, the lateral saphenous vein, the cephalic vein, and the auricular artery and veins.

TECHNIQUE. A butterfly catheter or a needle without a syringe attached is used to collect blood from the marginal ear vein or central ear artery. The ear vessels must be used with great caution. Rabbit veins are fragile and prone to hematomas. Damage to the ear vessel may lead to necrosis and loss of part of the pinna. Necrosis is also likely to occur if medications are administered through ear vessels.

Rabbit skin is easily torn by clippers and it is safer to pluck hairs from around the venipuncture site and/or use alcohol liberally to wet down the area. A 25 gauge needle attached to a 1 ml syringe is used for the small diameter veins such as the cephalic and lateral saphenous veins. For small rabbits, an insulin syringe attached to a 27 gauge needle is used for venipuncture of the cephalic vein. Rabbits are restrained for cephalic venipuncture in a manner similar to that used in a dog or cat.

The lateral saphenous vein is normally an easily accessible vessel for venipuncture. The rabbit is held on its side and the hindlimb held off around the quadriceps. The lateral saphenous vein has numerous branches that can be utilized.

A 22 gauge needle attached to a 3 ml syringe is used for the jugular vein. In dwarf breeds, a 25 gauge needle may be necessary. The rabbit is held in sternal recumbency on an edge of a table with its forelimbs pulled down and its head held up. The vein is in the

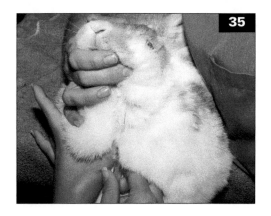

jugular groove and is superficial. In obese rabbits, there may be fat over the jugular vein, which decreases visualization (**35**).

Case 36: **Bloody vaginal discharge due to adenocarcinoma in a rabbit**

CLINICAL PRESENTATION. A six-year-old female intact rabbit has had a bloody vaginal discharge for the last two months. The patient has resided as the only pet in the same household since eight weeks of age. On physical examination a palpable caudal abdominal mass is noted and a PCV of 0.22 l/l (22%) found. At surgery, a diseased uterus was removed (**36**).

DIFFERENTIAL DIAGNOSES. The differentials for a diseased uterus include uterine adenocarcinoma, benign uterine hyperplasia, hydrometra, pyometra, cystic endometrial hyperplasia, uterine aneurysm, and a uterus enlarged with fetuses.

INVESTIGATION. Radiography is performed first to help define the location of the mass. Then, if needed, abdominal ultrasound can be used to further define the location and architecture of the mass. If malignancy is part of the differential diagnoses, the lungs and liver are examined radiographically for metastasis. A CBC and biochemistry panel should be performed to determine the overall health status of the patient. Varying degrees of a regenerative anemia are usually present with this disease.

DIAGNOSIS. Uterine adenocarcinoma.

PREVALENCE. Uterine adenocarcinoma is the most common cancer in pet rabbits and the most common reproductive disease of unspayed female rabbits over two years of age.

MANAGEMENT. If there is no evidence of metastasis, an ovariohysterectomy is performed. At surgery, the

mesenteric lymph nodes and liver are biopsied to rule out metastasis. If a rabbit is severely anemic from blood loss, blood transfusions should be considered. Some workers recommend radiographs and/or ultrasound of the patient after three months and again at six months to look for metastasis. Metastasis will rarely occur after an ovariohysterectomy when no metastasis was seen grossly at surgery. There are no chemotherapy protocols to treat uterine adenocarcinoma.

PROGNOSIS. If there is no tumor spread, then the prognosis for a normal life span is excellent. If there is metastasis, then the prognosis is very poor. If surgery to remove the uterus is not performed, the prognosis is poor. Because of blood loss, some rabbits are very debilitated and may not do well during anesthesia and surgery.

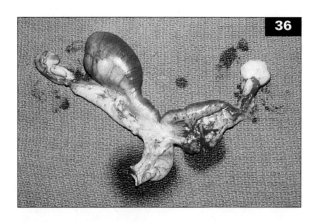

Case 37: **Rabbit with incisor malocclusion**

CLINICAL PRESENTATION. Incisor malocclusion is a common presenting problem in pet rabbits (**37**). This rabbit has been like this for two years and the owner wants to know what else can be done for this problem.

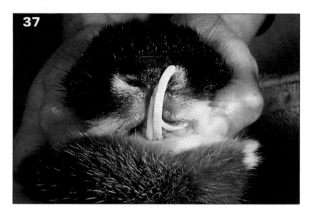

DIFFERENTIAL DIAGNOSES. Trauma, hereditary incisor malocclusion, or secondary to cheek teeth malocclusion.

INVESTIGATION. The condition of the cheek teeth should be throroughly examined and assessed. Clinical evaluation with palpation and visual examination, even under anesthesia, will only reveal about 50% of the dental or oral lesions present. Radiography is an essential part of the work up in these cases because it provides information about the tooth roots. It is essential to examine the tooth roots, as disease may first be apparent as abnormal growth of the roots. Lysis of the roots and the bone around the roots may be present and this is only found on imaging studies. A check is made for incisor tooth root deformity. Any enlargement of angulation toward the root apex will make extraction difficult.

DIAGNOSIS. Incisor malocclusion due to trauma.

PREVALENCE. Incisor malocclusion is a common problem in pet rabbits

MANAGEMENT. Overgrowth can be managed by trimming, but this procedure usually needs to be repeated at intervals throughout the patient's life. An alternative method of managing nonfunctional incisor teeth is extraction. Plasma biochemistry and hematology are performed to detect concurrent systemic disease. The dietary requirements following incisor extraction are

basically the same as for all rabbits; this includes good quality hay and fresh herbage. Bulky items such as carrot or celery are cut into thin strips so they can be picked up by the prehensile lips and fit into the rabbit's mouth. The tongue is then used to move the material to the cheek teeth for grinding. Most rabbits can graze normally and can manage long hay strands easily. Owners are advised to brush the rabbit's coat frequently to remove dead hair, because the loss of incisors prevents the rabbit from performing this grooming procedure.

PROGNOSIS. Incisor malocclusion due to trauma or genetic disease carries a good prognosis. Incisor malocclusion secondary to cheek teeth malocclusion leads to a variable prognosis. Early signs of cheek tooth overgrowth or root extension may be reversible, but if gross changes are seen on radiographs, the prognosis is poor.

Case 38: **Rabbit incisor removal**

CLINICAL PRESENTATION. The owners of the rabbit in *Case 37* decide that they want the incisors removed.

INVESTIGATION. The preoperative lateral radiograph should be examined to assess the length and curvature of the tooth roots. Preoperative hematology and biochemistry testing is carried out to assess the health status of the rabbit.

PREVALENCE. Incisor removal is a procedure occasionally performed in pet rabbits.

MANAGEMENT. The patient is anesthetized and the main incisors trimmed so that 5–10 mm of the crowns are visible. Any cheek tooth irregularities and oral mucosal lesions are treated at this time. The peg teeth are

extracted first because they are often fractured during extraction of the main maxillary incisors. The gingivae are cleaned with an antiseptic solution. A rabbit incisor dental elevator is worked around each peg tooth to sever carefully its periodontal ligaments. Leverage on the tooth crowns must be avoided because this can lead to root fracture. After the teeth are loosened, they are lifted out of their sockets using fingers or a small pair of forceps. No force should be used to remove the teeth. The marked curvature of the main incisors makes elevation of these teeth more difficult. A rabbit dental elevator is inserted medial to each of the teeth and slight lateral pressure is applied for a minute or two. This is repeated several times until the tooth is loosened. The crown of the tooth is gripped with fingers or forceps and the tooth rotated out of its socket along the line of eruption. The tooth sockets usually fill with blood, which clots rapidly. If hemorrhage persists or if the gingiva was torn, the wounds are closed with a fine absorbable suture material. The tooth socket is cultured and antibiotics administered in cases where tooth root infection is suspected. Analgesia is used postoperatively. Food and water are provided as soon as the patient is ambulatory. Soft food should not be used because it adheres to the wound area.

For the novice, root fracture is quite common, particularly affecting the peg teeth. The owner should be forewarned of this possibility. The best way to manage these cases is to extract the remaining incisors, leaving the fractured root in place. Within 6–8 weeks the tooth has usually regrown and is then extracted at a second procedure. If the tooth does not regrow, radiographs are obtained to check for impaction. If this has occurred, an osteotomy is performed to expose and remove the root remnant.

PROGNOSIS. Good if there are no surgical complications.

Case 39: **Anorexic rabbit due to dental disease**

CLINICAL PRESENTATION. A mature pet rabbit is anorectic for two weeks, is reluctant to take syringe feedings and is losing weight. There is a history of recurrent inappetence, which was previously managed by syringe feeding a slurry of liquidized rabbit pellets until the rabbit resumed eating. The rabbit was raised on a concentrated ration of pellets and grain without access to hay or fresh herbage. The rabbit has normal resting incisor occlusion, the tips of the mandibular incisors resting between the first and second maxillary incisors (**39**).

DIFFERENTIAL DIAGNOSES. Dental spikes (points), GI ileus (due to poor diet), any metabolic disease since anorexia is a nonspecific sign of disease.

INVESTIGATION. A complete diagnostic work up is recommended, but the first procedure should be a thorough oral examination. On examination, two spikes are observed on the cheek teeth

DIAGNOSIS. The most likely diagnosis is mucosal pain resulting from the enamel spikes on two of the cheek teeth causing buccal or lingual irritation. A concentrate ration (grain and/or pellets) requires much less chewing for each unit of energy intake when compared with dry or fresh herbage, resulting in inadequate wear to the cheek teeth.

ETIOLOGY. When eating natural foods, the lips are used for prehension and herbage is cut into manageable sections using the incisors. Rabbits use their incisor teeth in a lateral slicing action. The food is then crushed and ground using the cheek teeth prior to swallowing. The free end of the tongue is relatively thin and mobile and is used to assist the lips with prehension and the transfer of food from the incisor to the cheek teeth region. The body of the tongue is fairly solid, with a raised section between the cheek teeth arcades. It is used to move food between the grinding surfaces of the cheek teeth and form the ground material into a bolus for swallowing.

With a concurrent reduction in the degree of lateral jaw excursion during chewing, the buccal surfaces of the maxillary (see **34a**) and lingual surfaces of the mandibular cheek teeth (see **34b**) are worn least and sharp points or spikes of enamel form. Even very minor irregularities on the tooth surfaces may abrade or ulcerate the contacting lingual or buccal mucosa, causing significant pain. This leads to inappetence, dysphagia, quidding (food dropping from the mouth during chewing), excessive salivation, reduced food intake, and weight loss.

PREVALENCE. Common in pet rabbits, especially those on poor diets.

MANAGEMENT. The quickest treatment is grinding the spikes to relieve the pain. Further treatment includes periodic trimming.

PROGNOSIS. The owners need to know this may be a lifelong problem.

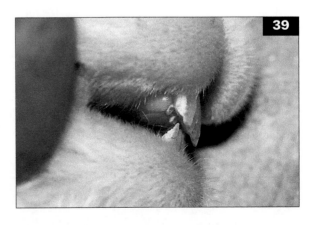

Case 40: **Rabbit with renal disease**

CLINICAL PRESENTATION. A seven-year-old intact male rabbit is lethargic, cachexic, and approximately 8% dehydrated. The kidneys are smaller than average. There has been a noticeable weight loss over the past two months and the rabbit has been anorectic for two weeks.

DIFFERENTIAL DIAGNOSES. Any metabolic disorder (e.g. renal disease, liver disease), dental disease, degenerative disease, and neoplasia.

INVESTIGATION. The plasma biochemistry and hematology results are shown below.

DIAGNOSIS. The presence of markedly elevated BUN and creatinine values in the face of isosthenuric (not concentrated) urine is diagnostic for renal failure.

ETIOLOGY. Chronic renal failure is more likely than acute renal failure in this rabbit because of the presence of small kidneys, hyperphosphatemia, and anemia, and the lack of hyperkalemia and oliguria. Causes for chronic renal failure in pet rabbits include infectious interstitial nephritis, pyelonephritis (bacterial, viral, fungal), glomerulonephritis secondary to immune complex deposition, neoplasia, *E. cuniculi*, and nephrotoxins.

PREVALENCE. Renal failure is an infrequent cause of disease in older rabbits.

MANAGEMENT. I/v or i/o lactated Ringer's solution should be administered immediately. The dehydration deficit is replaced over six hours and the diuresis continued. The patient is placed on standard maintenance fluids of 100 ml/kg/day once the BUN concentration approaches more normal values. Fluids can be given s/c once the dehydration is corrected and the patient is urinating normally. Serum potassium is monitored and any excesses or deficiencies corrected. Much of the acidosis is expected to be corrected by the fluid therapy. The anemia can be treated with ferrous sulfate (4–6 mg/kg p/o q24h). B complex vitamins are added to the parenteral fluids if needed. Although dosages are not established for rabbits, recombinant human erythropoietin therapy may be beneficial. The anorexia is treated with gavage or tube feeding until the patient is eating on its own. A safe broad-spectrum antibiotic with minimal nephrotoxicity is given while awaiting urine culture results. Enrofloxacin (15–20 mg/kg i/v or p/o q24h) is an excellent first choice. Trimethoprim/sulfa combinations, tetracyclines, and aminoglycosides should be avoided because of potential nephrotoxicity.

PROGNOSIS. If the rabbit shows minimal response to fluid therapy, the prognosis for long-term survival is grave.

Test	Patient value	Normal values
PCV	0.19 l/l (nonregenerative) (19%)	0.33–0.50 l/l (33–50%)
Plasma protein	74 g/l (7.4 g/dl)	54–83 g/l (5.4–8.3 g/dl)
WBCs	7.2×10^9/l (7.2×10^3/µl)	5.2–12.5×10^9/l (5.2–12.5×10^3/µl)
Calcium	3.0 mmol/l (12.0 mg/dl)	1.4–3.1 mmol/l (5.6–12.4 mg/dl)
Phosphorus	3.4 mmol/l (10.54 mEq/l)	1.3–2.2 mmol/l (4.03–6.82 mEq/l)
Glucose	5.6 mmol/l (100.8 mg/dl)	4.2–8.7 mmol/l (75.6–156.6 mg/dl)
Creatinine	689.5 µmol/l (7.8 mg/dl)	44.2–221 µmol/l (0.5–2.5 mg/dl)
BUN	68.2 mmol/l (191 mg/dl)	4.6–9.3 mmol/l (12.9–26.04 mg/dl)
Sodium	151 mmol/l (151 mEq/l)	131–155 mmol/l (131–155 mEq/l)
Potassium	6.4 mmol/l (6.4 mEq/l)	3.6–6.9 mmol/l (3.6–6.9 mEq/l)
ALT	63 u/l	48–80 u/l
Urine SG	1.010	1.003–1.036

Case 41: **Ferret with a GI foreign body**

CLINICAL PRESENTATION. A young ferret presented after two days of lethargy, anorexia, and diarrhea.

DIFFERENTIAL DIAGNOSES. GI foreign body, infection, parasites, metabolic and neoplastic disease of the intestinal tract.

INVESTIGATION. A lateral abdominal contrast radiograph is obtained (**41**). Frequently, GI foreign bodies are palpable during the physical examination. Most of the time, contrast radiographs are not necessary.

DIAGNOSIS. Radiopaque foreign bodies in the small intestine.

PREVALENCE. Ingestion of foreign objects is more common in ferrets under the age of one year. Older ferrets do not seem to eat foreign material.

MANAGEMENT. Abdominal exploratory surgery is performed, with careful palpation of the entire GI tract, including the stomach. This detects other foreign bodies not visible on the radiograph. If the foreign object is in the stomach, a routine gastrotomy is performed. If the object is in the intestinal tract and cannot be 'milked' into the stomach, an enterotomy is performed. The segment of bowel containing the foreign body is exteriorized and isolated by packing it off with moistened gauze sponges or laparotomy pads. The intestinal contents are gently milked away from the site, with an assistant 'finger clamping' the bowel. Sterilized 'bobby pins' (US) or hair grips are used in the absence of an assistant. An incision is made in the antemesenteric portion of the bowel just distal to the foreign body and the foreign body removed through this opening. Any necrotic bowel, if present, is removed and healthy tissue is anastomosed. The bowel is closed with 5-0 monofilament, nonabsorbable suture if there is severe infection; otherwise a monofilament, absorbable synthetic suture material can be used. It is not advisable to use chromic catgut. The bowel is lavaged and replaced in the abdomen. The sterile gloves and surgical instruments are changed, and the abdomen is lavaged with warm sterile saline. The abdomen is closed with 4-0 or 5-0 monofilament, synthetic absorbable suture. The ferret is fed within 12–24 hours after surgery. Peritonitis is rarely a complication of a GI foreign body in ferrets. If peritonitis is observed, the abdomen is cultured for aerobic and anaerobic bacteria, flushed copiously, and treated with drain placement or left as an open abdomen depending on the severity of the disease. Antibiotics are administered based on culture results if peritonitis is present. Otherwise, the ferret is given a broad-spectrum antibiotic post surgically. Ferrets should be caged unless supervised otherwise they will ingest objects that will cause a blockage of the GI tract.

PROGNOSIS. If the bowel is not necrotic and if severe peritonitis is not present, the prognosis is excellent.

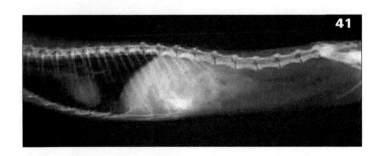

Case 42: **Ferret with heartworm disease**

CLINICAL PRESENTATION. A ferret living in the southern part of the US presents because of progressive episodes of coughing and dyspnea. On physical examination it is dehydrated and lethargic, with pale mucous membranes.

DIFFERENTIAL DIAGNOSES. Heartworm disease, cardiomyopathy (either dilated or hypertrophic). Other differentials include pneumonia (e.g. canine distemper virus), a severe case of influenza, or neoplasia.

INVESTIGATION. Thoracic radiographs reveal enlargement of the right ventricle and increased interstitial opacity throughout the lungs (**42a, b**). The ferret dies before any further diagnostics are performed.

Microfilarial tests may be performed when heartworms are suspected, but only 20% of heartworm infections in ferrets are microfilaremic. Also, plasma can be tested by one of the commercially available antigen detection kits that detect heartworm antigen in the plasma of dogs. While these tests are very specific and rarely give false-positives, ferrets may have too few worms in the heart to produce enough antigen to be detected. Therefore, false-negative results may occur when these tests are used for ferrets. Antibody tests are species-specific and cannot be used on ferret plasma to obtain an accurate answer. Cardiomegaly may be visualized on chest radiographs. Ultrasound is the best antemortem diagnostic procedure to detect the presence of worms.

At necropsy, two helminths measuring 100 mm and 65 mm in length are recovered from the right ventricle (**42c**).

DIAGNOSIS. Infection with *Dirofilaria immitis*, the dog heartworm.

ETIOLOGY. Ferrets are infected when mosquitoes bite them and deposit the infective third-stage larvae. The worms migrate into subcutaneous tissues and muscles. They reach the heart between 90 and 140 days post infection.

PREVALENCE. The prevalence of this disease is not known. Because most pet ferrets live indoors, and ferrets are not the natural host for this infection, dirofilariasis is very uncommon in pet ferrets. In the US, infection is mostly seen in ferrets that live in warm weather states with a longer mosquito season.

MANAGEMENT. A number of treatment protocols have been proposed, but if severe damage has been done to the heart and/or vena cava, treatment may be futile. Surgical removal should be considered if possible. The most common approach is to treat ferrets with heartworm disease in the same way as cats. Anti-inflammatory drugs such as prednisolone (2.2 mg/kg p/o q24h) should be given to keep the lungs 'happier' during worm death, and adult worms should not be treated with an adulticide. To prevent infection effectively, ferrets can also be placed on a monthly dose of ivermectin (6–50 µg/kg p/o). Keeping ferrets indoors and limiting exposure to mosquitos will decrease the chance of a pet ferret contracting this disease.

PROGNOSIS. If heart damage or vena caval damage is severe, the prognosis for survival is poor. If there is little damage, and the worms do not cause damage, the prognosis is good.

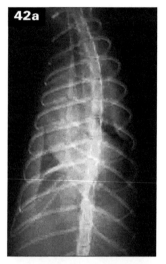

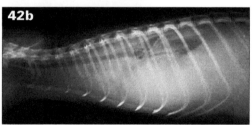

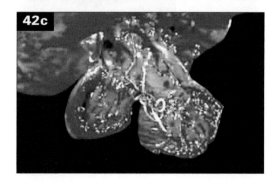

Case 43: **Ferret with a skin mast cell tumor**

CLINICAL PRESENTATION. A four-year-old ferret is brought into the hospital with a crusty, slightly raised red mass on its foot that has been there for three months (**43**). The ferret occasionally scratches the mass, which will then bleed.

DIFFERENTIAL DIAGNOSES. Mast cell tumors, sebaceous gland adenomas, squamous cell tumors, adeno-carcinomas, cutaneous lymphomas, and abscesses can present as skin masses in ferrets.

INVESTIGATION. An impression smear of the mass is made. Biopsy tissue for histology will provide a definitive diagnosis. If warranted, radiography and/or ultrasonography can be performed to look for the presence of organomegaly due to distant neoplasia.

DIAGNOSIS. Mast cell tumor.

ETIOLOGY. Cutaneous mast cell tumors in ferrets appear as papules or nodules and vary in color from tan, yellow, brown, or red. They are multiple or solitary and occasionally will resolve without surgical removal. Some are pruritic and are covered with dried blood. Some cause a localized area of hair loss. Lesions can occur anywhere. Mast cell tumors in the ferret are almost always benign, but metastasis to other organs should always be investigated.

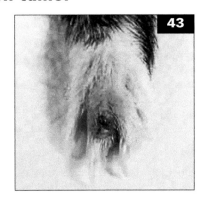

Since this disease is rarely systemic, the CBC and biochemistry profile usually do not reflect the changes caused by mast cell tumors.

PREVALENCE. This is the most frequent cutaneous neoplasm in ferrets.

MANAGEMENT. Treatment is by surgical excision. Some mast cell tumors may resolve on their own. Pretreatment with antihistamines is not indicated.

PROGNOSIS. The long-term prognosis for the majority of cases of mast cell tumor is good.

Case 44: **Ferret with insulinoma**

CLINICAL PRESENTATION. A ferret has been diagnosed with pancreatic beta cell tumors.

PREVALENCE. Insulinoma is is a very common disease in older ferrets in the US. Owners frequently seek advice on whether their ferret should be treated medically or surgically, or both.

MANAGEMENT. Surgery is primarily a debulking procedure, as it rarely removes all of the diseased pancreas. Medical treatment is aimed at controlling the signs but does not halt the progression of this disease. The owner should be advised that when insulinoma is diagnosed, the patient will require management of this disease for the rest of its life. A recent study revealed that ferrets receiving medical treatment for insulinomas lived an average of six months post diagnosis. However, some ferrets can live as long as two years on medical therapy alone. Medical treatment most often consists of prednisone and/or diazoxide. The owner should discontinue any sugary treats in the diet. The diet should consist of frequent feeding of a high-quality cat or ferret food. Medical treatment is begun when the blood glucose concentration is below 3.66 mmol/l

(65 mg/dl). All blood glucose concentrations should be based on a fasting sample, the ferret being fasted from two to no more than four hours.

If prednisone is given as the first line drug, the administration can be started at 0.10–0.50 mg/kg p/o q12h. Treatment should begin at the low end of the dosage range and gradually increased as dictated by the ferret's signs. Fasting blood glucose samples are obtained every 1–3 months. As the tumor spreads, it becomes increasingly resistant to the effects of the prednisone. The second commonly used medication is diazoxide (5–30 mg/kg p/o q12h), which prevents the release of insulin. Treatment is started with one medication and, as resistance increases, the other medication is added to the treatment regimen. There are no contraindications for giving the medications concurrently. Since prednisone theoretically increases the workload on the heart, it must be given cautiously to ferrets with heart disease. It is useful to screen ferrets for insulinoma by obtaining routine fasting blood glucose samples every six months once the ferret reaches three years of age. Food should always be available.

PROGNOSIS. Early detection and consequent treatment improve the long-term prognosis.

Case 45: **Ferret with dilated cardiomyopathy**

CLINICAL PRESENTATION. An acutely dyspneic six-year-old male castrated ferret, which is kept indoors, is responding well to oxygen therapy.

DIFFERENTIAL DIAGNOSES. Cardiac disease, neoplasia (particularly lymphosarcoma), and severe influenza infection are the most likely differential diagnoses. In certain geographical areas, heartworm disease should be considered.

INVESTIGATION. Radiographs (**45a, b**) reveal thoracic fluid. The pleural fluid is removed immediately via thoracocentesis and analyzed and cultured. Both sides of the thorax are drained using a 25 gauge butterfly catheter placed low in the chest wall. Multiple sites on either side of the chest are aspirated to remove as much fluid as possible. The ferret may need to be sedated for this procedure. Once the ferret is less dyspneic, repeat radiographs are obtained to view the thoracic contents more clearly. In this case a large heart is present, leading to a diagnosis of heart disease. To further characterize the heart disease, an echocardiograph is performed to determine the type and extent of heart disease present. The echocardiograph reveals left ventricle dilation, mitral and tricuspid valve regurgitation, and a poor shortening fraction. An ECG is also performed.

When the ferret is more stable, a CBC and biochemistry panel and urinalysis are performed. These tests will assess the metabolic condition of the ferret and help to direct treatment effectively.

DIAGNOSIS. Dilated cardiomyopathy.

PREVALENCE. Not uncommon in older pet ferrets. Hypertrophic cardiomyopathy is much less common and is seen in younger ferrets.

MANAGEMENT. While the ferret is in the hospital, it is given oxygen therapy as needed and the pleural effusion is removed as it accumulates. Long-term treatment is commenced in the hospital and continued at home. Furosemide (2.2 mg/kg p/o q8–12h), digoxin (0.01 mg/kg p/o q24h), and an ACE inhibitor such as enalapril (0.5 mg/kg p/o q48h) are administered.

PROGNOSIS. The prognosis depends on the response to treatment. Even ferrets with severe heart failure may do well for a period of time with treatment and have a good quality of life as long as they continue to respond to the medication.

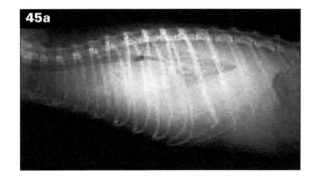
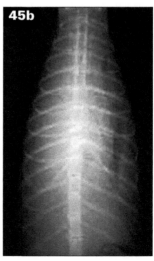

Case 46: **Ferret venipuncture**

INTRODUCTION. The prevalence of systemic disease in ferrets necessitates blood collection in most ferret patients. Blood can be taken from the cephalic vein, jugular vein, lateral saphenous vein, and ventral tail artery of ferrets using a 22, 25, or 27 gauge needle. Consideration should be given to sedating a difficult to handle ferret. Most ferrets can be phlebotomized fully awake with the aid of a trained handler once some experience is gained.

TECHNIQUE. To obtain blood from the cephalic vein, the ferret is restrained with one hand around the neck, the other hand holding off the vein with the thumb and the forearm restraining the patient's body (**46a**). 0.5–1.0 ml of blood can be collected from this site.

For jugular venipuncture, the ferret is scruffed and its body wrapped tightly with a towel, restraining the ferret's forelimbs against its chest. A scruff hold is maintained on the upper neck area and the ferret laid on its dorsum. Pressure is applied just lateral to the thoracic inlet and the jugular vein, which runs from the inlet to the base of the ear, is visualized or palpated. The hair is clipped if needed to aid in visualization. The jugular vein can also be accessed by holding the ferret in a similar manner as a cat, with its forelimbs pulled over the edge of the table and the neck hyperextended (**46b, c**).

The lateral saphenous vein is a short vein that yields up to 0.5 ml of blood. It is accessed by holding the ferret on its side with a scruff on the neck and firm pressure applied to the upper thigh.

A maximum of 1% of the body weight can be removed as blood volume in a healthy ferret. For example, a 1,000 g ferret can lose a maximum of 10 ml of blood safely.

Ferrets have no discernable blood types, therefore blood typing is not necessary and multiple donors may be used to transfuse a ferret patient.

The cephalic, lateral saphenous, and jugular veins are all suitable for intravenous catheterization using a 22, 24, or 26 gauge intravenous catheter. Jugular catheters (**46d**) are used only when a central line is necessary, as ferrets do not like their necks wrapped. Due to the thick ferret skin, a large gauge needle is used to prepuncture the skin before placing a catheter. The most common site for an intraosseous catheter is the femur, which can be approached through the trochanteric fossa using a 20 gauge spinal or regular hypodermic needle.

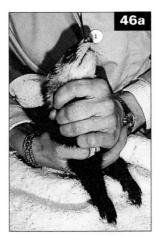
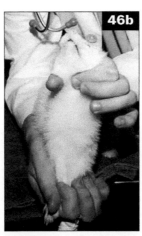
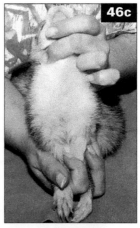

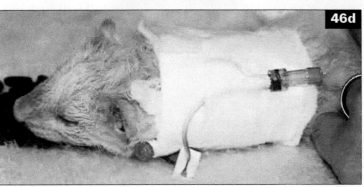

Case 47: **Ferret vaccines**

CLINICAL PRESENTATION. A two-year-old ferret living in the US is brought to the veterinary hospital for advice on vaccines and vaccination schedules. Ferrets in the US are routinely vaccinated against canine distemper virus and rabies virus, both of which cause a fatal disease.

ETIOLOGY. Canine distemper virus is common in certain canid populations in the US. Raccoons and skunks can also transmit this disease to ferrets. Rabies virus is endemic in certain areas of the US and any outdoor ferret could be exposed to this virus.

MANAGEMENT. In the US, one canine distemper virus vaccine is available that is licensed for use in ferrets. It is a modified live vaccine given subcutaneously. The first dose is administered at 6–8 weeks of age and repeat doses are given at three week intervals until the ferret is 16 weeks of age. Booster vaccination should then be administered annually. Ferrets over 16 weeks of age that have never been vaccinated receive two doses 2–3 weeks apart. A canine distemper virus vaccine that is propagated in a canine cell line must not be used, as it can induce clinical disease. A killed vaccine may not offer long lasting protection.

Vaccination against rabies virus is recommended in the domestic ferret (in the US). Although the risk of exposure is small in ferrets housed indoors, local animal control ordinances may require vaccination. In some areas an unvaccinated ferret that bites a human will be euthanized and the head submitted for rabies virus examination. Not every municipality will recognize vaccination. In the US the killed rabies virus vaccine licensed for use in ferrets is IMRAB-3. Ferrets are susceptible to rabies virus but are not natural reservoir hosts of the virus. Ferrets are vaccinated subcutaneously at three months of age and given boosters annually.

Ferrets do not need to be vaccinated against feline panleukopenia, feline leukemia, and feline infectious peritonitis viruses because they are not susceptible to these diseases.

PROGNOSIS. Ferrets that are vaccinated properly against canine distemper vaccine have only a remote chance of developing the disease. Ferrets that are exposed to canine distemper virus and contract the disease are likely to die from the disease. Ferrets that are properly vaccinated against rabies virus are highly unlikely to develop this disease. Ferrets that are exposed to the rabies virus and are not vaccinated will develop this fatal zoonotic infection.

Case 48: **Ferret with splenomegaly**

CLINICAL PRESENTATION. On physical examination a ferret is diagnosed with a large spleen, but it does not appear clinically ill.

DIFFERENTIAL DIAGNOSES. Splenomegaly, lymphosarcoma, or other neoplastic disease. Palpation of a 'lumpy' or 'hard' spleen is more likely due to neoplasia.

INVESTIGATION. Hematology and plasma biochemistry panels provide useful information. Alterations in the hemogram may be seen with neoplastic and infectious disease. Radiographs confirm the presence of splenomegaly. Ultrasound is used to determine the splenic architecture. Extramedullary hematopoiesis does not change the normal parenchyma of the spleen, whereas other disease, especially neoplasia, distorts the splenic architecture.

A percutaneous splenic aspirate should be collected to determine the cause of the splenomegaly. The ferret is scruffed and placed on a flat surface while isolating the spleen with one hand. The spleen is aspirated with a 25 gauge needle attached to a 3 ml syringe. If neoplasia is present, it is usually diffuse and found on an aspirate. If needed, the ferret can be sedated for this procedure. Ultrasound guided aspirates can also be attempted. The ultimate diagnostic procedure is exploratory laparotomy with splenic biopsy or removal.

ETIOLOGY. Extramedullary hematopoiesis is a common cause of splenomegaly. Splenomegaly due to extramedullary hematopoiesis is characterized by an enlarged spleen with rounded borders. Palpation of the organ reveals a smooth surface and a spongy consistency. No other organ enlargement is present. There is no known reason for this disease to occur in ferrets.

PREVALENCE. Splenomegaly due to extramedullary hematopoiesis is very common in older ferrets. Splenic neoplasia is much less common.

MANAGEMENT. Typically, removal of the spleen for extramedullary hematopoiesis is not necessary. Infrequently, splenomegaly causes the splenic volume to be so great as to cause displacement of other abdominal organs. If this displacement is severe, it may cause the ferret to be uncomfortable and even partially anorexic. This is an indication for splenectomy even if the cause is extramedullary hematopoiesis. In most instances the spleen should be removed if neoplasia is present. Successful treatment of lymphosarcoma may not depend on splenic removal.

PROGNOSIS. Excellent

Case 49: **Ferret with respiratory and neurologic signs due to canine distemper virus**

CLINICAL PRESENTATION. A four-month-old ferret is found wandering outside. It is weak, tachypneic, and sneezing. It has a copious mucoid nasal discharge, chin swelling, and crusting and thickened foot pads (**49**) The ferret is brought into a house where there are two other ferrets. Despite supportive care, the ferret develops ataxia and torticollis and is now comatose.

DIFFERENTIAL DIAGNOSES. Canine distemper virus (CDV) infection, a severe infection with influenza virus, bacterial pneumonia, or mycotic pneumonia. If only neurologic signs are apparent, rabies virus infection and listeriosis should be considered in the differential diagnoses, although these are rare diseases in ferrets.

INVESTIGATION. A fluorescent antibody test for CDV antigen should be performed on conjunctival smears, mucous membrane scrapings, or blood smears to diagnose CDV. This is useful only in the first few days of disease, usually before disease signs are apparent. Therefore, this is not generally a very practical method of diagnosis. The modified live viral strains used for vaccination do not interfere with this testing method. Hematology will aid in the diagnosis of CDV infection. As with other viral infections, a leukopenia can be observed. Radiographs characterize the extent of the pneumonia. A lung wash will determine the cause of the pneumonia. A secondary bacterial pneumonia is usually present and this can be responsible for the respiratory signs. Cytology on a cerebrospinal fluid tap will determine the cause of the neurologic signs. CDV infection is diagnosed definitively at postmortem. CDV inclusion bodies are generally found in the epithelial cells of the trachea, urinary bladder, skin, GI tract, lymph nodes, spleen, and salivary glands.

DIAGNOSIS. CDV infection is the diagnosis in this ferret.

ETIOLOGY. Although other diseases can cause severe respiratory infection, only CDV causes both respiratory and neurologic disease signs. CDV also causes chin swelling and crusting, which are cardinal signs of this disease and appear before thickened foot pads are apparent. Swelling and crusting may also be present in the perineal and inguinal area of ferrets infected with CDV. This ferret was found outside, where it likely came in contact with infected animals. The vaccine status of the ferret is unknown.

PREVALENCE. CDV infection is an uncommon disease for two reasons: many pet ferrets are vaccinated and most pet ferrets rarely come in contact with carriers of this virus.

MANAGEMENT. There is no treatment for CDV infection. Treatment for secondary bacterial infections only prolongs the inevitable.

PROGNOSIS. Grave.

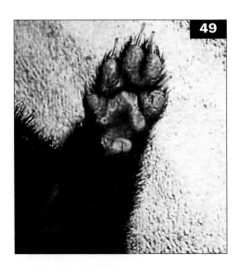

Case 50: **Ferret handling**

CLINICAL PRESENTATION. A young ferret is proving difficult to handle. What is the best way to handle this ferret and how should enteral and parenteral medications be administered?

MANAGEMENT. It is rarely necessary to use gloves or other hand protection when handling pet ferrets. Kits under four months of age tend to 'play bite' more frequently than adults. Ferrets have a very keen sense of smell and some odors on the hand, especially food or other ferret body odors, can precipitate a bite. Placing a drop of isopropyl alcohol on the gums of the biting animal will cause an immediate release. To examine the dorsum, the ferret's body is rested along the forearm. To inspect the ventrum, the patient is placed on its dorsum by cupping its head in the palm of the hand and securing the ferret between the forearm and body. A ferret can also be 'scruffed', which calms down some active patients and allows better access for palpation of the cranial abdomen (**50**). The ferret is grasped by the loose skin along the back of the neck and suspended over a table. Gently stroking downwards on its abdomen will aid relaxation. This hold is used for administering subcutaneous injections, cleaning ears, and trimming nails. Ferrets love sweet treats and these can be employed to handle a fractious patient. A sticky sweet substance, such as a cat hairball laxative, can be put on a tongue depressor and the ferret allowed to lick it when it is being weighed or given injections. For nail trimming without assistance, the ferret is set in a sitting position in the lap, and a small amount of a sticky sweet substance is placed on its lower abdomen and shown to the ferret. While the ferret is licking the treat, the nails can be trimmed on all four paws. The ferret's abdomen should

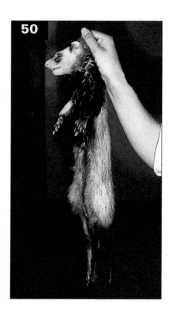

normally be relaxed and easy to palpate. The spleen, kidneys, stomach, intestines, and bladder are all palpable.

The easiest way to medicate a ferret orally is by masking the taste with a sweet or oily substance. Substances high in sugar content are contraindicated if the ferret is diagnosed with insulinoma. Sweet substances can be diluted with water and still maintain the taste desired. Subcutaneous injections are given in the neck area as the animal is scruffed or along the back or shoulders. Intramuscular injections are administered in the lumbar musculature or quadriceps.

Case 51: **Ferret with neurologic signs due to low blood glucose caused by an insulinoma**

CLINICAL PRESENTATION. A four-year-old spayed female ferret is found unable to walk. On physical examination there is no voluntary motor movement in the hindlimbs. All reflexes are assessed as normal and muscle atrophy is not apparent. The ferret has a blood glucose concentration of 1.68 mmol/l (30 mg/dl).

DIFFERENTIAL DIAGNOSES. Include hypoglycemia due to insulinoma, intervertebral disc disease, discospondylitis, other causes of hypoglycemia, myelitis, diffuse muscular disease, diffuse skeletal disease, neoplasia, heart disease, anemia, hyperthermia, metabolic disease, GI disease, and Aleutian disease.

INVESTIGATION. Hematology and plasma biochemistry are performed. Anemia is not seen with insulinoma, but if a low RBC count is observed, one cause to consider is hyperestrogenism as seen in unspayed ferrets that remain in estrus or, rarely, ferrets with adrenal gland disease. Severe GI ulcers can also cause anemia. Renal disease and any chronic disease can result in anemia. An elevated WBC count may indicate a severe infection or lymphoma leading to weakness. A low blood glucose concentration is highly indicative of a pancreatic beta cell tumor. A fasting blood glucose (2–4 hours) concentration below 3.92 mmol/l (70 mg/dl) is good evidence that an insulinoma is present, especially if the ferret is above the age of three years. Ferrets with insulinoma commonly present with hindlimb paresis. Other metabolic diseases should be ruled out based on the biochemistry results. Radiographs are obtained to rule out cardiac disease and/or abdominal disease. If necessary, spinal radiographs are taken or a myelogram performed to determine if disc disease is present.

DIAGNOSIS. Insulinoma due to low blood glucose.

ETIOLOGY. Insulinoma (beta cell carcinoma) is common in ferrets over the age of three years of age in the US. Collapse and hindlimb paresis can be a nonspecific sign of disease in ferrets. Therefore, many diseases are considered when a ferret shows signs of paresis. The differential diagnoses are not limited to neuromuscular disease processes. Diagnosis of hindlimb paresis requires a thorough history, examination, and possibly extensive testing.

PREVALENCE. Common disease of older ferrets.

MANAGEMENT. The ferret responded well initially to one dose of oral glucose and was then maintained on prednisone, starting at 0.1–0.5 mg/kg p/o q12h. Food should always be available and sugary treats are to be avoided.

PROGNOSIS. Ferrets can be maintained for months on medication, but surgical treatment is more likely to give a better quality of life.

Case 52: **Ferret with an acute vaccine reaction**

CLINICAL PRESENTATION. A seemingly healthy three-year-old ferret is vaccinated for CDV. Twenty minutes later, the ferret is battling for its life. The ferret is limp and is vomiting, and a bright red bloody diarrhea is evident.

DIFFERENTIAL DIAGNOSES. Due to the temporal sequence between vaccine administration and observance of signs, there are no other differentials to consider other than a vaccine reaction.

INVESTIGATION. The hematologic and biochemistry results will reflect a ferret in shock, with the GI system being the 'shock organ'. Initially, the picture is one of dehydration. Later, the results may reflect anemia and electrolyte imbalance.

ETIOLOGY. Both canine distemper and rabies virus vaccines have been implicated in causing severe vaccine reactions. Most anaphylactic reactions occur within 15–30 minutes of vaccine administration. A variety of signs can be seen including clear to blood-tinged vomit, bloody diarrhea, dyspnea, cyanosis, tachycardia, and collapse.

PREVALENCE. The prevalence of these reactions is unknown. It is likely that the incidence rate of this problem is low. It is unknown if ferrets that have had previous vaccine reactions are more likely to have another reaction. Some authors suggest not vaccinating ferrets that have had a vaccine reaction.

MANAGEMENT. If the patient is not immediately treated, severe reactions can lead to seizures, coma, and finally death. Oxygen should be administered by endotracheal tube or facemask and an intravenous catheter placed. Epinephrine (0.25–1.0 ml of a 1:10,000 dilution i/v) and diphenhydramine hydrochloride (1–2 mg/kg i/v) should be given. In addition, either hydrocortisone sodium succinate (25–40 mg/kg i/v) or prednisolone sodium succinate (5 mg/kg i/v) should be given along with lactated Ringer's solution with added dextrose at a shock rate. If the i/v route cannot be established, the above medications can be given by the intraosseous route. A high rate of fluids must be maintained as hypovolemia is common. Owners should be advised to remain with their animal at the veterinary hospital for at least 30 minutes following vaccination to observe for anaphylactic reactions. Some authors have suggested either premedicating with diphenhydramine hydrochloride at least one hour before vaccination or separating the CDV vaccine administration from the rabies virus vaccine administration by at least one week. Both of these suggestions are unproven.

PROGNOSIS. If treated immediately, the prognosis is excellent for a full recovery. If the ferret is not treated and shows severe signs of shock, it may die. Most ferrets respond quickly to treatment and do not need to spend an extensive period of time in the hospital.

Case 53: Ferret unable to urinate due to prostatomegaly secondary to adrenal gland disease

CLINICAL PRESENTATION. A four-year-old male castrated ferret was examined because of progressive stranguria and urinary incontinence of two weeks duration. The ferret also had a two-month history of dorsal pruritus. Physical examination revealed a large, painful bladder that was difficult to express.

DIFFERENTIAL DIAGNOSES. The differential diagnoses for stranguria associated with a large bladder in ferrets include prostatomegaly due to adrenal gland disease, urinary tract calculi, urinary tract infection, neoplasia, and constriction of the urethral passageway due to diseased prostatic tissue along the urethra caused by infection, cysts, hyperplasia, or cancer.

INVESTIGATION. In this case, radiography (53) revealed the presence of a large bladder. Urine should be collected by cystocentesis for urinalysis and bacterial culture. The plasma concentration of adrenal gland hormones should be determined to aid in the diagnosis of adrenal gland disease. Abdominal ultrasound will detect the cause of the enlarged bladder and any adrenal gland enlargement. In this case, abdominal ultrasound revealed a large left adrenal gland and a swelling along the urethra just distal to the bladder. Determination of plasma concentration of adrenal gland hormones revealed high androstenedione and estrogen, which is consistent with adrenal gland disease in ferrets. Determining the metabolic status of these ferrets is extremely important. A CBC and plasma biochemistry profile should be performed. The longer the bladder is blocked, the more deranged the metabolic health of the ferret becomes. The blockage needs to be relieved, but just as important is reversing any metabolic changes caused by the inability to urinate.

DIAGNOSIS. Prostatomegaly leading to urinary tract blockage.

ETIOLOGY. Urethral stricture in male ferrets with adrenal gland disease is caused by enlargement of the prostatic tissue surrounding the urethra.

PREVALENCE. Unknown in the general ferret population and unknown in the population of ferrets with adrenal gland disease.

MANAGEMENT. Initial treatment includes administration of antibiotics and placement of a urinary catheter and collection system under anesthesia. Once stable, an exploratory laparotomy is performed to remove the enlarged adrenal gland. In this case the periurethral tissue was bilaterally swollen just distal to the bladder. Incisional biopsy of the mass revealed cystic prostatic tissue. No attempt was made to remove this tissue, because without the presence of infection the swelling dissipates when the adrenal gland is removed. The entire diseased left adrenal gland was removed. The ferret recovered uneventfully, and the urinary catheter system was removed 12 hours after surgery.

PROGNOSIS. If the entire diseased adrenal gland is not removed, the prognosis is guarded because prostatic enlargement may not subside. If the entire diseased adrenal gland is removed, the prognosis is good.

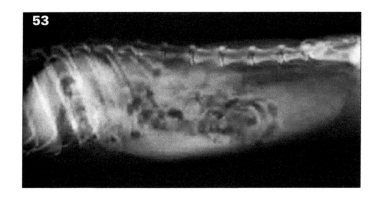

Case 54: **Ferret with signs of hypoglycemia due to insulinoma**

CLINICAL PRESENTATION. A seven-year-old ferret has numerous episodes of lethargy, ptyalism, and collapse over a six-month period. On physical examination, nothing unusual is found apart from the ferret appearing slightly weak. A blood glucose evaluation shows that the blood glucose is below the normal range.

DIFFERENTIAL DIAGNOSES. The three causes of low blood sugar in ferrets are insulinoma, liver disease, and sepsis.

INVESTIGATION. Hematology and plasma biochemistry values are usually normal in ferrets with an insulinoma, except for the blood glucose. In this ferret the blood glucose was 2.8 mmol/l (32 mg/dl).

DIAGNOSIS. A pancreatic beta cell tumor or insulinoma.

ETIOLOGY. Inappropriate insulin concentrations result in hypoglycemia leading to episodic weakness. In the ferret, ptyalism may be a sign of nausea.

PREVALENCE. Very common in pet ferrets.

MANAGEMENT. Medical treatment includes frequent feeding, prednisone, and diazoxide. Although surgery is the treatment of choice, as it prolongs the ferret's life, it is not always possible. If the ferret has systemic disease (e.g. decompensated heart disease), if the owner cannot afford surgery, or if there are other extenuating circumstances, then the ferret can be maintained with medical therapy. Owners need to realize that with either medical or surgical treatment, malignant beta cells will eventually spread to other organs and thus prevent glucohomeostasis.

In this case an abdominal exploratory laporatory was performed and a mass found on the pancreas (**54**). When performing an exploratory laparotomy, careful inspection of all the abdominal organs is vital. The pancreas is palpated gently, feeling for discrete, firm nodules. More than one insulinoma may be present in the pancreas. Insulinomas can be as small as 1–2 mm in size. Occasionally, only diffuse pancreatic thickening may be present. A nodulectomy in the body of the pancreas is performed by shelling out the nodules. A partial pancreatectomy should be carried out if tumors are located in the right or left limb. Hemostatic clips are used for a partial pancreatectomy. Bleeding is minimal. The liver and any abnormal lymph nodes are biopsied. The abdomen is closed using a 4-0 monofilament, synthetic absorbable suture material. Post surgically, the blood glucose concentration is moinitored until the ferret is euglycemic. Infrequently, ferrets will need to be maintained on either prednisone and/or diazoxide in the immediate post-surgical period. The ferret is rechecked 7–10 days after surgery and the fasting blood glucose level evaluated at that time.

PROGNOSIS. Because surgery is rarely curative, it will be necessary to monitor the fasting blood glucose at regular intervals for the rest of the ferret's life.

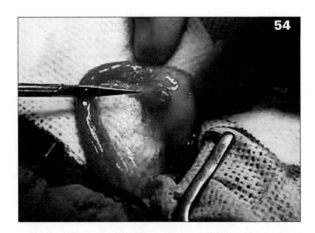

Case 55: **Ferret adrenal gland disease: lack of treatment?**

CLINICAL PRESENTATION. A six-year-old ferret has a two-year history of an enlarged vulva, vulvar discharge, and hair loss.

DIFFERENTIAL DIAGNOSES. With these signs and signalment, only adrenal gland disease should be considered.

INVESTIGATION. Signalment, history, and physical examination are used to diagnose this disease. More definitive diagnostic tests include abdominal ultrasound and adrenal androgen concentration measurements.

DIAGNOSIS. Adrenal gland disease.

PREVALENCE. Unknown, but appears common in pet ferrets.

MANAGEMENT. Abdominal exploratory surgery to remove the diseased adrenal gland is the recommended treatment, but in this case the owner opts for medical care. Medical treatment is still equivocal in regards to long-term prognosis, although great strides have been made. Mitotane is no longer recommended. Numerous other drugs are now recommended including anastrozole (Arimidex), flutamide (Eulexin), melatonin implants, and leuprolide acetate (Lupron).

PROGNOSIS. If the owner elects not to treat this disease, the ferret will likely continue to lose hair and the vulva may continue to grow in size. In younger ferrets the alopecia and enlarged vulva may resolve and recur spontaneously over time. However, these are essentially cosmetic problems. Is it worth the morbidity and mortality that accompanies surgery when treating a disease that may only cause cosmetic problems? More serious complications of adrenal gland disease include estrogen-induced bone marrow suppression leading to anemia and pancytopenia. This is a rare complication of prolonged adrenal gland disease in ferrets, but it is life threatening. Adrenal gland disease can lead to intense pruritus in approximately 30% of ferrets with this disease. Although not a health complication, it is a quality of life issue that is difficult to control in a ferret without treating the adrenal gland disease. A large adrenal gland, especially right sided, can increase in size and put pressure on the vena cava. Finally, in male ferrets a syndrome is recognized where the prostatic tissue around the urethra near the neck of the bladder increases in size under the influence of the androgens produced by the diseased adrenal gland. This is a fatal complication if the blockage is not relieved.

Treating adrenal gland disease in ferrets can be expensive and is not without risk. As many ferrets only develop the cosmetic signs of this disease, it is not wrong to question whether all ferrets with adrenal gland disease should be surgically treated. Unfortunately, there is no method yet devised to determine which ferrets will develop life-threatening complications and which will only have cosmetic signs. It is, therefore, risky not to treat ferrets with this disease.

Case 56: **Surgical treatment of ferret adrenal gland disease**

CLINICAL PRESENTATION. A five-year-old ferret is brought to the veterinary hospital for bilaterally symmetrical alopecia. The owner also notes the ferret is pruritic and has an increase in body odor. A slightly enlarged vulva is also observed.

DIAGNOSIS. Diseased adrenal gland.

PREVALENCE. Adrenal gland disease is a common problem of ferrets in certain countries (e.g. the United States).

MANAGEMENT. Both medical (see *Case 55*) and surgical options are available. In this case the owner chose surgery. An exploratory laparotomy is performed and both adrenal glands are visualized and palpated. Normal adrenal glands are 5–8 mm long, 4–5 mm wide, and 3–4 mm thick. The left adrenal gland is located craniomedial to the cranial pole of the kidney and is usually surrounded in fat. The main blood supply to the left adrenal gland is the phrenicoabdominal vein, which courses ventrolaterally across it. When removing the left adrenal gland, this vein is ligated using hemostatic clips, as the tissues are friable and may not hold sutures well. The phrenicoabdominal vein is clamped medial and lateral to the left adrenal gland. The gland is dissected gently away from the retroperitoneal tissues. Capillary bleeding is controlled with a hemostatic sponge. A tumor of the right adrenal gland is present in the abdomen of this six-year-old ferret (**56**). The right adrenal gland is more difficult to remove since it is partially under the liver and is adherent to the caudal vena cava, craniomedial to the cranial pole of the right kidney. Attempts to 'tease' the adrenal gland off the vena cava usually result in tearing of the vessel. The adrenal gland is removed by placing hemostatic clips between it and the lateral wall of the vena cava and carefully cutting away the gland. Alternatively, the adrenal gland is debulked by incising its lateral surface and scooping it out of the subcapsular contents. However, this method can result in severe bleeding and death if venous sinuses are present. If both adrenal glands are abnormal, the larger of the two is removed and a subtotal adrenalectomy performed on the other gland. The liver and any abnormal abdominal structures are biopsied. The pancreas is examined for evidence of insulinoma. The abdomen is closed in a routine manner. The ferret is maintained·on i/v fluids post surgically until stable. Postoperative steroids are administered if more than one adrenal gland is removed or if the ferret is lethargic with no obvious cause.

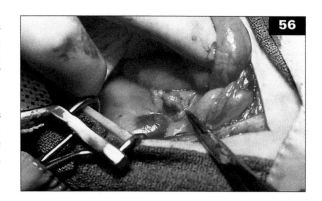

PROGNOSIS. The prognosis is dependent on whether the entire diseased adrenal gland tissue is removed or only debulked.

Case 57: **Guinea pig intubation**

INTRODUCTION. Endotracheal intubation in the guinea pig patient is very challenging. The caudal aspect of the oral pharynx of a guinea pig is shown (**57a**). (Photo courtesy S Jahn). The central circular opening is called the palatal ostium.

TECHNIQUE. In the guinea pig the soft palate extends down to the base of the tongue. The small palatal ostium is the only opening between the oral pharynx and the more proximal aspects of the pharynx. It is difficult to pass either a stomach tube or an endotracheal tube through this small opening. Trauma to the soft palate can cause bleeding and subsequent asphyxiation of the animal.

The mouth of the guinea pig is long and narrow and does not open very wide. Access to the glottis is achieved by passing through the small palatal ostium. Prominent cheek teeth limit the space available for placement of a laryngoscope blade. The tongue is large, only the tip is freely movable, and food material often accumulates at the base. This can obstruct visualization of the palatal ostium and result in aspiration and airway obstruction. To overcome this problem, the food at the back of the mouth is removed with cotton swabs after anesthetic induction. Fasting a guinea pig prior to anesthesia may result in GI ileus.

For short procedures, a guinea pig may be satisfactorily maintained under inhalant anesthesia using a small mask and appropriate gas flows. Endotracheal intubation is necessary when ventilatory support and control of the airway is required. A number of different techniques are described for endotracheal intubation of the guinea pig. Small laryngoscope blades (e.g. size 0 Miller blades) are tapered to a narrow point to facilitate visualization of the glottis. In another technique, a lighted otoscope with a 3–4 mm cone is used. The anesthetized guinea pig is placed in sternal recumbency. The lighted otoscope cone is introduced into the mouth, passed over the tongue, and used to hold the ostium open, thus allowing visualization

of the glottis. A 3.5 Fr urinary catheter is introduced into the larynx (**57b**). (Photo courtesy S Jahn). The otoscope cone is withdrawn, leaving the catheter in place. The endotracheal tube is advanced over the catheter and the stylet removed. A tracheal tube placed over a narrow endoscope can also be used. Endotracheal tubes used in guinea pigs include 1.5–2.5 mm Cole or straight tubes. Modified intravenous catheters (14 gauge) or other atraumatic tubing are also used.

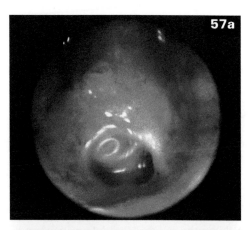

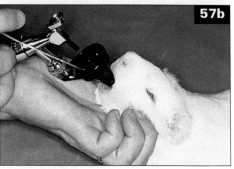

Case 58: **Guinea pig dystocia due to late age breeding**

CLINICAL PRESENTATION. A two-year-old guinea pig is bred for the first time. She presents to the hospital with a fetus protruding from her vagina (**58**). The fetus is dead and the sow is weak and in shock.

DIFFERENTIAL DIAGNOSES. Causes of dystocia include first time breeding over the age of eight months, nutritional deficiencies, anatomic disorders, and infection.

INVESTIGATION. A CBC and biochemistry profile allows the clinician to determine the metabolic status of the patient. This is important if surgery is recommended. Radiographs are important to rule out more than one fetus.

ETIOLOGY. The most common cause of dystocia in sows is the inability of the pubic symphysis to expand under the influence of the hormone relaxin. It then does not separate as needed just prior to parturition. In addition, older, obese sows have larger fat pads in their pelvic canals that can impede parturition.

PREVALENCE. Dystocia commonly occurs in guinea pigs bred for the first time after the age of eight months.

MANAGEMENT. Initially, the guinea pig is treated for shock and appropriate supportive care administered. An intravenous or intraosseous balanced electrolyte solution with 5% dextrose is given immediately, and this is followed with i/v antibiotics. The hypothermia is corrected.

Venipuncture (see *Case 60*) should be performed as soon as possible. This can be difficult as venipuncture is stressful even in healthy guinea pigs. Attempts are made gently to manually extract the fetus. An emergency cesarean section is performed if the fetus is wedged in the birth canal. An assistant retropulses the fetus carefully through the birth canal while the surgeon gently applies traction from within an opened uterus. An ovariohysterectomy is performed at this point if the sow is stable. The best way to manage this problem is to prevent its occurrence. Owners and breeders should be recommended not to breed guinea pigs for the first time over the age of eight months.

PROGNOSIS. Poor unless medical attention is sought immediately.

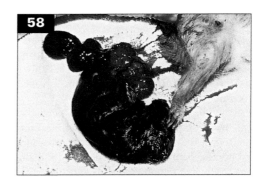

Case 59: **Guinea pig dental disease due to overgrown teeth**

CLINICAL PRESENTATION. Bridging of the tongue by the mandibular premolars is seen in this guinea pig, which has not eaten for two days (**59a**). The tooth on the left has bridged across the top of the tongue and is markedly discolored, while the overgrowth of the premolar on the right side is much less obvious.

INVESTIGATION. An oral examination is performed during the initial visit. With the guinea pig awake, an otoscope is introduced into the mouth. More information can be gained from an oral examination done while the guinea pig is sedated. For even more information, skull radiographs and/or a CT scan help treatment planning and disease prognosis.

ETIOLOGY. The guinea pig is a hystricomorph (porcupine-like) rodent and a true herbivore. Healthy rodents typically have yellow/orange pigmented enamel on their incisor teeth. Guinea pigs do not. The guinea pig has the same dental formula as the chinchilla, yet there is a more significant rostrocaudal divergence of

the guinea pig's dental arcades. Guinea pig cheek teeth are also markedly curved, compensating for a wider degree of anisognathism and resulting in the occlusal planes being angled at about 30 degrees to the horizontal plane (**59b**). Additionally, the occlusal planes pass directly through the mandibular condyles and the tips of the incisor teeth.

As the cheek teeth overgrow and the mandible is forced forwards, the mandibular premolars no longer occlude, resulting in overgrowth. This eventually leads to bridging over the tongue. Until bridging develops, the guinea pig usually shows no signs; therefore, the problem is rarely detected early.

Cheek tooth overgrowth tends to prevent the dental arcades from being brought fully into occlusion. It also prevents the mouth from closing fully in the normal resting jaw position. As a result, the mandible is held in a more prognathic position. This results in secondary malocclusion and overgrowth of the incisors.

PREVALENCE. Dental disease is common in pet guinea pigs.

MANAGEMENT. Under anesthesia, the crown height of all the teeth is reduced to approximate normal occlusion. Analgesics and assisted feeding are used after trimming until the patient eats on its own. Patients should be re-examined every 2–3 months because recurrence is common. A diet high in grass hay and herbage is provided to encourage frequent chewing and a natural level of tooth wear. Adequate supplementation with vitamin C must be provided, as deficiency affects collagen production and maintenance. Scurvy causes weakening of the periodontal ligament and may be a primary factor in cheek tooth malocclusion. Guinea pigs prone to dental disease should not be used for breeding.

PROGNOSIS. Once disease has caused bridging, it may be difficult to control this problem even with reduction of the height of the cheek teeth.

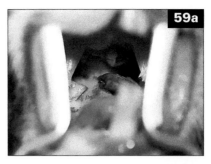

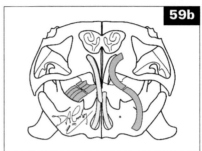

Case 60: **Guinea pig venipuncture**

INTRODUCTION. The owner of a five-year-old guinea pig asks that a CBC and plasma biochemistry profile be performed to make sure that the pet is in good health. It is not appropriate to scruff a guinea pig, as is done with hamsters and ferrets, to restrain it and aid in examination. Guinea pigs do not have excess skin over the nape to allow scruffing. The skin is tightly attached to the underlying tissues, particularly the subcutaneous fat pad over the nape of the neck. Guinea pigs appear to be more sensitive than other species and exhibit a painful response to scruffing. In addition, guinea pigs become distressed when they are placed in dorsal recumbency. When examining the ventrum of the awake patient, the head must always be kept elevated. Some guinea pigs will become so stressed that they will become unconscious during an examination or when a diagnostic procedure is attempted. Oxygen must always be available for these situations and the owner advised of potential underlying problems, such as cardiac disease, pulmonary disease, or anemia.

TECHNIQUE. The cephalic, lateral saphenous, femoral, and jugular veins can be accessed in guinea pigs in order to perform venipuncture. Depending on the condition and cooperation of the patient, it may be necessary to use sedation to obtain the sample.

The procedure for bleeding from the cephalic, femoral, or lateral saphenous vein is very similar to that for other species. The lateral saphenous vein is shown (**60**). The vein is raised manually or with a tourniquet and a 25–27 gauge needle and insulin syringe are used to obtain the sample. Once blood is observed in the hub of the needle, the pressure on the vein is released to allow more blood to enter the area. Gentle traction on the plunger of the syringe is used to avoid collapsing the vein. An alternative method is to use the needle without a syringe attached and allow the blood to flow directly from the hub into a collecting tube.

The jugular vein is approached with the sedated patient in dorsal recumbency. It is difficult to palpate the vein due to the thick and muscular neck of the guinea pig. The jugular vein lies in a furrow running from the thoracic inlet to the base of the ear. The vein is raised at the level of the thoracic inlet and a 22–25 gauge needle attached to a syringe used to draw the blood sample.

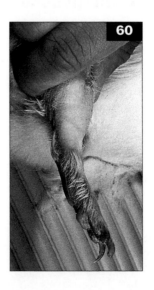

Case 61: **Guinea pig with dermatologic signs consistent with a mite infestation, *Trixacarus caviae***

CLINICAL PRESENTATION. A six-month-old male guinea pig has alopecia accompanied by crusting and flaking skin (**61**). The patient appears to be intensely pruritic and uncomfortable.

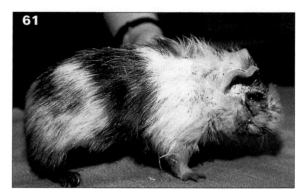

DIFFERENTIAL DIAGNOSES. Ectoparasites, including, *Trixacarus caviae*, endocrine alopecia, and fungal dermatitis.

INVESTIGATION. Skin scrapings or examination of the hairs from affected areas will reveal the mite in its various life stages. The scrapings do not have to be very deep to find this organism. Other mites are ruled out by the appearance of the mite under the microscope. It is very unusual not to find this mite on skin scrapings.

DIAGNOSIS. The likely diagnosis is infestation with the sarcoptiform mite *Trixacarus caviae*, as this is found on skin scrapes. The sarcoptic mite of dogs, *Sarcoptes scabiei*, can also affect guinea pigs in a similar manner. In severe infestations the guinea pig is so pruritic that seizures can occur.

PREVALENCE. Disease due to ectoparasites are common in pet guinea pigs.

MANAGEMENT. Ivermectin (0.4–0.8 mg/kg s/c) is administered and repeated twice more at seven-day intervals. This treatment is effective for the eradication of either *T. caviae* or *S. scabiei*. Cage mates are treated and the owner must clean the cage and cage furniture thoroughly after each treatment. The owner must be advised of the potential for zoonotic disease in the case of *S. scabiei*.

Although it is usually unnecessary to provide topical therapy for these cases, because ivermectin is very effective, some patients are in extreme discomfort from the intense pruritus or have a secondary bacterial dermatitis. In these cases the majority of skin crusts can be gently softened and removed with a warm bath. A topical antibiotic preparation appropriate for guinea pigs is applied sparingly. Topical preparations that include steroids must not be applied. The *T. caviae* mite is usually only contagious to other guinea pigs, but there have been reports of it causing urticaria in humans. *S. scabiei* may affect a variety of species, including humans.

PROGNOSIS. The prognosis for a cure of these ectoparasites is excellent. Treatment failure usually occurs when not all the guinea pigs in the house are treated or when the environment is not properly cleaned.

Case 62: **Guinea pig with pododermatitis**

CLINICAL PRESENTATION. A guinea pig has difficulty walking and physical examination reveals this lesion (**62**). The guinea pig is housed in a commercial wire cage that has a 1 × 2 cm mesh bottom with a piece of carpet placed in one corner. The diet consists of pellets and fresh vegetables. Water is available from a sipper tube.

DIFFERENTIAL DIAGNOSES. Pododermatitis, other causes of lameness, metabolic disease.

INVESTIGATION. Pododermatitis is almost always a secondary problem, usually due to poor husbandry. Therefore, a thorough review of the husbandry might reveal the primary problem. Both hematologic and biochemistry panels should be performed to delineate the metabolic condition of the patient. Radiographs are necessary to rule out additional disease associated with osteomyelitis.

DIAGNOSIS. This guinea pig has pododermatitis.

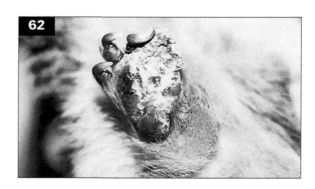

ETIOLOGY. Predisposing factors to this condition include rough cage flooring, unsanitary cage conditions, obesity, foot lacerations, hypovitaminosis C, and any debilitating disease. *Staphylococcus aureus* is commonly isolated from these lesions, but is usually secondary to these other factors. The feet appear swollen and discolored, and the foot pads are often cracked.

PREVALENCE. Common with poor husbandry conditions.

MANAGEMENT. Uncomplicated cases (no cracks or fissures in the foot pads) can be managed with topical antibiotics, clean bedding, and any additional husbandry improvements. Protective ointments with a heavy petroleum base are used to keep these lesions moist and prevent cracks. Severe lesions are treated more aggressively. In severe cases, systemic antibiotics should be administered, the lesions debulked surgically, the bandages changed daily, and affected limbs soaked in a hypertonic or astringent solution. Emphasis should be placed on cleanliness of the cage area. If the cage has a mesh bottom, it should be of correct size. Finally, vitamin C supplementation should be adequate.

PROGNOSIS. If left untreated, pododermatitis can lead to cellulitis, osteomyelitis, and eventual death of the animal.

Case 63: **Guinea pig alopecia due to cystic ovaries**

CLINICAL PRESENTATION. A four-year-old pet female guinea pig has progressive hair loss for one year (**63a**). Repeated skin scrapings are negative for parasites. Areas of thinning and alopecia are bilaterally symmetrical over the flank area and the skin appears grossly normal.

DIFFERENTIAL DIAGNOSES. Endocrine alopecia including ovarian follicular cysts, ovarian neoplasia. A number of ectoparasites should be considered including *Chirodiscoides caviae*, *Trixacarus caviae*, *Gliricola porcelli*, and *Gyropus ovalis*. Other causes of alopecia include dermatophyte infection (*Trichophyton mentagrophytes*), bacterial skin infection, and malnutrition. Though less likely in guinea pigs, self-barbering should be considered.

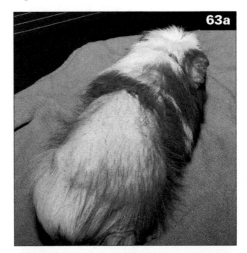

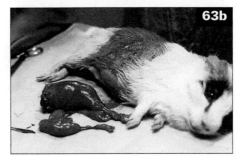

INVESTIGATION. Skin scrapings, hairs, and skin debris should be examined microscopically for dermatophytes as well as parasites. Material for a fungal or bacterial culture should be submitted as indicated. A skin biopsy is performed if scrapings are negative and other physical findings are normal. Careful abdominal palpation often reveals abnormal enlargements of the ovaries or uterus. Radiography and ultrasonic examination of the abdomen is useful if ovarian or uterine disease is suspected.

DIAGNOSIS. The cause of the hair loss in this guinea pig is hyperestrogenism caused by cystic ovaries. The ovarian cysts were palpated during the physical examination. They were confirmed by ultrasonic evaluation.

PREVALENCE. Alopecia in guinea pigs caused by cystic ovaries is a common problem in older intact female pet guinea pigs.

MANAGEMENT. Cystic ovaries are managed both medically and surgically. Surgical removal of the ovaries and uterus will cure the problem. In this case there were cystic ovaries and uterine fibrosarcoma (**63b**).

Medical management includes at least one or two injections of human chorionic gonadotropin. Percutaneous aspiration of the cystic ovaries may also help alleviate the signs of this disease.

PROGNOSIS. The haircoat usually returns to normal within three months after performing an ovariohysterectomy. If neoplasia of the genital tract is involved, the prognosis, even with surgery, is poor. If benign cystic follicular ovarian disease is present, then the prognosis is improved.

Case 64: **Hypovitaminosis C in a guinea pig**

CLINICAL PRESENTATION. A two-year-old male guinea pig is anorectic and reluctant to walk (**64**). Pain is elicited during joint palpation and it moves with a stiff gait. The incisors appear normal, but the guinea pig has difficulty prehending its food. The skin has petechial hemorrhages present on the right side of the neck and over the tarsal/metatarsal joints.

DIFFERENTIAL DIAGNOSES. Vitamin C deficiency, sepsis, arthritis, dental disease.

INVESTIGATION. History will elucidate if appropriate amounts and types of vitamin C are being given to the guinea pig. Radiographs reveal if arthritis is present. An oral examination will determine if dental disease is present.

DIAGNOSIS. Hypovitaminosis C, also known as scurvy.

ETIOLOGY. Guinea pigs, like humans, do not produce their own vitamin C and require a dietary source. Signs of vitamin C deficiency are consistent with damage to connective tissue and include swollen painful joints and costochondral junctions, resulting in reluctance to move, crying in pain when touched, poor coat condition, dysphagia, and hemorrhage around joints, muscles, and skin. The angle of the teeth may change as they become loosened, resulting in malocclused and overgrown molars and a resultant inability to prehend food. Some guinea pigs present with chronic mild upper respiratory signs and increased ocular secretions, while others may present with diarrhea and inappetence.

PREVALENCE. One of the most common guinea pig husbandry errors.

MANAGEMENT. The minimum daily requirement for vitamin C in the guinea pig is 10 mg/kg/day in the nonbreeding animal and 30 mg/kg/day in the pregnant and lactating sow. The diet is a crucial factor in this case. Owners are either unaware of the vitamin C requirement of guinea pigs or believe that commercial guinea pig pellets are an adequate diet. Vitamin C is a water soluble vitamin and its potency decreases rapidly in the feed, particularly if exposed to excessive heat or moisture. Most commercial guinea pig pellets lose their vitamin C potency within 90 days after milling; therefore, it is important to determine the age of the food being fed. It is equally important to know how the feed is stored. Pellets should be stored in a cool, dry area away from direct sunlight. Rabbit or other rodent pellets are inappropriate as the sole diet for guinea pigs because they do not contain supplemental vitamin C. The best way to ensure vitamin C supplementation is to give vitamin C-rich foods daily (e.g. kale, other dark leafy greens, citrus fruits, or tomatoes).

PROGNOSIS. Good if caught early and disease signs are mild. Guarded if long-standing, as signs may not be reversible, especially dental changes.

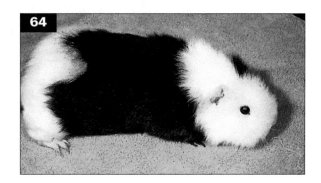

Case 65: Guinea pig with signs of urinary tract disease due to urinary calculi

CLINICAL PRESENTATION. A four-year-old female guinea pig has a history of five days of stranguria, hematuria, and lethargy. She is on a diet of guinea pig pellets, vitamin C in the water, and alfalfa cubes.

DIFFERENTIAL DIAGNOSES. Urinary tract calculi, urinary tract infection.

INVESTIGATION. Radiography of the abdomen revealed a 1 × 2 cm radiopaque object in the urinary bladder (65). Urinalysis via cystocentesis revealed the results shown below.

DIAGNOSIS. Calculi in the urinary bladder and right distal ureter.

ETIOLOGY. Most urinary tract calculi in guinea pigs are composed primarily of calcium carbonate. The cause of urinary tract calculi in guinea pigs is unknown.

PREVALENCE. This is an infrequent problem in pet guinea pigs.

MANAGEMENT. Exploratory laparotomy is the treatment of choice for this problem. Hematology and plasma biochemistry panels should be obtained prior to surgery in order to evaluate renal function. The ureters are palpated for calculi. Attempts to dislodge a calculus into the bladder are usually not successful. A ureterotomy may be performed to remove a calculus, but postoperative strictures can occur. If the ureteral calculus has caused unilateral hydronephrosis, the kidney and ureter should be removed. A cystotomy is performed to remove the calculus from the urinary bladder. The bladder is exteriorized and packed off with moistened gauze sponges. An incision is made in the apex of the bladder and the calculi removed. The bladder wall is cultured and the bladder and urethra lavaged. The bladder is closed with 5-0 or 6-0 monofilament, absorbable synthetic suture in a continuous, one or two layer inverting pattern. The bladder wall is very thin and care should be taken not to place any sutures in the lumen. The abdomen is lavaged and closed with 4-0 or 5-0 synthetic absorbable suture in a routine pattern. Post-surgical management should be aimed at reducing the calcium in the diet, ensuring adequate fluid intake, pain relief, and treating any underlying bacterial infections. An antibiotic that is safe for guinea pigs and is consistent with the culture and sensitivity results should be given. If no culture was taken or there was no growth, an antibiotic such as trimethoprim/sulfadiazine (30 mg/kg p/o q12h) or enrofloxacin (20–30 mg/kg p/o q24h) is given for a minimum of three weeks post surgically.

PROGNOSIS. Even with this therapy some guinea pigs will develop urinary tract calculi again; therefore, the prognosis should be guarded. Frequent rechecks are recommended, with complete urinalysis. Periodic abdominal radiographs should be obtained.

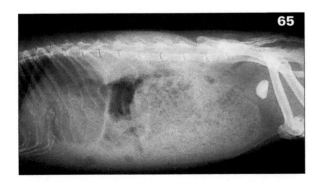

Urinalysis:	
Color	Red
Appearance	Opaque
SG	1.020
pH	9.0
Protein	3+
Glucose	Negative
Ketone	Negative
Bilirubin	Negative
Hemoglobin	4+
Urine sediment:	
Epithelial cells	Transitional
Casts	None
Crystals	Amorphous and calcium carbonate (moderate amount)
RBCs	50–60/high power field
WBCs	10–20/high power field
Bacteria	Few

Case 66: **Urethral calculi in a guinea pig**

CLINICAL PRESENTATION. A five-year-old intact male guinea pig is thin, painful on abdominal palpation, and has had a decreased appetite for one month. There is a urethral plug visible (**66**).

DIFFERENTIAL DIAGNOSES. Urinary tract calculi, inspissated secretions from the vesicular glands.

INVESTIGATION. Abdominal radiographs. Most calculi in guinea pigs are formed from calcium or magnesium salts and are therefore radiopaque. Calculi are found in all areas of the urinary tract. Concretions in the vesicular glands can also appear radiopaque, but they will be located outside the areas of the ureters or bladder. Urinalysis and urine culture on urine obtained by cystocentesis will evaluate for an infectious cystitis. A plasma biochemistry profile will evaluate the metabolic status of the guinea pig.

DIAGNOSIS. Urethral calculi.

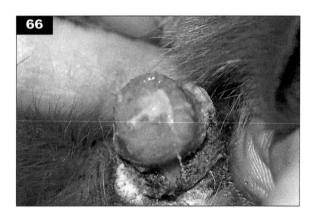

PREVALENCE. An infrequent problem in guinea pigs.

MANAGEMENT. Before any treatment is started, the radiographs should be checked to be certain no other calculi are present in the urinary tract. The obstruction is relieved using a water-soluble lubricating jelly and gentle digital pressure. A normal stream of urine should be observed as the bladder is gently expressed. If urethral patency is questionable, the guinea pig is sedated with isoflurane and a small, soft catheter passed into the urethra, which is then flushed with sterile saline. Analgesics are necessary post catheterization to prevent urethral spasm and reduce pain.

In cases where the obstruction cannot be relieved quickly, cystocentesis is performed with a 25–27 gauge needle to reduce the pressure in the bladder. If the urethra remains obstructed, the guinea pig is stabilized metabolically and a cystotomy performed to allow retrograde flushing and removal of the plug. Many obstructions are associated with a bacterial infection, therefore appropriate antibiotics should be given. Secretions from the prepuce and perineal area are cleaned gently with a mild antiseptic solution once a week. The guinea pig is put on a healthy diet that contains free-choice grass hay, limited pellets, and a minimum of a half cup daily of dark leafy greens to provide essential dietary vitamin C. Vitamin C should not be added to the drinking water. It has a bitter taste and is inactivated in less than 24 hours. A bitter taste in the water may decrease water consumption, which is not desirable in an animal with potential renal disease.

PROGNOSIS. Even if treatment is successful, owners need to know that urinary tract calculi can recur at any time.

Case 67: **Traumatic injury to a pet hamster**

CLINICAL PRESENTATION. A pet golden hamster has fallen off a table and fractured its incisor teeth (**67**). The pulp cavity is not visibly exposed.

INVESTIGATION. An oral examination with the hamster sedated will allow a more accurate prognosis and treatment planning. Also, dental radiographs and/or skull radiographs may be required to determine the extent of the injury.

DIAGNOSIS. Fractured right lower incisor. Traumatic injuries, such as falls, commonly cause dental disease in hamsters.

MANAGEMENT. Treating the fractured incisor starts with administering analgesics, such as an NSAID (e.g.

meloxicam at 0.1–0.3 mg/kg p/o q12–24h), immediately post trauma. No other immediate treatment is needed if the pulp chamber has not been exposed. The right upper incisor should be shortened at regular intervals (avoiding iatrogenic pulp exposure) until the lower tooth has grown back into normal occlusion. Unfortunately, in some cases the trauma damages the germinal tissues at the root apex of the damaged tooth and it does not regrow. In these cases the opposing tooth should continue to be trimmed or be extracted. A dental burr in a high-speed dental hand piece is used to trim the incisors. (NB: Rodent or rabbit teeth must not be trimmed with nail cutters. This practice commonly leads to iatrogenic pulp exposure, which can ultimately result in more serious tooth root disease.) If the hamster is not eating, assisted feeding may be necessary. It is important to discuss the cage and environment with the owner in order to prevent the hamster suffering further falls.

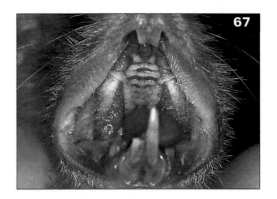

PROGNOSIS. Good if the germinal tissue is not damaged and periodic trimming is maintained.

DISCUSSION. The dental formula of the golden hamster is I 1/1, C 0/0, P 0/0, M 3/3. Some sources classify the first cheek teeth as premolars not molars. Hamsters have brachyodont cheek teeth similar to rats and mice. Also, like rats and mice, hamsters are granivorous rather than herbivorous.

Case 68: **A depressed hamster infested with the tapeworm** *Hymenolepis nana*

CLINICAL PRESENTATION. An anorectic, depressed hamster is brought to the surgery. It has not eaten or defecated in two days. The hamster was recently purchased from a pet store. Other hamsters in the store are reported also to have died and appeared emaciated.

DIFFERENTIAL DIAGNOSES. The signs of this hamster are nonspecific and any disease can be considered. An infectious bacterial, viral, or parasitic disease should be considered, as other hamsters in contact with this one have been affected.

INVESTIGATION. A fecal floatation finds the eggs of *Hymenolepis nana* (**68**). These eggs (30–50 mm) have internal hooks and filamentous processes. If a fecal floatation is negative for parasites, further investigations in a non-specifically sick hamster could include a CBC, biochemistry profile, urinalysis, radiographs, and fecal cultures.

DIAGNOSIS. Tapeworm (*Hymenolepis nana*) infestation.

ETIOLOGY. In large numbers, *Hymenolepis nana* causes intestinal occlusion, impaction, and death. The parasite has a direct and an indirect life cycle. The adult tapeworms live in the small intestine. In the direct life cycle, gravid proglottids detach from the body and disintegrate in the intestine, releasing eggs that are immediately infective when passed in the feces. Hamsters ingest these eggs, which hatch in the small intestine, and the onchospheres (embryos) penetrate into the mucosa and lie in the lymph channels of the villi. They develop into metacestodes (cysticercoids), which emerge from the villi in five or six days, attach to the intestine, and mature into adult tapeworms.

In the indirect life cycle, the eggs are ingested by insects (grain beetles, fleas, cockroaches) and develop into the next larval stage (cysticercoid/metacestode). The hamster is infected by ingesting these insects.

Finally, autoinfection is also possible. Some of the eggs that are released when the proglottids disintegrate in the intestine may hatch in the hamster and the onchospheres penetrate the intestinal villi. Cysticercoids emerge in five or six days and develop into adult tapeworms without ever leaving the hamster.

Hymenolepis nana also infects humans. Only a moderate number of parasites are needed to produce diarrhea, anorexia, and abdominal pain in children.

PREVALENCE. Infrequent disease in large hamster colonies or pet stores.

MANAGEMENT. Praziquantel (5 mg/kg s/c or 10 mg/kg p/o q14d for 2 treatments) is active against both the larval and adult stages. The bedding and feces should be incinerated to prevent the spread of the eggs, and the hamster cage cleaned and sterilized, or replaced. The life cycle of the tapeworm is broken by sanitation and insect control. Rodent control is essential, since wild rodents may also be a source of contamination.

PROGNOSIS. Usually poor unless disease found early and intensive supportive care is given.

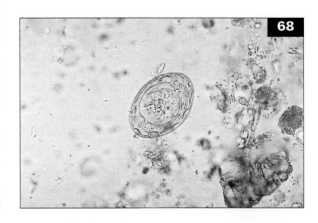

Case 69: **Wet tail disease in hamsters**

CLINICAL PRESENTATION. Any condition in hamsters that results in a wet perineal area is often referred to as 'wet tail' by pet owners. It is not uncommon for these animals to be treated with a variety of over-the-counter medications before presentation to the veterinarian.

DIFFERENTIAL DIAGNOSES. Debilitated animals or those with overgrown incisors may have soiled perineums because they cannot groom themselves. An older hamster with polyuria caused by renal disease or endocrinopathies may have a urine-soaked perineum. Damp and dirty bedding can cause the fur to become wet and matted. Cystitis or cystic calculi can result in urine scald. Uterine neoplasia or infection can cause a mucoid, foul-smelling discharge that soils the perineum. Enteritis in hamsters can also be caused by the use of antibiotics inappropriate for hamsters. Potentially fatal enterotoxemia caused by *Clostridium* species results when the antibiotic destroys the delicate balance of bacterial flora in the GI tract.

INVESTIGATION. Fecal cultures and floats can rule in or rule out other diseases. Radiographs and ultrasound can also rule out other diseases. Wet tail is usually diagnosed based on history (recent stress) and eliminating other diseases.

ETIOLOGY. Classic 'wet tail' is proliferative ileitis caused by *Lawsonia intracellularis* and resulting in a watery or mucoid diarrhea. It is primarily a disease of recently weaned hamsters. The most common cause of perineal staining is diarrhea from bacterial enteritis. In the laboratory this disease can be created by infecting hamsters with chlamydial or campylobacter-like organisms. Conditions that can predispose a hamster to this disease include overcrowding and shipping stress. The mature single household pet is not likely to develop this disease.

PREVALENCE. Common in recently shipped or purchased young hamsters.

MANAGEMENT. The cause of the bacterial enteritis needs to be determined and corrected. The administration of 'unsafe' antibiotics should be stopped (some antibiotics [e.g. amoxicillin and first-generation erthyromycin] are believed to destroy the normal bacterial flora and therefore allow abnormal flora to proliferate), the environment cleaned, and the patient isolated. Warmed s/c fluids should be given, taking care to avoid the cheek pouches. Oral electrolyte solutions are administered along with syringe feeding of a bland diet. Enrofloxacin (20 mg/kg p/o q24h), trimethoprim/sulfadimethoxine (30 mg/kg p/o q12h), or tetracycline (10 mg/kg p/o q12h) are used as antibiotic treatment. In severe cases, assisted feeding and administering i/v fluids should be considered. Wet tail can be prevented by decreasing stress in hamsters during weaning and shipping times.

PROGNOSIS. Intussusception and rectal prolapse are severe sequelae to this disease. The hamster often chews the prolapsed tissue and dies from secondary complications.

Case 70: **Hamster with food stored in cheek pouch**

CLINICAL PRESENTATION. A five-month-old male hamster has a firm swelling on the left side of its face. The owner noticed this two nights ago and is now concerned because the swelling appears to be getting larger. In addition, the pet is eating and drinking less than normal. The owner wants the swelling investigated.

DIFFERENTIAL DIAGNOSES. The most common cause of facial swelling in hamsters is an enlarged cheek pouch due to normal food hoarding, food impaction, or a cheek pouch abscess. Abnormalities of the jaw or teeth can also result in facial swelling. Cheek pouch neoplasia, tooth root abscess, molar malocclusion, abscess, or neoplasia of the mandible can also lead to facial swellings.

INVESTIGATION. The most useful diagnostic tool is oral cavity examination. This can be done with the hamster awake, but is best done under sedation. A swab can be used to invert the cheek pouch for better examination. If necessary, skull or dental radiographs are used to elucidate tooth or bony changes. If needed, cultures and biopsies will help determine the etiology.

ETIOLOGY. Hamsters possess well-developed cheek pouches, which may appear as bulges on the sides of the face when normally filled with food or when diseased. Hamsters hoard food by filling their cheek pouches and then hiding their food in a secure location for later consumption. The physical examination of this patient revealed food in the cheek pouch, with no other abnormalities noted.

Hoarding behavior is amplified when a hamster is stressed or moved to a different environment. Other stressors that may result in this behavior include exposure to new cage mates, rearranging of cage furnishings, or provision of excess food after a period of food deprivation. This animal was recently moved to a new cage and then placed in a different area of the house. The resulting insecurity probably caused the hamster to hoard food more vigorously.

PREVALENCE. A common presentation in pet hamsters. In most cases this is normal food hoarding and not associated with disease.

Case 71: **A combined fungal dermatitis and ectoparasite infestation in a hamster**

CLINICAL PRESENTATION. These two adult pet hamsters have developed chronic, nonpruritic generalized alopecia with scaling and crusts most evident around the ears and feet (**71**). The child in the household plays with the hamsters and was recently treated for dermatophytosis.

DIFFERENTIAL DIAGNOSES. *Demodex* species (*Demodex aurati, D. criceti*) and *Trichophyton mentagrophytes* can occur simultaneously. Other rule outs include low-protein (under 16%) feed, bedding abrasion, systemic disorders associated with ageing (including renal amyloidosis and renal neoplasia), staphylococcal pyoderma, adrenocortical neoplasia, and other endocrine disease.

INVESTIGATION. A deep skin scraping should be examined microscopically. A mineral oil or KOH wet-mount is prepared to assess for fungal hyphae. The skin and hair are cultured for fungal and bacterial pathogens and the diet and husbandry practices are evaluated. Further diagnostic tests are performed as needed, including radiography, ultrasonography, hematology, urinalysis, and a plasma biochemistry panel.

DIAGNOSIS. A heavy infestation of *Demodex* species was identified in this case. Additionally, abundant growth of *T. mentagrophytes* was observed on dermatophyte test medium.

ETIOLOGY. Usually, *Demodex* species become clinically apparent when there is underlying primary disease such as adrenal gland disease, neoplasia, severe environmental stress, malnutrition, and other systemic disease. Demodocosis is not zoonotic. *T. mentagrophytes* or *Microsporum canis* are the most common causes of dermatophyte infections in hamsters. Dermatophyte infections on hamsters can be zoonotic.

PREVALENCE. Both dermatologic diseases are common in pet hamsters.

MANAGEMENT. Attempts should be made to treat the demodectic mange with ivermectin (0.2–1.0 mg/kg s/c, repeated twice at 10–14 day intervals). This treatment often does not work because ivermectin may not be effective. The use of amitraz is dangerous in hamsters because even when diluted it is extremely toxic to this species. Dermatophytosis can be treated with griseofulvin (25–30 mg/kg p/o q24h for 3–4 weeks) or ketoconazole (10 mg/kg p/o q24h for 3–4 weeks). Localized infections can be treated with a topical antifungal cream or lotion. The cage must be thoroughly cleaned and nontoxic pelleted bedding should be used. Gloves should be worn when handling affected hamsters and hands washed with a germicidal hand soap afterwards.

PROGNOSIS. Dependent on the underlying condition. If the infestation is a primary problem, the prognosis is good if the disease is controlled by medication.

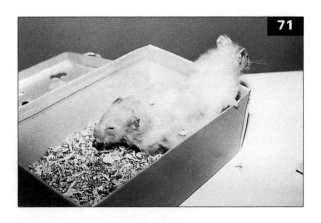

Case 72: **Proper handling of hamsters**

CLINICAL PRESENTATION. An eight-month-old female hamster has nonspecific signs of lethargy and ataxia of 24–36 hours duration. Since hamsters hoard food, the owner is not sure about its appetite, but the hamster appears to be in normal body condition and approximately 3–5% dehydrated.

DIFFERENTIAL DIAGNOSES. In this hamster, any disease can cause these nonspecific signs (e.g. infectious disease, metabolic conditions [particularly renal or hepatic disorders], neoplastic disease, digestive disorders [dental malocclusion, gastric foreign bodies], trauma, pneumonia, cardiac disease, and toxicity) and no specific organ system can be identified. Therefore, further investigation is necessary and the ability to examine the hamster is integral to determining the cause of disease.

INVESTIGATION. A physical examination is the first place to start. Further diagnostics might include fecal examination, a CBC, a plasma biochemistry profile, whole body radiographs, and ultrasonic examination of both body cavities. It is important to be able to handle hamsters appropriately to perform these diagnostics.

PREVALENCE. It is not uncommon for sick hamsters to present with nonspecific signs of illness that are not easily elucidated by history and a cursory observation. Most pet hamsters that are sick require a physical examination, diagnostics, and treatment.

MANAGEMENT. If the hamster is relatively tame or debilitated, it should be scooped up gently in a cupped hand. To avoid being bitten by a fractious patient, it can be scooped into a can or small box. Hamsters must not be picked up when they are sleeping, since many will bite in response to being surprised. Once the hamster is captured, it should be carefully scruffed by grasping the large skin fold over the nape of the neck. This skin is loose and plentiful, and if a sufficient amount is not grasped, the pet can turn and bite. Your hold should be repositioned as needed to minimize pressure that may cause the eyes to bulge. Due to the sometimes fractious nature of some hamsters, both when healthy or sick, it is tempting to wear gloves for protection when handling hamsters. This should be avoided, as it is difficult to clean the gloves and destroy potential infectious diseases. Also, hamsters may be even more aggressive when being handled with gloves.

PROGNOSIS. The prognosis for a complete recovery decreases if the hamster cannot be handled for examination and procedures.

Case 73: **Normal skin anatomy of the hamster and hair loss due to a poor diet**

CLINICAL PRESENTATION. The owners of a hamster have noticed a black oval 'lesion' on the hamster's flank (**73**). They want to know what this is. They also want to know why the hamster is losing its hair.

DIFFERENTIAL DIAGNOSES. Alopecia due to a diet low in protein. Alopecia can also be due to ectoparasites, dermatophytes, and endocrine disease. The black area is a normal scent gland, but the differential diagnoses should include dermatitis and neoplasia such as melanoma.

INVESTIGATION. History will rule out poor diet. Skin scrapes and bacterial and fungal skin cultures should be carried out and biopsies performed to rule out neoplastic disease.

DIAGNOSIS. The 'lesion' is a flank or scent gland. It is normal.

ETIOLOGY. Flank or scent glands are most prominent in mature male hamsters and they become visible with hair thinning. Prominent scent glands are found in many rodent species kept as pets. Gerbils possess a prominent patch of sebaceous glands on the mid-ventral abdomen; they are used for territorial marking and identifying the pups, and are larger in male gerbils. Guinea pigs have

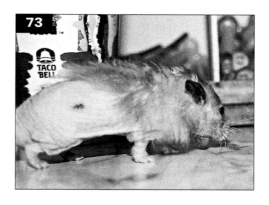

prominent sebaceous glands, which produce waxy secretions used for territorial marking, around the anus and over the rump. The glands are common sites of cysts, abscesses, hyperplasia, and neoplasia in these species. The scent gland serves as a means for olfactory marking of territory, individual identification, and, possibly, sexual attraction. The hair loss in this particular hamster is due to a poor diet. The owners purchased a cheap, store brand of food. The label specified the protein content as 12%. If the protein content is not at least 16%, alopecia can ensue.

PREVALENCE. Scent glands are found in all hamsters. Most hamsters are fed a diet adequate in protein, so alopecia due to low protein is uncommon.

MANAGEMENT. Scent glands are normal and no treatment is required. The hamster needs to be put on a diet higher in protein. Once the diet is changed, hair will begin to regrow. If there is any concern, owners should always be asked to bring in the label from the food to check the contents.

PROGNOSIS. Excellent with a diet change.

Case 74: **A hedgehog with *Caparina triplis* infestation**

CLINICAL PRESENTATION. An adult European hedgehog with erythema and pruritus of the haired areas of the skin is presented. There is some quill loss over the spine, but the condition is most obvious on the face, where the skin is thickened and crusted with dried serum (**74**).

DIFFERENTIAL DIAGNOSES. *Caparina triplis* infestation, other ectoparasites, fungal skin infection.

INVESTIGATION. Microscopic examination of a skin scraping from the affected areas will confirm the cause. Close examination with the naked eye or using a hand lens allows direct visualization of *Caparina* mites moving at the base of the spines. Although less than 0.5 mm across, they are white and contrast markedly with the dark skin of the hedgehog.

DIAGNOSIS. A skin mite infestation.

ETIOLOGY. This severe disease may have taken as little as three months to develop. Three species of mites are implicated in this disease. In continental Europe and New Zealand, the most common species found is the psoroptid mite *Caparina triplis*, whereas in the UK, *Sarcoptes* species and *Notoedres* species are more frequently isolated. *Trichophyton erinacei* has been isolated from the feces of some skin mites, and damage to the skin may predispose the hedgehog to this or other dermatologic disease. In addition, serum accumulation on the skin may attract flies and the risk of myiasis. Studies in New Zealand concluded that hedgehogs with skin mite infestation were less likely to survive hibernation.

PREVALENCE. Ectoparasites are common cause of disease in hedgehogs.

MANAGEMENT. Ivermectin (0.2–0.4 mg/kg s/c) is the treatment of choice. Injections are repeated at 2–3 week intervals for up to three total treatments. It is important to clean the environment in the case of hedgehogs held in captivity.

PROGNOSIS. Prognosis is excellent if the pet and its environment are treated properly.

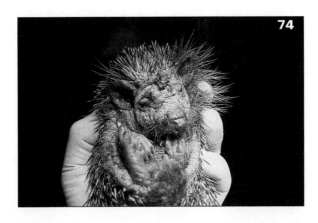

Case 75: **Hedgehog venipuncture and catheter techniques**

INTRODUCTION. An African hedgehog has rolled tightly into a ball and has stayed in this position for some time (**75**). This is normal behavior for a healthy hedgehog. Some highly socialized pet hedgehogs will not role into a ball when handled. Also, when hedgehogs are very sick, even the least socialized of hedgehogs, will not roll into a ball.

TECHNIQUE. As most pet hedgehogs roll into a ball when in the surgery, it is usually necessary to anesthetize a hedgehog to obtain a blood sample. Isoflurane anesthesia is preferred for short procedures, although injectable anesthetics can also be used. The superficially located lateral or medial saphenous vein should be visualized. Blood is collected either by lancing the vein with a needle and collecting the free flow of blood, or by drawing blood directly into a syringe. Small gauge needles (25–27 gauge) should be used. Insulin syringes with the needle attached work well. The femoral vein is also a good collection site. This vein can be palpated on the medial aspect of the thigh as pressure is applied at its proximal end. The delicate cephalic vein collapses easily and is a poor choice for venipuncture. The jugular vein is very short and lies deep beneath subcutaneous fat in the hedgehog, making it difficult to palpate. It runs from the thoracic inlet to the base of the ear. Pressure should be applied just lateral to the thoracic inlet on the preferred side of venipuncture. Toe nail clipping should not be used as a routine method of blood collection in the hedgehog. It is painful and yields a very small, potentially contaminated, sample.

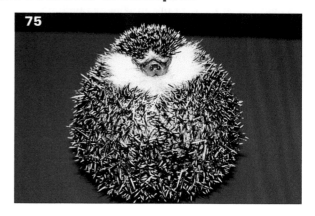

It is sometimes necessary in sick hedgehogs to administer parenteral fluids. Intravenous catheterization can be difficult in the hedgehog; therefore, the intraosseous route is sometimes used. An intraosseous catheter is placed in the femur, with the approach through the trochanteric fossa using a 20–22 gauge hypodermic needle of appropriate length. Administering a systemic antibiotic should be considered while the catheter is in place and for at least three days afterwards. Intravenous catheters can be placed in the cephalic or lateral saphenous veins.

Case 76: **Hedgehog with respiratory disease caused by a lungworm infection**

CLINICAL PRESENTATION. In late autumn, a juvenile European hedgehog weighing 300 g exhibits marked dyspnea with open mouth breathing. There is some foam visible at the lip commissures and the oral mucous membranes are cyanotic.

DIFFERENTIAL DIAGNOSES. Lungworm infestation (*Crenosoma striatum* and *Capillaria aerophilia*) is the most likely diagnosis. A thorough history should establish if paraquat poisoning, the most likely other diagnosis, is possible. The finding of *Capillaria* eggs in the feces does not rule out paraquat poisoning, because intestinal *Capillaria* can produce such findings. Other causes of dyspnea include heart disease, bacterial pneumonia, and thoracic neoplasia.

INVESTIGATION. In heavy infestations, direct examination of a wet preparation of feces under the microscope may reveal *Crenosoma* larvae. Most commercial laboratories that examine bovine or ovine species should be able to

analyze hedgehog feces. Radiographs are used to rule out other forms of thoracic disease. If possible, a tracheal wash or lung wash can be used to examine for eggs, cells, and bacterial organisms.

DIAGNOSIS. Lungworm infestation. In European hedgehogs this is usually a mixed infestation of *Crenosoma striatum* and *Capillaria aerophilia*.

PREVALENCE. Not uncommon in European hedgehogs.

MANAGEMENT. An oxygen cage or chamber should be used to minimize stress when treating cyanosis. Furosemide (2.5–5.0 mg/kg s/c) is administered, plus an injectable antibiotic such as amoxicillin to cover the potential for secondary bacterial infection. Often there is a respiratory infection superimposed on the lungworm infection. *Bordetella bronchiseptica* is frequently isolated at post mortem. To maximize the chances of successful treatment, the course of antibiotic therapy should be continued. Once the patient is stable, ivermectin (0.2–0.4 mg/kg s/c) or, alternatively, levamisole hydrochloride (10–20 mg/kg s/c) can be given. A hedgehog weighing 300 g is too small to hibernate, so it will need to be overwintered in a warm environment and provided food on a daily basis. To prevent a recurrence

of the respiratory disease, the ivermectin or levamisole injection should be repeated at monthly intervals.

PROGNOSIS. Prognosis is dependent on the response to treatment and if a severe secondary bacterial infection has occurred.

Case 77: **A wild hedgehog with ringworm**

CLINICAL PRESENTATION. A wild European hedgehog is picked up out of the backyard by a concerned home owner (77). It has a number of nonpruritic, scaling lesions, most prominently on the head.

DIFFERENTIAL DIAGNOSES. The most likely differentials include ringworm, ectoparasites, and bacterial skin infection.

INVESTIGATION. Superficial and deep skin scrapes did not reveal any organisms or eggs. An examination of the quills under the microscope did not reveal any organisms. The lesions did not fluoresce under a Wood's lamp. Some material from a scab taken from one of the skin lesions was placed on dermatophyte test medium. A heavy growth of *Trichophyton erinacei* was cultured within one week.

DIAGNOSIS. This is a case of ringworm caused by *T. erinacei*.

ETIOLOGY. *T. erinacei* can be transmitted to dogs and humans. In dogs the lesions appear on the lips or muzzle either from investigating hedgehogs found while walking or by eating leftover food from a bowl at which an infected hedgehog has been feeding. The lesions on humans can be intensely pruritic, but they may not

resemble classic ringworm and therefore not be recognized by a medical practitioner. People working with wild hedgehogs can contract dermatophytosis without having encountered an animal with obvious lesions due to the presence of asymptomatic carriers.

PREVALENCE. About 25% of wild hedgehogs of this species are asymptomatic carriers of *T. erinacei*.

MANAGEMENT. Griseofulvin (15–50 mg/kg p/o q24h) or ketoconazole (10 mg/kg p/o q24h) should be administered for several weeks. If there are other hedgehogs in the house, consideration should be given to treating them as well, as they might be asymptomatic carriers. For wild hedgehogs accustomed to feeding from a bowl, the home owner should be advised to give the daily dose of medication in a little food. A chocolate flavored pediatric elixir of griseofulvin is particularly well accepted by hedgehogs. For captive hedgehogs, a solution of enilconazole can be sprayed onto the lesions to assist in clearing up the infection and reduce the infectivity of the hedgehog to others. This can be done once every 3–4 days for 3–4 applications. Enilconazole solution can also be used to treat the environment to prevent transmission of the infection to dogs and humans.

PROGNOSIS. Response to treatment is usually good.

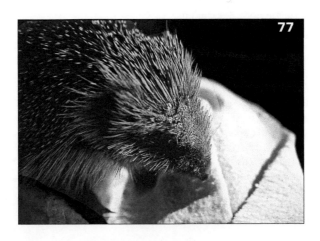

Case 78: **Hedgehog anesthesia**

CLINICAL PRESENTATION. An African hedgehog requires anesthesia for removal of a mass on the foot. Physical examination reveals an otherwise healthy animal.

MANAGEMENT. As a rule, it is safest to obtain blood results before anesthetizing a patient. In practical terms, this is not usually possible in hedgehogs, as they roll into a ball when handled. Owners need to be warned that the metabolic status of the patient will likely not be known before anesthesia is performed due to the shy nature of hedgehogs. Hedgehog are commonly anesthetized for examination and procedures.

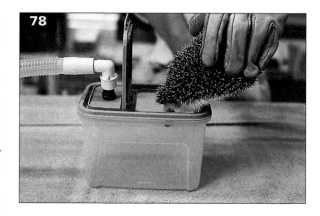

Isoflurane provides the easiest and most effective means of achieving anesthesia in hedgehogs. An induction chamber with 100% oxygen and an isoflurane concentration of 3–5% is used (**78**). Once induced, the hedgehog is maintained with either an endotracheal tube or face mask at an isoflurane concentration of 0.5–3.0%. Although not generally needed, atropine (0.02–0.04 mg/kg i/m or s/c) can be used as a premedication. Injectable anesthetic agents produce more prolonged and, sometimes, more difficult recovery times than inhalant anesthesia. One choice is ketamine (5–20 mg/kg i/m) either alone or with diazepam (0.5–2.0 mg/kg i/m). Another combination is tiletamine/zolazepam (1–5 mg/kg of the combined drug i/m). There is a large amount of subcutaneous fat over the dorsum in hedgehogs. Injection into this area can result in unpredictable absorption.

Case 79: **Hedgehog with dental trauma**

CLINICAL PRESENTATION. European hedgehogs are frequently victims of road traffic accidents and are commonly presented for treatment for head injuries.

DIFFERENTIAL DIAGNOSES. Dental trauma, skull fractures, soft tissue damage.

INVESTIGATION. An oral examination under sedation should be carried out and skull and dental radiographs taken for improved detail.

PREVALENCE. Dental trauma is common in injured wild European hedgehogs. Damage to the oral cavity is common. Occasionally, it is necessary to stabilize a bilateral mandibular fracture so that it remains in normal occlusion.

MANAGEMENT. If road accident casualties are to be released back into the wild, it is important to ensure that they will be able to survive. The adult dental formula for European hedgehogs is I 3/3, C 1/1, P 4/4, M 3/3. If a tooth is fractured, it should be treated in the same manner as for carnivores. Minor surface damage should be smoothed and polished, but if there is pulp exposure, affected teeth should be extracted. Endodontic treatment is theoretically possible, but is impractical in such small teeth.

The fractures are reduced and the mouth checked for occlusion. If there are sufficient teeth on either side of the fracture line to provide anchorage, intraoral acrylic splints can be formed *in situ* in the mouth. As the acrylic is setting, a check should be made that normal occlusion is maintained. Splints can be carefully broken away from the teeth once the jaw has healed. As an alternative approach, enamel bonded composite restorative material can be used between intact rostral teeth to fix the mandible and maxilla together until the fractures have healed (**79**). The rostral mandible is fixed in a slightly open position while still maintaining occlusion. The natural gap between the maxillary first incisors, plus the slightly open jaw position, provide space for the tongue to function, reducing the need for hand feeding. The composite material is removed carefully and the teeth polished once the fractures have healed. The animal is released back into its natural habitat if the jaw functions adequately and all other injuries have healed.

PROGNOSIS. Good with proper reduction and supportive care.

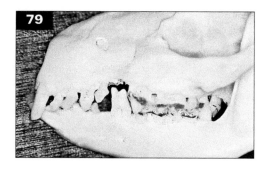

Case 80: **Hedgehog handling**

CLINICAL PRESENTATION. This African hedgehog is displaying normal defensive behavior (**80a**). When threatened, a hedgehog will draw its body tightly into a ball using the powerful orbicularis and panniculus carnosus muscles, thus making examination difficult.

PREVALENCE. Very common defensive behavior.

MANAGEMENT. To coax a hedgehog to uncurl, the first thing to do is to simply leave it undisturbed for several minutes on the table; it may then uncurl and try to escape. If that doesn't work, the curled hedgehog is held in a gloved hand and stroked heavily from front to back over the caudal half of the body. Another method is to hold the hedgehog's head downwards over a flat surface and it may unroll to reach for that surface. It is also possible to bounce the pet gently in cupped hands. Finally, some workers recommend placing the hedgehog in a shallow (2.5 cm deep) container of warm water. This method should not be used if the pet is exhibiting any respiratory signs.

Once the awake hedgehog uncurls, it can be scooped up off the table in open hands; it will not usually curl up again. If all else fails, general anesthesia is induced with either injectable drugs or inhalants. Isoflurane introduced with a face mask or anesthetic chamber works well with rapid induction and recovery times.

Hedgehogs have spines that do not come out when handled. However, the spines are quite irritating when held firmly erect in a defensive position. It is useful to protect your hands with latex examination gloves or lightweight leather gloves (**80b**).

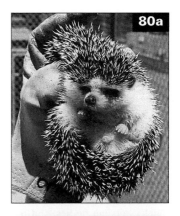

If the hedgehog is tractable or debilitated, the loose skin behind the ears can be grasped and the patient suspended over a table. This prevents the hedgehog from rolling up and allows access to the mouth for administration of oral medications or feedings.

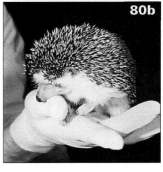

In hedgehogs that are difficult to handle, injectable drugs that can be given s/c can be used. Hedgehogs have an extensive subcutaneous space that contains a large amount of fat. Subcutaneous injections are given even when the pet is tightly curled into a ball. It is often not necessary to remove the animal from its cage. Oral medications should be masked with sweet flavors and put in the patient's food; however, some pets will stop eating altogether if they sense there is a change in their diet.

Case 81: **Hedgehog dietary requirements**

INTRODUCTION. Obesity is the most commonly observed diet-related disease in wild and pet hedgehogs. Secondary problems due to obesity include lowered fertility rates and poor survivability of neonates. Other diet-related illnesses include hepatic lipidosis, dental disease, poor spine and hair condition, heavy scaling of the skin, nutritional secondary hyperparathyroidism, and hypervitaminosis A and D. There is a poor understanding of the dietary requirements of hedgehogs.

MANAGEMENT. What is an appropriate diet for a pet African hedgehog at our present level of knowledge? In the wild, hedgehogs feed on a wide variety of insects, small animals, fruits, and vegetables. In captivity, an average adult hedgehog should be maintained on a daily diet consisting of 25 g of dry reduced-calorie cat food or mixture of dry and canned food, and 10 g of mixed fresh or thawed frozen vegetables. Five grams (3–5 insects) of live crickets or mealworms should be added 3–4 times a week. Since hedgehogs can easily become overweight, it is important to monitor the animal's weight frequently and adjust the amount fed appropriately. Feeding light or reduced-calorie cat food helps to maintain the animal's weight without compromising the nutritional quality of the diet. Live insects provide variety and behavioral enrichment for hedgehogs. The dietary requirements of the captive African hedgehog are still poorly understood. Exercise is vitally important for the hedgehog species kept in captivity. A large area in which the pet can exercise must be provided. Alternatively, a large exercise wheel, with a piece of wire or plastic mesh fitted on to the inner surface to prevent the feet from slipping through and to provide traction, can be used.

PROGNOSIS. If obese hedgehogs become ill, the ensuing hepatic lipidosis will result in a poorer prognosis.

Case 82: **Chinchilla with diarrhea due to *Giardia* infection**

CLINICAL PRESENTATION. A chinchilla has diarrhea for several days after purchase from a pet store. There is now a rectal prolapse. Other chinchillas from the pet store have similar problems.

DIFFERENTIAL DIAGNOSES. Giardiasis, GI bacterial overgrowth, intestinal roundworms, inappropriate use of antibiotics, other protozoal organisms.

INVESTIGATION. A zinc sulfate flotation of the feces is performed and organisms measuring 15 mm in length are found (**82**). This is a cyst of a *Giardia* species. It is identified by its size, the oval shape, and the presence of nuclei, median bodies, and flagella within the cyst. Zinc sulfate flotation is the test of choice to recover *Giardia* species from feces. A direct fecal smear is usually insufficient and multiple very fresh samples need to be evaluated.

DIAGNOSIS. Giardiasis.

ETIOLOGY. Infection with *Giardia* may produce diarrhea in many species of animals including chinchillas. Other signs associated with giardiasis include anorexia and lethargy. *Giardia* organisms are found in both healthy and sick chinchillas and their role in disease is not totally elucidated. Stress, poor husbandry, and crowding are all possible triggers to clinical disease associated with increased numbers of organisms on fecal examination.

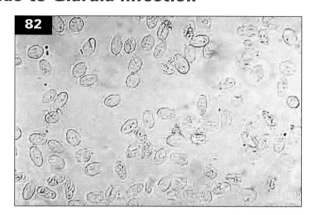

PREVALENCE. Possibly more common in fur-ranched chinchillas than in individual pet chinchillas.

MANAGEMENT. Fenbendazole (25–50 mg/kg p/o for 3–5 days) is the drug of choice for treatment, although metronidazole has also been used. The zoonotic implication of *Giardia* infection in chinchillas is unknown. It is best to be safe and advise clients that there is a slight potential zoonotic risk.

PROGNOSIS. Unless the predisposing causes leading to overgrowth of *Giardia* organisms are identified and resolved, the prognosis for reversal of signs is poor.

Case 83: **Chinchilla venipuncture**

INTRODUCTION. Chinchillas commonly present to the veterinarian with nonspecific signs of disease. History and physical examination does not always elucidate a cause. Frequently, hematology and biochemistry results are necessary to determine the etiology of the disease. Venipuncture is challenging in chinchillas due to their anatomy.

TECHNIQUE. The thick fur coat and relatively short forelimbs make venipuncture in chinchillas challenging. In the laboratory, orbital sinus bleeding using a hematocrit tube is an efficient method for collecting small quantities of blood. This technique is effective but should only be carried out under general anesthesia, as there is always the potential of damage to the orbital sinus if performed incorrectly. This technique should not be used on client owned animals.

In pet chinchillas, the small cephalic vein is located on the dorsum of the antebrachium. The fur is moistened with a small amount of alcohol rather than shaved. The lateral saphenous vein, which runs diagonally across the cranial aspect of the tarsus, is perhaps the most convenient vein to access for both venipuncture and catheterization. If needed, large quantities of blood can be collected from the jugular veins. This can be a challenge due to the chinchilla's short neck, thick fur, and difficulties with restraint. Sedation or anesthesia may be necessary. A 25 gauge needle attached to a 1 or 3 ml syringe is used.

Case 84: **Normal chinchilla dentition**

CLINICAL PRESENTATION. A chinchilla is brought to the surgery because the owners are concerned that it has incisor occlusion (**84a**). They want to know if this is normal.

INVESTIGATION. Oral examination in awake chinchillas gives a limited view of their dental health. The examination should be performed with the chinchilla sedated or anesthetized. Further examination requires imaging techniques including radiographs and CT scans. Skull radiographs are used to assess the dentition. The occlusal plane is horizontal in chinchillas. It can be demonstrated on lateral and rostrocaudal radiographs. A distinctive radiographic feature of the chinchilla is the large tympanic bulla. The lateral radiograph (**84b**) clearly shows the curvature and extent of the incisor teeth and the cheek tooth occlusal planes. Even with superimposition of the two sides, the position and length of the cheek teeth can be identified. Note the normal radiolucent germinal areas at the root apices. The rostrocaudal view (**84c**) demonstrates the temporomandibular articulations.

DIAGNOSIS. This is normal dentition.

ETIOLOGY. Unlike rabbits, the majority of rodents maintain their jaws in a retrognathic position when at rest. In this position the cheek teeth are usually in occlusion. When gnawing, the jaw is brought forward and then moved in a dorsoventral direction. As many rodents have a relatively large normal range of rostrocaudal jaw movement, they can compensate for even quite dramatic jaw length discrepancies. The chinchilla is a true herbivore, with typical rodent incisor dentition: I 1/1, C 0/0, P 1/1, M 3/3.

Epiphora is a common indication of dental disease in rabbits and herbivorous rodents. The nasolacrimal ducts, which pass next to the root apices of the premolars and incisors, frequently become obstructed when the roots of these aradicular hypsodont teeth elongate or develop other periapical pathology. In addition to primary eye disease, a purulent ocular discharge may originate from lacrimal duct infection secondary to either simple obstruction or a tooth root abscess.

PREVALENCE. Dental disease is a common problem in pet chinchillas.

MANAGEMENT. Chinchillas with dental disease may require frequent examination and treatment. Treatment may consist of periodic grinding of teeth and incisor removal. Periodic supportive care includes fluids, nutritional support, and pain relief.

PROGNOSIS. Dental disease may be considered a terminal illness that is controlled with periodic examinations and treatment.

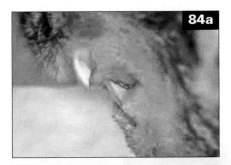

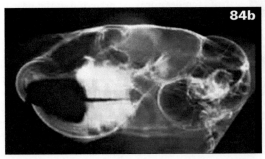

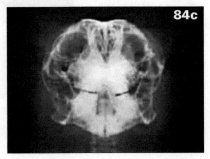

Case 85: **Chinchilla with alopecia due to self-barbering**

CLINICAL PRESENTATION. A two-year-old intact female chinchilla presents with areas of partial alopecia on the lateral aspects of the limbs of four weeks duration. She is caged alone and her owner has just started full-time employment.

DIFFERENTIAL DIAGNOSES. Self-barbering, dermatophytosis, fur slip. Ectoparasite infestation is uncommon in chinchillas.

INVESTIGATION. Epilated or plucked hairs from the affected area are examined microscopically. The distal tips of the hairs will be broken and damaged in cases of fur chewing. With fur slip, the hairs appear normal because almost complete shedding occurs. Plucked hair from dermatophytosis cases may be frayed or damaged. The hairs are mounted either in mineral oil or KOH to assess for fungal hyphae or spores. Hairs should also be placed on fungal culture. Finally, a skin scrape for ectoparasites should be done for completeness.

DIAGNOSIS. Self-barbering.

ETIOLOGY. This chinchilla was self-barbering due to the change in the household schedule caused by the owner going back to work. Predisposing factors to self-trauma in the chinchilla include stress, chronic disease, malnutrition, and the absence of dust baths. Examples of stress include gestation, cage mate death or disease, overcrowding, or moving into a new cage or location. There is also a theory that in some undiagnosed cases there may be an inherited behavioral trait or endocrine disease.

PREVALENCE. Common problem in pet chinchillas and a serious problem in chinchillas raised for fur production.

MANAGEMENT. When a chinchilla is found to be self-barbering, the cause needs to be elucidated, usually by a thorough history. Changes are recommended based on the cause of the self-barbering. In this case the owner was advised to spend more time with the chinchilla.

PROGNOSIS. The prognosis is good if environmental changes are made as directed. If the source of stress to the chinchilla is not removed, the self-barbering may continue.

Case 86: **Normal chinchilla biology**

INTRODUCTION. Chinchillas have only recently become highly popular as pets (**86**). The chinchilla is a hystricomorph rodent originally found in the high Andes Mountains of South America. This species was hunted to near extinction in the early 1900s and 11 animals were brought to California in 1923. Many of the chinchillas in the US are descended from these 11 animals. Until recently, chinchillas were mainly bred for their pelt or for medical investigation (hearing research and studies of Chagas disease). The majority of chinchillas are now bred for the pet trade.

86

In females the cone-shaped clitoris is easily confused for a penis. The female has four mammary glands, one at each inguinal region and one on each lateral rib. There are two uterine horns opening into one cervix. A membrane closes the vaginal vault except during estrus and parturition.

In the male there is no true scrotum. The testicles are located in the inguinal canal area and are palpated just beneath the skin. This necessitates closure of the inguinal canal when castration is performed. The sex of young chinchillas is determined by measuring the length of the perineal distance, which is longer in males than in females.

MANAGEMENT. Although chinchillas survive in a variety of environments, they do best in cool, dry conditions. Cold temperatures are preferred in the pelt industry, as it stimulates a thick coat. Heat stroke is a significant problem, especially in humid environments. Wire cages are commonly used, but solid flooring in a portion of the cage reduces foot problems. Since chinchillas enjoy climbing and jumping, a multilevel cage is recommended for pet animals or for research animals that are kept for long periods of time. Commercially raised chinchillas are typically caged in polygamous groupings. If a single large cage is used, escape boxes are provided to protect other chinchillas from the aggressive behavior of the dominant females. Chinchillas require a dust bath to keep their fur coat groomed. If they are deprived of this, the coat will appear oily and matted and the chinchilla may become depressed and anorectic. A mixture of silver sand and Fuller's earth (9:1) is placed in a small container in the cage for a short period of time each day. If left in the cage, the bath will be soiled with feces and food.

Case 87: **Mammary gland tumors (fibroadenomas) in a female rat**

CLINICAL PRESENTATION. A two-year-old female intact pet rat develops these two large tumors on its abdomen (87).

DIFFERENTIAL DIAGNOSES. Benign fibroadenomas, malignant mammary gland tumor, abscess.

INVESTIGATION. A fine needle aspirate of the masses will determine whether this is a tumor or an abscess; however, the aspirate may not be of good enough quality to determine the tumor type. Radiography should be performed before surgery to rule out metastatic disease.

DIAGNOSIS. A mammary gland fibroadenoma.

ETIOLOGY. Mammary tumors are common in rodents. In rats these tumors are usually benign mammary fibroadenomas, and metastasis is rare. If metastasis does occur, it is generally to regional lymph nodes, abdominal viscera, or lungs. Mammary gland tumors are found in most pet rodents.

In contrast to rats, mammary tumors in mice are frequently malignant, invasive, and difficult to remove. They are associated with infection by the mouse mammary tumor virus.

In guinea pigs, about 70% of mammary gland tumors are benign fibroadenomas and 30% are mammary adenocarcinomas. Male guinea pigs are more likely to have malignant mammary gland tumors as opposed to female guinea pigs.

PREVALENCE. This is a common problem in older pet rats.

MANAGEMENT. Ovariohysterectomy at a young age may decrease the incidence of mammary gland tumors and should be recommended to owners of female pet rats. During surgical removal of mammary tumors, regional lymph nodes should be collected and biopsied to stage the disease. Unless ulcerated or suspected to be malignant, the skin overlying the tumor should not be removed. Any blood vessels supplying the tumor are ligated and closure is routine. A subcuticular suture pattern or skin staples are used because rodents frequently chew and may remove the sutures. An Elizabethan collar is used as needed. There is evidence that ovariohysterectomy at the time of tumor removal may decrease the chance of tumor recurrence, even in benign tumors.

PROGNOSIS. The prognosis for recovery is good unless there is metastasis.

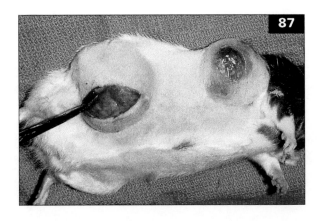

Case 88: **Laboratory rat with corneal ulceration**

CLINICAL PRESENTATION. Several rats from a large research facility have developed the ocular lesion shown (88). A technician working with these rats has been anesthetizing them for two hours daily for a skeletal loading experiment. The protocol consists of using a standard xylazine/ketamine dosing regimen.

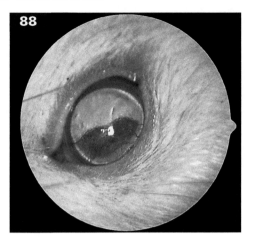

DIFFERENTIAL DIAGNOSES. Corneal ulceration from exposure, infection, or trauma.

INVESTIGATION. A complete ocular examination may determine the cause of the ulceration. In this case, history is also important. Are the researchers placing a lubricant in the eyes of the sedated rats? Fluorescent dye is used to delineate the extent of the ulcer and to indicate if it is an on-going or an older ulcer. A slit lamp examination will give a more detailed view of the ulcer. Cytology and culture of the ulcerated cornea may help determine the etiology.

DIAGNOSIS. There is a vascularized area of corneal ulceration in the central interpalpebral zone of the cornea.

ETIOLOGY. This occurred because the animals had their eyes wide open during anesthesia with these anesthetic agents. Dehydration of the cornea plays a major role in the development of this lesion.

PREVALENCE. Common if the cornea is not protected while the rat is sedated or anesthetized.

MANAGEMENT. The problem can be solved by taping the lids closed during surgery. Consideration should be given to protecting the eyes in this manner during any long procedure under anesthetic where ocular drying and subsequent trauma may occur if the eyes remain open. Alternatively, a sterile ophthalmic ointment may be placed in the eyes to keep them lubricated. The ulcer needs time to heal, but an ocular antibiotic ointment can be applied to prevent secondary infections.

PROGNOSIS. The prognosis is good if the lesion is identified quickly and the cause of the lesion is removed.

Case 89: **A fatal case of murine (rat) mycoplasmosis**

CLINICAL PRESENTATION. A two-year-old pet female rat exhibits wheezing respiratory sounds and dyspnea. Despite treatment with oxygen, the rat dies and the lungs are examined. Grossly (89a), the lungs show bronchopneumonia and areas of atelectasis due to bronchial occlusion. The pleural surface is unevenly elevated due to bronchiolectasis. Histopathologically (89b), the lung tissue reveals peribronchial lymphoid hyperplasia and neutrophil exudation within the bronchial lumina.

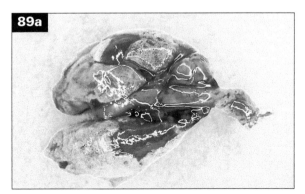

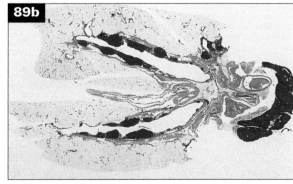

DIFFERENTIAL DIAGNOSES. *Mycoplasma pulmonis*, other causes of bacterial pneumonia, primary viral pneumonia, cardiac disease.

INVESTIGATION. The agent may be isolated from tracheal washings; however, special enriched medium is required and subculturing is often necessary. Most laboratories are not equipped to isolate *M. pulmonis*. A positive antibody titer to *M. pulmonis* is indicative of infection. Radiography will aid in determining the extent of pulmonary involvement and the prognosis.

DIAGNOSIS. Murine respiratory mycoplasmosis caused by *M. pulmonis*.

ETIOLOGY. Infection is transmitted both horizontally and vertically and is chronic for the life of the animal. It is enzootic in many rat colonies unless they have originated from hysterectomy derivation. The disease may lie dormant for varying periods and asymptomatic carriers exist.

PREVALENCE. Common, especially in pet stores and in laboratory animal facilities without proper surveillance.

MANAGEMENT. Rats with suspected *M. pulmonis* infection are treated with one or a combination of these antibiotics: enrofloxacin (20–30 mg/kg p/o q24h), chloramphenicol (50 mg/kg s/c q8h or 1 g/l drinking water), tetracycline (20 mg/kg p/o q12h), oxytetra-cycline (60 mg/kg s/c q72h), or tylosin (10–20 mg/kg i/m q24h or 100 mg/kg p/o q8–12h). It is difficult to achieve a complete cure and relapse is common. When treating a colony, it is important always to check for an underlying primary viral infection.

PROGNOSIS. The prognosis for controlling mild disease in a young rat is good. The success of treatment decreases as the age of the rat, the duration of the disease, and the likelihood of secondary infection increase.

Case 90: **Rodent venipuncture**

INTRODUCTION. A definitive diagnosis would not be possible for many diseases in small rodent pets without appropriate laboratory samples.

TECHNIQUE. Blood collection from the orbital sinus is not acceptable in the pet rodent because of complications such as nasal or ocular blood draining or blindness.

Mice, rats, and gerbils all have large lateral tail veins (**90**); hamsters have a ventral caudal tail artery, which is more accessible in the female. The jugular veins and femoral arteries, while not easily visualized, are equally as large as the tail veins. The cephalic and lateral saphenous veins are more easily visualized, but are smaller in diameter. A toe nail clip must not be used to collect blood as it is painful and stressful and the blood can mix with tissue fluids, leading to inaccurate results.

It may be necessary to anesthetize some patients for successful phlebotomy. Excessive restraint in debilitated animals can have fatal results. The patient should be warmed slightly before venipuncture to dilate the vessels. The blood volume to be collected is calculated. In a hydrated, healthy animal, 6–10% of the body weight in grams is the total blood volume. A maximum of 10% of the total blood volume may be taken in whole blood. An insulin syringe is used to reduce blood waste in the needle hub and prevent excessive negative pressure on the vessel. The suction on the syringe is broken and the syringe coated with heparin before use. Blood is allowed to flow into the syringe, without pulling on the plunger, until the vein has time to fill again. Hemorrhage is considered as part of the total collectible volume. Pressure is applied to the vein until hemostasis is achieved.

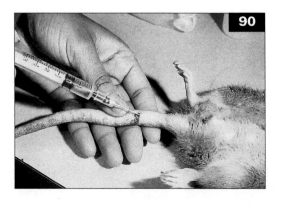

Case 91: **Sialodacryoadenitis virus (SDAV) infection in a adult rat with porphyria**

CLINICAL PRESENTATION. An adult male rat in a pet shop has what appears to be blood coming from his eyes (**91**). Two other adult males in the same cage are sneezing and sitting hunched in the corner, with rough appearing hair coats. There is a total of six large rats in the 75-liter glass tank, which has fresh pine shavings for bedding. There is red staining around the rat's eyes.

DIFFERENTIAL DIAGNOSES. SDAV, other causes of porphyria including infections caused by Sendai virus, P3 virus, and corona virus. Organisms such as *Pasteurella pneumotropica* and *Mycoplasma pulmonis* can act as common bacterial secondary invaders.

INVESTIGATION. Diagnosis is usually made by a combination of history, response to treatment, and necropsy results.

DAIGNOSIS. Sialodacryoadenitis.

ETIOLOGY. A common viral agent, SDAV is frequently responsible for this highly contagious condition. SDAV is an RNA virus (coronavirus) that replicates in the epithelial cytoplasm of the respiratory tract and travels along the ducts into the glands of the head. It has a special predilection for the Harderian gland. Younger animals are more severely affected and the virus usually resolves in a week. The red staining around the eyes is from porphyria. It occurs when the rat's Harderian gland becomes inflamed and secretes porphyrin-pigmented tears.

PREVALENCE. Common in pet store rats and in rat colonies with poorly controlled security.

MANAGEMENT. It is advisable to treat most cases with antibiotics following appropriate culture and sensitivity testing. In some cases the porphyria persists due to

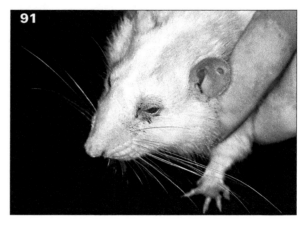

permanent damage to the Harderian gland. Bedding such as cedar or pine shavings or cypress mulch can predispose rats to respiratory disease, as it contains the volatile oil thujone. Thujone is a respiratory irritant and may be tumorogenic. Thujone can cause convulsions and cortical brain lesions if there is prolonged exposure. In addition, volatile oils are strongly scented and may mask feces and urine odors in the cage. In an aquarium or other enclosed environment, ammonia and other toxic gases, which are heavier than oxygen, sink to the floor where the animals are living. This disastrous situation may cause respiratory conditions to deteriorate rapidly. Hardwood shavings or pellets are a much better choice for cage litter, with no sanitary compromise. Other predisposing factors include overcrowding, high environmental temperatures and inadequate nutrition.

PROGNOSIS. The prognosis is dependent on treatment response, disease severity, and other secondary infections.

Case 92: **Rodent male reproductive surgery**

INTRODUCTION. Owners with rodent breeding colonies occasionally need to have the males castrated or vasectomized. Therefore, it is important to know how to perform a castration and vasectomy in a rodent. Vasectomy procedures are important when mating is required without pregnancy.

TECHNIQUE. The inguinal rings remain open throughout life in male mice, rats, guinea pigs, and hamsters. Inguinal hernias are prevented by using castration techniques that functionally close the inguinal rings. Rats, guinea pigs, and hamsters have a large fat pad associated with each testis and

spermatic cord. These structures make visualization and ligation of structures within the cord difficult. A standard closed castration technique is used in smaller rodents. In larger rodents such as the guinea pig, one approach is to perform an open castration technique modified to close the inguinal ring. The anesthetized guinea pig is placed in dorsal recumbency and an incision made longitudinally over the scrotum. The testis is exteriorized with the tunic intact (**92a**). A length of suture is placed around the tunic and the cord as close to the superficial inguinal ring as possible. The suture is left untied as it will later identify and ligate the tunic. The tunic is incised distal to the untied

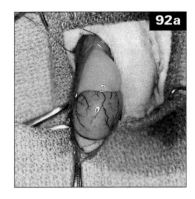
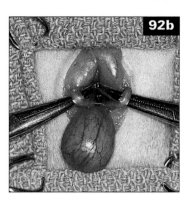

suture, as shown. The structures of the spermatic cord are clamped, ligated, and removed distal to the ligatures. Synthetic absorbable suture is used. The ligated stumps are allowed to slip back into the abdomen. The suture that was previously placed proximally around the tunic is tied. This functionally closes the superficial inguinal ring. The distal tunic is excised. The procedure is then repeated on the other side. The scrotal incisions are left open or are closed with synthetic absorbable suture in a buried continuous intradermal pattern or with skin staples or tissue adhesive.

Vasectomy in rodents is performed through bilateral scrotal incisions or via a suprapubic ventral midline incision. A small (2–3 cm) incision is made in the ventral midline just cranial to the pubis, taking care to avoid injury to the bladder. The bladder is reflected caudoventrally, revealing the two vas deferens (**92b**).

Each vas is double ligated and a section removed between the ligatures. The linea alba is closed with 4-0 or 5-0 synthetic absorbable suture. The skin is closed with the same type of suture material in a buried continuous intradermal suture pattern, using Michel clips or skin staples.

Case 93: **Rat dental anatomy**

CLINICAL PRESENTATION. A dental abnormality is seen as an incidental finding during a preoperative examination on a pet rat prior to excision of a mammary tumor. One of the rat's mandibular second molar teeth is missing.

DIFFERENTIAL DIAGNOSES. Absence of molar teeth may be congenital, the result of periodontal disease, or post extraction. Caries is not likely to be the cause because it is rare in rodents unless they are fed an unnatural diet and are exposed to cariogenic bacteria. Loss of molars from external trauma is also unlikely because they are protected by a thick layer of masseter muscle laterally.

INVESTIGATION. Imaging is key to a complete description of this problem. Skull radiographs or dental films are recommended. If possible, a CT scan will give superior detail compared with radiographs and dental films. A lateral radiographic view of the patient's skull is shown (**93**).

DIAGNOSIS. Absence of molar teeth.

ETIOLOGY. Anisognathism of rodents differs from that in carnivores, rabbits, horses, and cattle. In rodents the maxilla is narrower than the mandible, providing space for the large masseter muscles, which are required for gnawing. In carnivores and herbivores, such as rabbits, horses, and cattle, the jaw width relationship is reversed, with the mandible being narrower than the maxilla.

The dental formula for rats and mice is I 1/1, C 0/0, P 0/0, M 3/3. The dentition of rats and mice differs from that of guinea pigs and chinchillas. Rats and mice are granivorous rather than herbivorous like chinchillas and guinea pigs. The granivore diet is nutritionally concentrated, is relatively nonabrasive, and requires little grinding before it is swallowed. The cheek teeth are reduced in number and size compared with the herbivorous species. Rats and mice have brachyodont molar teeth that stop growing once they have erupted and the roots are fully formed. In contrast, the incisors in these species grow continuously.

In this case the absence of the molar tooth was considered congenital, as no other problems were noted.

PREVALENCE. Not common.

MANAGEMENT. No treatment was recommended as no disease was found to be associated with this finding.

PROGNOSIS. Excellent.

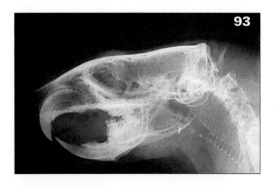

Case 94: **Mouse with skin lesions due to *Sarcoptes* species mites**

CLINICAL PRESENTATION. A mouse develops pruritus and hair loss over its dorsum. The skin appears reddened, with multifocal crusts and patchy alopecia. Another mouse in the same cage is asymptomatic. There is also a 10-year-old Yorkshire Terrier recently diagnosed with allergic dermatitis living in the same household.

DIFFERENTIAL DIAGNOSES. The causes of pruritus and alopecia in the mouse include ectoparasites, dermatophytosis, bacterial infections, barbering, pinworms, and neoplasia. The more common ectoparasites include the parasitic mites *Myobia musculi* and *Myocoptes musculinus*. Less common species of mites include *Radfordia affinis*, *Psorergates simplex*, *Otodectes bacoti*, *Sarcoptes scabiei*, *Notoedres muris*, and *Trichoecius romboutsi*. Other ectoparasites include fleas, primarily in households with dogs and cats. The louse, *Polyplax serrata*, is also considered. Dermatophytosis is an uncommon cause of pruritus in the mouse. *Trichophyton mentagrophytes* can be isolated from 60% of clinically normal pet shop mice. Bacterial dermatitis (e.g. *Staphylococcus* species) is not typically pruritic, but it may cause skin crusting. Severe, secondary bacterial dermatitis can be associated with pruritus and ulceration. Barbering, due to stress and overcrowding, causes alopecia but not pruritus. Pinworms cause a localized perianal pruritus. Neoplasia (e.g. epitheliotrophic lymphoma) occasionally causes alopecia and pruritus, but generally is associated with scaly skin.

INVESTIGATION. Skin scrapings, fungal cultures, and skin biopsies should be performed to determine the cause.

DIAGNOSIS. This *Sarcoptes* mite (**94**) was found after a skin scraping.

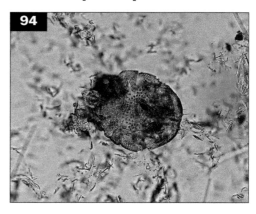

PREVALENCE. Ectoparasites are common in mice, but this particular mite is not the most frequently encountered mite.

MANAGEMENT. Two to three injections of ivermectin (0.4–0.8 mg/kg s/c q7d) is usually sufficient to cause resolution of the signs. Insecticidal dips may be too toxic, even when diluted, for mice. Any insecticide product should be used in mice with great caution. The other mouse is considered an asymptomatic carrier and should also be treated with ivermectin. Since the dog may not be suffering from allergic dermatitis, but rather a mite infestation, it is important to examine all household pets and people for mites. The household environment should be thoroughly cleaned.

PROGNOSIS. Good if the mites are controlled, the environment cleaned, and secondary bacterial infections treated.

Case 95: **Mouse with pinworm parasites**

CLINICAL PRESENTATION. A company that sells 'germ-free mice' to researchers is receiving complaints that the mice are infected with worms. The company assures the researchers that fecal flotations performed weekly are negative for eggs, larvae, cysts, and oocysts. The company maintains that the mice are negative when they leave the facility and become infected when they arrive at the research facility. The mice are 28 days old when they arrive at the research facility.

INVESTIGATION. One of the researchers performs a 'tape test' on a newly arrived group of mice and recovers eggs measuring 118–153 × 33–55 mm (**95a**). On sugar flotation, a second kind of egg is found that measures 89–93 × 36–42 mm (**95b**).

ETIOLOGY. Both figures show pinworm eggs; **95a** shows the common mouse pinworm *Syphacia obvelata*, and **95b** is of the mouse pinworm *Aspisculuris tetraptera*. Note the flattened side of the *S. obvelata* egg.

The tape test is necessary to find the eggs of many pinworms, including *S. obvelata*, because the female worms do not deposit eggs in the intestine. *S. obvelata* eggs are not usually recovered on fecal flotations. The female worm crawls through the anal opening and cements eggs to the perianal skin. The adhesive side of a clear piece of cellophane tape should be pressed against the anus and perianal skin. The tape is stuck to a slide for microscopic examination. *S. obvelata* adults live in the colon. The life cycle is direct and the larvated eggs deposited by the female are the infective stage. The prepatent period of *S. obvelata* is 8–15 days.

PREVALENCE. Pinworms are ubiquitous in mice.

MANAGEMENT. Why are eggs found on the flotation performed at the research institution but not at the breeder? *A. tetraptera* adults live in the anterior colon and cecum, where females deposit eggs rather than attach them to the perianal skin. Eggs, therefore, are present on flotation. As with *S. obvelata*, the life cycle is direct and larvated eggs are infective. The prepatent period, however, is approximately 23 days and eggs larvate to the infective stage in approximately six days. The breeding facility was performing fecals on the young mice and the worms were not old enough to produce eggs. In addition, the breeding facility was not performing the tape test.

PROGNOSIS. Pinworms are considered nonpathogenic, but they could lead to rectal prolapse if straining is continual. In a research colony, these may be undesirable.

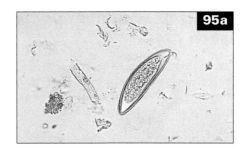

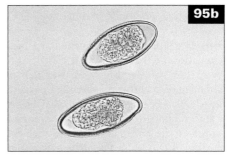

Case 96: **Squirrel that is unable to walk due to poor nutrition**

CLINICAL PRESENTATION. A juvenile male squirrel, cared for by a wildlife rehabilitator, is no longer able to walk. On palpation, there is pain and swelling in the left shoulder. The squirrel's diet consists of only fruits and nuts.

DIFFERENTIAL DIAGNOSES. Lack of sufficient quantities of dietary calcium, lack of vitamin D, other causes of pathologic bone disease, trauma.

INVESTIGATION. A detailed history, especially diet, is essential is establishing a diagnosis. Radiographs (**96a, b**) elucidating the lack of bony mineralization is diagnostic for dietary disease. A plasma biochemistry profile usually reveals a low total calcium.

DIAGNOSIS. The squirrel can no longer walk because of compression fractures of the proximal left humerus and of the second lumbar vertebra. There is also a general decrease in cortical thickness in all the long bones.

ETIOLOGY. The fractures are pathologic due to nutritional secondary hyperparathyroidism. Fruits and nuts are low in calcium and relatively high in phosphorus. The result of a diet with a reverse calcium:phosphorus (Ca:P) ratio is metabolic bone disease.

PREVALENCE. Common when inexperienced handlers attempt to raise wildlife.

MANAGEMENT. The overall goal of treatment is to place the animal on a proper plane of nutrition by correcting the diet, specifically the Ca:P ratio. Parenteral calcium is administered once, followed by oral calcium supple-

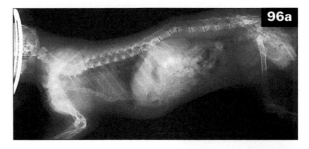

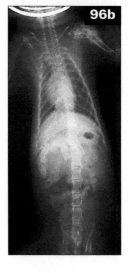

mentation. The diet is corrected. Stabilization is not recommended for the fractures, as the bones are too soft to hold implants. Pins often tear through the bone and wires can collapse the bone. The squirrel is confined to a small cage and handled with great care. Generally, pathologic fractures due to nutritional secondary hyperparathyroidism heal rapidly once the diet is corrected. Remodeling of malunion fractures generally results in a functional outcome.

PROGNOSIS. In a compression vertebral fracture, if pain perception is present, the prognosis is fair to good for a complete recovery. It must be emphasized that gentle handling and restricted activity is vital, as well as an improved diet.

Case 97: Squirrels with neurologic disease secondary to *Baylisascaris procyonis*

CLINICAL PRESENTATION. Two squirrels were hand raised as part of a rehabilitation program. After a week in an outdoor dirt floored pen, they exhibit ataxia, tremors, and torticollis. A year ago, the pen had previously housed a young raccoon.

DIFFERENTIAL DIAGNOSES. *Baylisascaris procyonis* infection, toxins (e.g. lead, pesticides), trauma.

INVESTIGATION. The squirrels were euthanized and histologic examination of their brain and spinal cord performed. A recent soil sample from the pen is examined by sedimentation and reveals larvated parasite eggs measuring 63–70 × 53–58 mm (**97a**). The thorax and abdomen are examined for larval granulomas and brain sections for larvae and characteristic malacic inflammatory lesions. A portion of the brain is placed in two layers of cheese cloth and suspended in a conical-shaped tube filled with warm saline for approximately 12–24 hours. The sediment is then examined microscopically for *Baylisascaris* larvae.

DIAGNOSIS. Cerebral larva migrans caused by *B. procyonis* larvae is the most likely diagnosis. The diagnosis of *B. procyonis* is confirmed at necropsy as antemortem tests are not possible.

ETIOLOGY. The eggs are viable in the environment for years and were probably deposited by the raccoon that was in the pen previously. This can be confirmed by examination of the soil for parasite eggs. *B. procyonis* eggs resemble those of *Toxocara* species (**97b**).

PREVALENCE. This disease can be found in any area inhabited by raccoons.

MANAGEMENT. Control of this disease is difficult and it includes environmental decontamination. The soil remains contaminated with viable eggs for years. Eggs can be transported to the surface during gardening or by earthworms and insects. Bleach has little to no effect on the viability of the eggs. Small areas of contamination on resistant surfaces are treated with a 1:1 mixture of xylene:ethanol. Metal cages and small items are autoclaved or flamed. Large areas of soil or concrete can be flamed with a portable flame gun. The soil should be turned, raked, and flamed several times. Any raccoons are treated with either pyrantel pamoate (10 mg/kg p/o), fenbendazole (50 mg/kg p/o q24h for 3 days), or mebendazole (25–40 mg/kg p/o q24h for 3–5 days). After treatment, feces are burned with the expelled worms. The raccoons are treated weekly or biweekly for four weeks. Because of the zoonotic potential of *B. procyonis*, clients are advised to discourage the presence of raccoons in their yards and homes.

PROGNOSIS. This disease causes severe morbidity and mortality and is usually fatal.

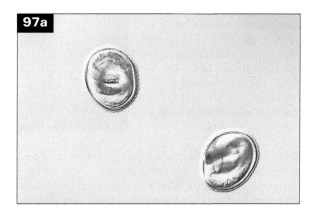

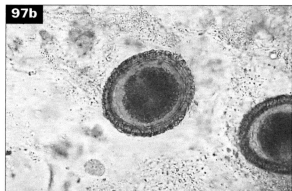

Case 98: **Gerbil with ocular disease due to Harderian gland infection**

CLINICAL PRESENTATION. A two-year-old male gerbil has crusts around the eyes, is depressed, and is anorectic (**98**). The perinasal area is erythematous, with patches of alopecia. Both front paws are denuded medially and the hair coat over the entire body is matted.

DIFFERENTIAL DIAGNOSES. Harderian gland disease, ocular infection.

DIAGNOSIS. Harderian gland disease.

ETIOLOGY. The cause of the perinasal changes is disease of the Harderian gland. This is a periocular lacrimal gland found in many small rodents. It drains into the nose and, when inflamed, its secretions increase. The lacrimal secretions contain a porphyrin pigment (red-orange in color) that is irritating to the skin. Alopecia on the face and forelimbs is caused by the gerbil trying to clean the excessive secretions from its eyelids and nose. In addition, overgrown, sharp, or broken toenails can cause ocular damage including corneal lacerations. Secondary loss of ocular or periocular integrity allows bacterial invasion, resulting in conjunctivitis. The gerbil becomes weakened and depressed when it can no longer see or smell its food.

PREVALENCE. Not uncommonly seen in gerbils.

MANAGEMENT. The crusts and skin debris are gently removed and the face cleansed with a mild antiseptic solution. It may be necessary to use anesthesia in severe cases. The nails are trimmed to prevent further abrasions. A nonsteroidal ophthalmic antibiotic ointment is applied to the affected areas at least twice daily. The minimum amount of topical medication should be used because gerbils will ingest any excess during grooming. Separating compatible gerbils for an extended period of time should be avoided, because they may fight when reunited. It is important to make sure owners follow the husbandry guidelines. The husbandry factors contributing to nasal dermatitis in the gerbil include:
- Bedding that is too rough or too shallow. Gerbils live in burrows and spend a great deal of time digging. Perinasal tissue integrity is lost when thin layers of bedding or substrates, such as sand or rough shavings, are used. *Staphylococcus* species and *Streptococcus* species infections are often secondary invaders.
- The gerbil is a desert dwelling species and they tolerate poorly a humidity level above 50%.
- Bedding containing volatile oils, such as cedar shavings.
- Primary or secondary mycoplasma infections, as well as some viral infections, contribute to disease of the respiratory tract, which may lead to increased nasal and Harderian gland secretions.
- Stress. Common causes of stress are dirty cages, improper or inadequate diet, or an incompatible cage mate.

It is important to change the bedding to a soft, nontoxic material such as hardwood shavings or pellets, cellulose pellets, or newspaper products. At least a 5 cm depth of bedding should be provided.

PROGNOSIS. Excellent with appropriate treatment and husbandry changes.

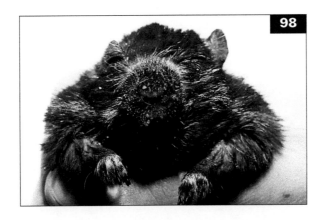

Summary questions and answers

Q1. Describe a proper diet for rabbits. What happens if fiber is too low?

Q2. What is the cause of dental points in rabbits, and how are they treated?

Q3. What is the best treatment for adrenal gland disease in ferrets?

Q4. What is the best treatment for insulinoma in ferrets?

Q5. How does the dental anatomy of rats and mice differ from that of guinea pigs and chinchillas?

Q6. Radiographs reveal calculi in a rabbit's urinary tract. How is this managed?

Q7. What are the differentials for a rat with respiratory disease, and how is the condition managed?

Q8. A hedgehog is reported to be losing quills. What are some differentials, and how is this problem diagnosed and managed?

Q9. Two rabbits live together but only one is losing hair. What are some differentials, and how is this problem diagnosed and managed?

Q10. What is the likely etiology of a rabbit mandibular abscess, and how should it be managed?

Q11. Describe how to take blood from rabbits, ferrets, chinchillas, and guinea pigs.

Q12. Describe how to hold a rabbit to minimize the chance of trauma to its back?

Q13. How would you hold a hedgehog for a physical examination?

Q14. What is the best protocol for anesthetizing a rabbit?

A1. Although replicating the 'wild' rabbit diet in captivity is not possible, the goal is to feed a diet high in fiber. Not only should the diet be at least 20% fiber, but also the fiber should be in a form that includes long stems. If fiber is too low, gastrointestinal disease can ensue, leading to ileus, a bacterial flora imbalance, and intermittent soft stools.

A2. It is not clear whether genetics or diet, or a combination, is the cause of dental points in rabbits. Treatment consists of periodic examination, along with removing the points as necessary. Long-term treatment includes improving the diet, usually with the addition of the correct amount and type of fiber.

A3. There is no one method that can be considered the best treatment. Only surgical removal offers the possibility of a cure. Medical treatment may be the best option for some ferrets. The best treatment will always be an individual decision for the owner and patient.

A4. As with adrenal gland disease, the best treatment is surgical. Although surgery will rarely cure this disease, in general it extends the life of the ferret longer than medical treatment alone will.

A5. The cheek teeth and incisor teeth of guinea pigs and chinchillas grow throughout the life of these animals, whereas only the incisors of rats and mice continue to grow. The dental problems of guinea pigs and chinchillas usually require much more veterinary attention than dental issues of rats and mice. Diet plays a much bigger role in the dental health of guinea pigs and chinchillas than in that of rats and mice.

A6. Managing calculi depends upon where they reside in the urinary tract. Ureteral, bladder, and urethral stones usually require surgical management, especially if clinical signs are present. Renal calculi are usually left in place unless severe clinical disease due to the calculi is present. Diuresis and diet change are possible medical aspects of treatment.

A7. Respiratory disease in rats is a complex problem with a multitude of causes. Bacterial, fungal, and viral agents have all been implicated. This disorder is usually complicated by less than ideal husbandry conditions. Management of this disease is based on improving husbandry and medical treatment. The ultimate course of treatment is based on the signalment of the patient and whether it is a solitary pet or belongs to a colony of rats.

A8. The loss of quills in a hedgehog should be considered in the same way as the loss of hair. Quill loss, like hair loss, can be caused by metabolic disorders, parasitic dermatitis, bacterial dermatitis, fungal dermatitis, and neoplasia, and it can even be self-induced. Diagnosis is much like it is with hair loss, with a combination of skin scrapings, microscopic examination, cultures, and biopsies. Diagnosis dictates how this problem is managed.

A9. Although hair trauma due to either self-barbering or cage mate barbering appears to be a likely differential, parasitic and fungal causes of hair loss should be considered. Diagnosis will be based on such tests as skin scrapings, microscopic evaluation, cultures, biopsies, response to treatment, and even separation of the two rabbits. Management of this condition is based on the findings of the diagnostics.

A10. It is now assumed that most mandibular abscesses in rabbits are caused by dental disease. Tooth root elongation with disruption of the tooth socket allows oral bacteria to colonize the bone around the tooth root. The abscess can be treated with medication. The preferred treatment is surgical removal of all diseased tissue and affected teeth, along with long-term antibiotics. Improved dental health and husbandry are also essential.

A11. The key to venipuncture in these patients is practice, good restraint, proper equipment, and the realization that the available blood volume that can be safely removed is small. The most common and easiest places for venipuncture in each species include:
- Rabbits: lateral saphenous, jugular vein.
- Ferrets: lateral saphenous, jugular vein, cranial vena cava.
- Chinchillas and guinea pigs: lateral saphenous, jugular vein.

A12. During some procedures, rabbits need to be held as securely as possible. This includes transporting the rabbit around the hospital and performing diagnostic tests such as venipuncture. Wrapping a rabbit tightly in a towel, 'burrito' fashion, does not guarantee a risk-free event, but it greatly reduces back fractures. Whatever method is used, the most important aspect is not to allow the hindlimbs to 'kick' with any force.

A13. Only very sick hedgehogs or extremely well socialized hedgehogs can be examined without chemical restraint. The typical hedgehog examination includes immobilization, usually by isoflurane induced by a 'whole-body' face mask.

A14. This is individual, based on the medications available at the hospital, the patient status, the length of the procedure, and the risk of the procedure. The main points of anesthesia are to keep the rabbit anxiety free, to prevent hypotension, to support respiration, and to minimize pain. The anesthesia protocol usually involves premedicants to reduce anxiety, reduce pain, and sedate the patient prior to anesthesia. Induction can be by face mask or intravenous medication. Maintenance is usually performed by gas anesthesia via a face mask or endotracheal intubation.

Bibliography

Textbooks

Carpenter JW (2005) *Exotic Animal Formulary* (3rd edn). WB Saunders, Philadelphia.

DeForge DH, Colmery BH (2000) (eds) *An Atlas of Veterinary Dental Radiology*. Iowa State University Press, Ames.

Fox JG (1998) (ed) *Biology and Diseases of the Ferret* (2nd edn). Williams & Wilkins, Baltimore.

Fox JG, Anderson LC, Loew FM, Quimby FW (2002) (eds) *Laboratory Animal Medicine* (2nd edn). Academic Press, London.

Harcourt–Brown F (2002) *Textbook of Rabbit Medicine*. Elsevier, Philadelphia (Butterworth-Heinemann, Oxford, Boston).

Harkness JE, Wagner JE (1995) *The Biology and Medicine of Rabbits and Rodents* (4th edn). Lea & Febiger, Philadelphia.

Lewington JH (2007) *Ferret Husbandry, Medicine, and Surgery* (2nd edn). Elsevier, Philadelphia.

Meredith A, Flecknell P (2006) (eds) *Manual of Rabbit Medicine and Surgery* (2nd edn). British Small Animal Veterinary Association, Gloucester.

Meredith A, Redrobe S (2002) (eds) *Manual of Exotic Pets* (4th edn). British Small Animal Veterinary Association, Gloucester.

Oglesbee BL (2006) *The 5-Minute Veterinary Consult: Ferret and Rabbit*. Blackwell Publishing, Oxford.

Percy DH, Barthold SW (2007) (eds) *Pathology of Laboratory Rodents and Rabbits* (3rd edn). Iowa State University Press, Ames.

Popesko P, Rajtova V, Horak J (2003) *Colour Atlas of Anatomy of Small Laboratory Animals, Volumes 1 and 2*. WB Saunders, Philadelphia.

Quesenberry KE, Carpenter JW (2004) (eds) *Ferrets, Rabbits, and Rodents: Clinical Medicine and Surgery* (2nd edn). WB Saunders, Philadelphia.

Richardson VCG (2000) *Diseases of Domestic Guinea Pigs* (2nd edn). Blackwell Science, Carlton.

Richardson VCG (2003) *Diseases of Small Domestic Rodents* (2nd edn). Blackwell Science, Oxford.

Silvermann S, Tell LA (2005) *Radiology of Rodents, Rabbits, and Ferrets: An Atlas of Normal Anatomy and Positioning*. WB Saunders, Philadelphia.

Suckow MA, Douglas FA (1997) *The Laboratory Rabbit*. CRC Press, Boca Raton.

Section 2
BIRDS

Neil A Forbes

Classification of cases by species

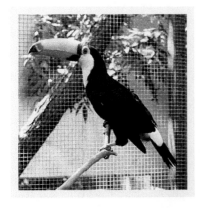
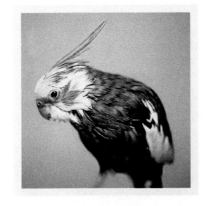
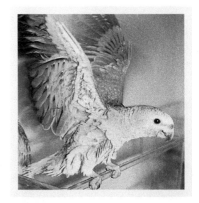

Introduction

Avian medicine is an exciting and challenging field. It is a young science and is, as such, developing and progressing at a staggering rate. It is essential for veterinarians continually to update and maintain their state of knowledge. Over 9,000 species may be presented, ranging in size from ostriches to humming birds, originating from differing climatic zones (from the Arctic and Antarctic Circles to the equator), eating a variety of diets (from nectar, fruit, vegetables, and cereals to crustaceans, fish, and meat), and ambulating by walking, flying, running, or swimming. Many of the species are globally challenged populations, so talking about any bird that is presented becomes a real challenge.

It is often suggested that some 75% of 'avian illness' is related to poor husbandry, management, or nutrition. Often, owners 'impulse purchase' a 'pretty bird' and either have no knowledge as to how it should be kept or, at best, were advised by a poorly trained, part-time, school-aged assistant in a pet store. The clinician must not only find out how the bird is being kept and what it is currently being fed on, but he/she must also know how the species is normally kept and what it is normally fed in captivity, at the same time contrasting this information with how it would survive in the wild and what it would normally eat there.

Birds typically have a high metabolic rate because of their general small size and high surface area to body mass ratio. The metabolic rate of all birds is also higher in comparison with other animals of similar size.

The vast majority of birds are still ostensibly wild creatures and, as such, maintain many of the intrinsic behavioral patterns of wild birds. They have learnt over the passage of time that if you look ill, you get predated upon. As a consequence, birds do not readily show signs of illness, particularly when first arriving in a strange situation and being looked at by unfamiliar people. Birds are often ill because of the unnatural way they are being kept; typically, no one knows a bird is ill until disease is significantly advanced. Once ill, pathogenesis is rapid and death may ensue quickly if the clinician is unable to intervene in an accurate and timely manner.

Avian clinicians should train clients to present their birds for new bird and well-bird checks so that husbandry, nutrition, and training deficits can be addressed prior to there being any adverse effects on the bird. Owners should be trained in good captive bird husbandry and care: regular monitoring of weight, condition, behavior, and feces; early disease recognition; and prompt presentation to an experienced avian clinician at the first sign of any transgression from normality. Clients should be given the opportunity to attend an urgent appointment, if possible bringing their bird in its own uncleaned cage. Avian appointments should be seen outside normal companion animal consulting hours, as each case will take longer and the already sick bird will not want to be further stressed by confinement close to predators such as cats and dogs.

The clinician must be familiar (or rapidly become so) with the natural ecology and captive management of the species presented. A full, lengthy, and detailed history must be collected, allowing time for the bird's natural reserve to become relaxed so that it visually demonstrates just how sick it is, prior to it being handled. As with all patient groups, 'common things occur commonly'. While investigating any disease, the clinician should be mindful of the common disease incidence and presenting signs for the genera, as well as being open to the challenge of the unexpected.

The consultation commences with a full thorough visual examination (of bird, cage, feces, and contents) and observation of the bird, its movements, and its interaction with the environment, while conducting the history collection. If fecal examination is to be performed, this should ideally be carried out prior to handling the bird, so that the clinician is as fully informed, equipped, and prepared as possible.

Birds should be handled with a fresh clean towel for each bird (rather than gloves). Prior to catching the bird, consideration should be given to what the bird's weapons are (beak, talons, or both). If the bird has to be physically caught, this should be achieved with minimal stress to bird or handler and in a darkened room (except owls and other nocturnal species). If catching a bird from a cage, all extraneous perches, toys, mirrors, and other objects that complicate catching the bird should be removed. Attempts should not be made to try and catch a bird through a small door in a cage side; instead, the base of the cage should be removed, the cage turned on its side, and the bird caught with two hands through this improved access. The first point of danger (i.e. talons, beak) should always be caught and restrained first, followed by the body and wings. Once restrained, the patient is subjected to a thorough and systematic physical examination, done in a minimally stressful manner, which, in the author's opinion, is best achieved under volatile anesthesia.

However much the clinician is drawn to one part of the bird's body, it is important to use a consistent approach, checking in turn: head, eyes, sinuses, nares, beak, mouth, choana, tongue, and ears; followed by neck, crop, condition (as assessed by degree of prominence of the carina of the keel amidst the pectoral muscles), shoulders (triossuem), and wing (shoulder, humerus, elbow, ulna, radius, carpus and metacarpals, propytagium, and flight feathers). The extension and flexion of each joint is checked and one extended wing is assessed against the other for comparison. Moving onto the body, the plumage, stage of moult, skin condition, dorsal spine, abdomen, preen gland, and each limb (acetabulum, femur, stifle, tibiotarsus, intertarsal joint, tarso-metatarsus, metatarso-phalangeal joint, and digits) is checked. The condition of the plantar aspect of each foot is carefully assessed. Any limb band is looked at to ensure that it moves easily around the limb and that there is no build-up of dead skin and detritus between the ring and the limb. The tail flight feathers are assessed for condition and signs of fret marks or bars, and the cloaca is checked. Particular attention is paid in those species prone to cloacal papilloma (Amazon parrots and macaws); the cloacal mucous membrane is everted (using a cotton bud) and assessed.

Recognizing normal behavior and conformation for each different species, even those that are closely related, is important; otherwise, false and inaccurate conclusions will be made. While dealing with a sick bird, the clinician must be prepared at the same time to collect suitable clinical pathology samples (swabs, aspirates, cytologic samples, feces, and blood), together with radiographs (in at least two views) and, if indicated, endoscopy. One per cent of the bird's body weight in volume of blood can be collected safely; therefore, a 200 g bird can have 2 ml of blood removed, although the clinician must always consider not just the volume that is being removed, but any further volume that might be lost in a post-sampling hematoma.

Any sick or injured bird will benefit from fluid therapy, which may be given subcutaneously (the addition of hyaluronidase will assist fluid uptake), orally (via gavage tube), intravenously (via the superficial ulna [basilica], medial tarsal, or jugular vein), or intraosseously (via the distal ulna or proximal tibiotarsus). Such birds will benefit from 10–20 ml/kg body weight of warmed saline. The fluid maintenance requirement of the average bird is 50 ml/kg/day.

Avian anatomy and physiology is markedly different to mammals or reptiles, and a full understanding of the differences is mandatory. The revolutionary respiratory system not only permits a far more efficient gaseous exchange system, it is also designed with the avian veterinarian in mind, as the air sacs readily facilitate full endoscopic examination of all internal organs (and biopsy if necessary).

In view of the patient's typically rapid disease pathogenesis, clinical pathology samples should where possible be processed in-house, with back up and verification where necessary from external laboratories. In all cases, if at all possible, a specific diagnosis should be made at the time of initial presentation. If this is not possible, nursing, support, and symptomatic therapy may need to be administered pending arriving at a specific diagnosis. Not only do birds get sick quickly, they also require the appropriate medication at higher doses (per kg body weight) and more frequently than most other patients. Many owners are unable to handle their birds or administer appropriate medication (e.g. 3–4 times daily). Because of this, avian clinicians must be prepared to hospitalize patients and provide exemplary standards of high dependency nursing.

There is a range of high quality, referenced avian formularies available. These should be referred to for dose rates and frequencies of administration, as these can vary greatly between apparently similar species.

A sick patient coming into a foreign environment will often not feed adequately enough to maintain its body weight. It is essential that the sick bird is maintained at a suitably high ambient temperature (23.8–29.4°C [75–85°F]), with appropriate fluid and nutritional support, so that body and soul are maintained pending response to therapy. In the author's opinion, more avian patients will be saved by appropriate fluid and nutritional support than any other medical or surgical therapy. Hospitalized birds must be weighed daily and, if not maintaining their body weight, must receive supplementary feeding, typically by gavage feeding. Smaller birds with a higher metabolic rate can survive without food for a shorter period. For example, a small parakeet such as a budgerigar should never be deprived of food for more than three hours. Therefore, the time from withdrawl of food prior to surgery to voluntary feeding post surgery must not exceed three hours. If the bird is not eating voluntarily at the three hour point, gavage feeding is essential. The proper use of analgesia and the provision of foods with which the bird is familiar, as well as maintenance of the bird in a low stress surrounding, will facilitate natural feeding.

The care and therapy of avian patients is further 'spiced' by the common presence of significant zoonotic infections (e.g. chlamydophilosis, salmonellosis, cryptococcosis, campylobacteriosis, avian influenza, and tuberculosis). Until the results of all diagnostic tests are returned, clinicians should consider any sick (or well) bird to be potentially infectious for other patients as well as for themselves and their staff.

In the field of avian medicine, veterinarians are currently plagued by many highly infectious and contagious pathogens, such as those that cause proventricular dilation syndrome of (predominantly) psittacine species, psittacine beak and feather disease (circovirus), and Pacheco's disease (herpesvirus), where, on occasions, such pathogens are highly contagious and can be very resistant and hence persistent in the environment. When such birds are examined in the clinician's own premises, the clinician must take on the responsibility of fully testing for these infectious and contagious diseases and to put in place biosecurity measures to ensure that veterinarians, as health care professionals, are not inadvertently propagating such diseases from case to subsequent case. In the author's opinion, any avian facility should maintain hospitalized patients in their own air space (i.e. a solitary compartment), from which air is extracted and temperature and humidity maintained. This compartment must be readily cleanable and must be resistant to the destructive nature of some patients, and birds must be easy to catch and restrain when removing them from the accommodation. However, even if birds are maintained in separate air space, the 'common areas' (i.e. areas where birds are handled, treated, examined, radiographed, etc.) must also be regularly disinfected so as to avoid cross contamination. Disinfection may be achieved by wet wiping with effective disinfectants, although there is added benefit in disinfecting by 'fogging' so that other areas (nooks and crannies where air borne pathogens may be harboured) are also disinfected.

So, the key elements are:

- See avian patients early.
- Make a thorough assessment using all diagnostic methodologies in order to reach a specific diagnosis on day one. Review and assess the patient over successive days.
- Provide appropriate medication, using a safe and effective agent at the correct rate and frequency.
- Ensure sufficient fluid and nutritional support is provided to maintain body condition.
- Maintain good biosecurity within the veterinary facility.
- Consider the stress of hospitalization on the patient and assess if the owner can effectively medicate and feed the patient; most patients will do better in their own home environment.
- Encourage avian owners to insure their pets against veterinary fees, as the realistic cost of providing comprehensive veterinary care for a sick bird is considerable.

English and Latin names

African grey parrot	*Psittacus erithacus*
Ariel toucan	*Ramphastos ariel*
Barred rock (chicken)	*Gallus gallus*
Black-necked aracari	*Pteroglossus aracari*
Blue and gold macaw	*Ara ararauna*
Blue-fronted Amazon parrot	*Amazona aestiva*
Blue-winged teal	*Anas discors*
Budgerigar	*Melopsittacus undulatus*
Buzzard	*Buteo buteo*
Canada goose	*Branta canadensis*
Canary	*Serinus canaria*
Carolina (wood) duck	*Aix sponsa*
Channel-billed toucan	*Ramphastos vitellinus*
Chestnut-eared aracari	*Pteroglossus castanotis*
Choco toucan	*Ramphastos brevis*
Cockatiel	*Nymphicus hollandicus*
Dove	*Columbia livia (domestica)*
Eclectus parrot	*Eclectus roratus*
Emerald toucanet	*Aulacorhynchus prasinus*
European sparrowhawk	*Accipiter nisus*
Festive Amazon parrot	*Amazona festiva*
Flamingo	*Phoenicopterus* species
Gabar goshawk	*Micronisus gabar*
Gyr falcon	*Falco rusticolus*
Harris' hawk	*Parabuteo unicinctus*
Hawaiian (Nene) goose	*Branta sandvicensis*
Hyacinth macaw	*Andorhynchus hyacinthus*

Keel-billed toucan	*Ramphastos sulfuratus*
Lanner falcon	*Falco biarmicus*
Lesser sulphur-crested cockatoo	*Cacutua sulphurea*
Lovebird	*Agapornis* species
Lugger falcon	*Falco jugger*
Macaw	*Ara* species
Mallard	*Anas platyrhynchos*
Meyer's parrot	*Poicephalus meyeri*
Moluccan (salmon-crested) cockatoo	*Cacatua moluccensis*
Muscovy duck	*Cairina moschata*
Mynah bird	*Gracula religiosa*
Northern goshawk	*Accipter gentilis*
Orange-winged Amazon parrot	*Amazona amazonica*
Ostrich	*Struthio camelus*
Pale-mandibled aracari	*Pteroglossus erythropygiu*
Peacock	*Pavo* species
Peregrine falcon	*Falco peregrinus*
Pheasant	*Phasianus colchicus*
Pigeon	*Columbia livia*
Plate-billed mountain toucan	*Andigena laminirostris*
Prairie falcon	*Falco mexicanus*
Red-billed toucan	*Ramphastos tucanus*
Red-breasted toucan	*Ramphastos tucanus*
Red-fronted macaw	*Ara rubrogenys*
Red-tailed hawk	*Buteo jamaicensis*
Rose-breasted cockatoo	*Eolophus roseicappillus*
Saffron toucanet	*Baillonius baillioni*
Salvin's Amazon parrot	*Amazona autumnalis salvini*
Saker falcon	*Falco cherrug*
Skua	*Catharacta skua*
Solomon Island eclectus	*Eclectus roratus solomomensis*
Spectacled Amazon parrot	*Amazona albifrons*
Spot-billed toucanet	*Selenidera maculirostris*
Tawny owl	*Strix aluco*
Toco toucan	*Ramphastos toco*
Umbrella cockatoo	*Cacatua alba*
White-winged wood duck	*Cairina scutulata*
Yellow-naped Amazon parrot	*Amazona ochrocephala auropalliata*

Case 99: **Lead poisoning in an Amazon parrot**

CLINICAL PRESENTATION. A six-year-old yellow-naped Amazon parrot presented with blood in its droppings (**99**). No significant abnormalities were found on physical examination. While discussing options with the owner, the bird had a seizure.

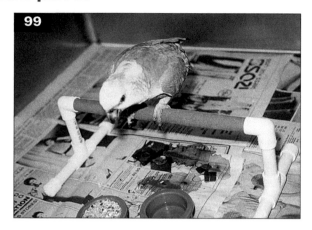

DIFFERENTIAL DIAGNOSES. Heavy metal poisoning, primarily lead.

INVESTIGATION. The owner was questioned about possible exposure to any sources of lead. Radiographs were taken and blood lead levels and hematology/blood chemistries were evaluated. The absence of lead particles on radiographs does not rule out heavy metal toxicosis. Blood lead concentrations >0.9652 µmol/l (>20 µg/dl) are suggestive, levels >2.413 µmol/l (>50 µg/dl) are diagnostic. D2 aminolaevulinic acid dehydratase and protoporphyrin concentrations may be used to confirm a diagnosis.

DIAGNOSIS. Lead poisoning.

ETIOLOGY. The clinical signs of lead toxicity are multisystemic and involve depression, weakness, vomiting, polyuria/polydipsia, seizures, hemoglobinuria, and diarrhea.

MANAGEMENT. The bird's seizures must be controlled prior to performing any diagnostic investigations (i.e. treat the patient not the toxin). If suspicions are high for lead poisoning, chelation therapy may be commenced prior to laboratory confirmation. Therapy includes CaEDTA (35 mg/kg i/m q12h until 48 hours after the cessation of clinical signs). Alternative oral chelation treatment for long-term therapy includes d-penicillamine (55 mg/kg p/o q24h) or DMSA (25–35 mg/kg q24h for 5 days out of every 7 days for 3 weeks). Surgery to remove particulate lead is rarely indicated; however, if clinical signs recur or if there are large pieces of lead present in the GI tract, then ventricular gavage under general anesthesia will usually facilitate lead removal by a low-stress, noninvasive method.

Case 100: **Skin pigmentation in an African grey parrot chicks**

CLINICAL PRESENTATION. An African grey parrot chick presented with dark skin (**100**).

DIFFERENTIAL DIAGNOSES. Normal pigmentation for this species; indicates stunting and dehydration; suggests that the chick is not actually an African grey parrot; is only visible due to the lack of normal feathering.

DIAGNOSIS. This chick is normal.

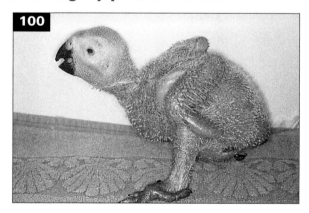

Case 101: **Seizures in African grey parrots**

CLINICAL PRESENTATION. An African grey parrot presented because it was having a seizure ('fitting') (**101**).

DIFFERENTIAL DIAGNOSES. The main differential diagnoses of seizures and their causes are listed below:
- Hypocalcemia. This is particularly common in young (2–5-year-old) African grey parrots that have been fed on a poor (e.g. sunflower seed-based) diet. These birds are deficient in calcium and vitamin D_3 or UV light. A viral condition affecting the parathyroid glands has also been implicated, but to date has not been proven. Blood calcium is protein bound, so hypocalcemia is more likely in hypoalbuminemic birds.
- Heavy metal poisoning. This is most commonly caused by lead or zinc and should be considered in any bird showing nervous signs. The signs demonstrated are dependent on the quantity of lead ingested and the chronicity of ingestion. Diagnosis comprises whole body radiography and blood lead analysis. Lack of radiographic evidence does not exclude lead poisoning. The diagnosis may be suspected if a dilated proventriculus and distal esophagus is present. Nonenteric lead is generally considered to be nonpathogenic. Zinc poisoning most commonly occurs in new flights or aviaries, where galvanized wire, wire clips, or other parts have been used. Poisoning is typically acute and metal particles are usually still evident on abdominal radiographs.

- Hypoglycemia. This is caused by starvation, severely impaired liver function, infection, or endocrine disorders.
- Hepatic encephalopathy. This is caused by any severe liver disease.
- Pesticide poisoning. This is caused by malicious or accidental poisoning through acetylcholinesterase inhibitors (e.g. carbamates, malathion, dichlorvos, or organophosphates).
- Drug toxicities (e.g. dimetronidazole, levamisole).
- Meningitis, through bacterial, viral, parasitic, or fungal infections.
- Chlamydophilosis: cases may rarely present with CNS signs.
- Proventricular dilatation: a small percentage of proventricular dilatation disease cases present with CNS signs, even in the absence of GI tract signs.
- Idiopathic epilepsy.
- Trauma.

INVESTIGATION. Rapid diagnostic laboratory results are essential in cases involving fitting birds. A full hematology and biochemistry profile should be performed, as well as radiography and blood lead and zinc analysis. The most diagnostically important parameters are the hemogram (which may show evidence of infection), blood calcium and blood glucose levels, serology or antigen tests for clamydophilosis, and radiography for proventricular dilatation.

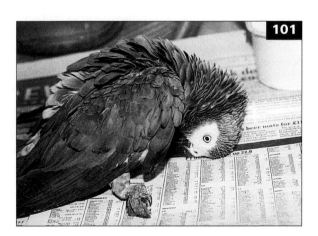

Case 102: 'Pattern picking' in an African grey parrot

CLINICAL PRESENTATION. A two-year-old hand-reared African grey parrot presented that was clinically normal in all respects except for its plumage. The feathers on the head were totally normal, but only down feathers remained on the body (**102**). Feather picking, which only occurred in the presence of the owner, had been ongoing for one year. On occasion, during intimate 'cuddling sessions', the bird regurgitated on its owner.

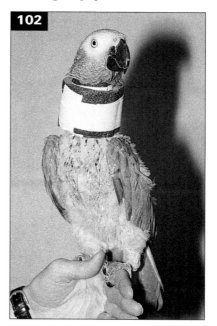

INVESTIGATION. All the bird's blood parameters were normal. Bacterial, fungal, parasitic, viral, chlamydophilial, and metabolic etiologies for feather plucking were ruled out.

DIAGNOSIS. 'Pattern picking'.

ETIOLOGY. Reproductive hormonal pressure (sexual frustration) often begins to cause feather picking in young birds that are bonded to their owner even before reaching what is thought to be their natural reproductive age. The hormonal drive provides a natural incentive for the young bird to try to achieve a status in the dominance hierarchy of the flock. This will lead to success in obtaining a mate, holding territory, and having access to adequate food, so that the bird is able to reproduce. Captive birds often mature earlier than wild birds, especially when the owner is providing all the necessary advantages as well as stimulating it with a close bond. Consequently, the bird reaches reproductive maturity, but the 'mate' is not responding in a manner that will result in the production of offspring. This often leads to 'displacement behaviour' such as feather picking, screaming, or aggression.

MANAGEMENT. Some success has been achieved with the administration of progesterones to decrease the hormonal pressure, but some treated birds become obese, suffer from polyuria/polydipsia or diabetes mellitus, or develop hepatic lipidosis. Recently, human chorionic gonadotrophin (HCG) (500–1000 IU/kg i/m) and leuprolide acetate (100 iu/kg i/m on 3 occasions at 2-week intervals) have shown promise in providing effective, short-term resolution, especially in African grey parrots and cockatoo hens. There have been no reports of adverse reactions with this treatment, but it is not always reliable. Tranquillizing agents, such as haloperidol, and psychotropic agents, such as clomipramine and fluoxetine (Prozac), have shown some limited effectiveness in some individual cases. These medications can only provide a temporary solution and they should be used in combination with behavior modification techniques and changes in the bird's environment to provide a more reliable response. Petting on the bird's back and intimate cuddling should be reduced or eliminated. Foraging enrichment should be added as part of the bird's daily routine.

For the owner to assert dominance the bird should be maintained below human chest height. The cage may be moved to a location away from the main traffic area to reduce the anxiety of seeing the owner without being cuddled. The length of the day may be shortened by covering the cage earlier in the evening. In females, surgical removal of the oviduct may provide the best long-term solution. In some cases the picking becomes a habit, even though the original cause is resolved, and long-term, anticompulsive medication may be indicated.

Case 103: **Poxvirus infection in an Amazon parrot**

CLINICAL PRESENTATION. A blue-fronted Amazon parrot presented because of a problem with its eyes (**103a, b** – early stages; **103c** – more advanced stage).

DIAGNOSIS. The bird has conjunctivitis purulenta (**103a**) and blepharitis crustosa (**103b**) due to poxvirus infection. Confirmation of the diagnosis includes the demonstration of intracytoplasmic Bollinger inclusion bodies from biopsy material or culturing the virus from the feces.

ETIOLOGY. Local cutaneous and mucosal forms of avipox infections are the most important viral infections in avian ophthalmology. The disorder progresses more or less rapidly, depending on the virulence of the poxvirus strain, and usually affects several birds at the same time. In the early stage, purulent conjunctivitis is diagnosed followed by typical conjunctivitis crustosa. Serious sequelae, which may also be attributable to secondary bacterial eye infection, are ulcerative keratitis and panophthalmitis, as well as severe palpebral lesions with scar retraction and epiphora following damage to the lacrimal and drainage apparatus.

MANAGEMENT. There is no specific therapy. Multivitamins, in particular vitamin A, can be given and systemic antibiotic cover provided to prevent secondary infections. Topical antibiotic-containing irrigation solutions and tear replacement fluid can be instilled. Early removal of cutaneous crusts around the lid is absolutely contraindicated in order to prevent scar retraction, which can lead to narrowing of the palpebral fissure and, in extreme cases, to ankyloblepharon (**103c**).

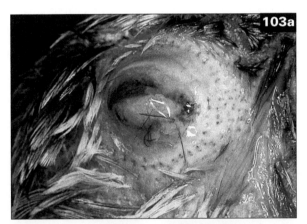

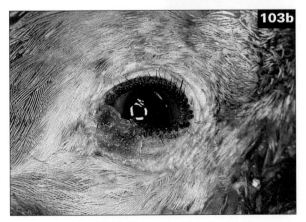

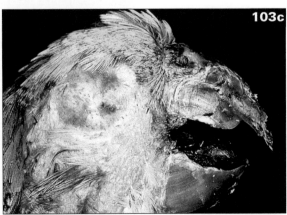

Case 104: **Chlamydophilosis in an Amazon parrot**

CLINICAL PRESENTATION. A recently purchased five-year-old Amazon parrot presented with diarrhea and weakness. The bird had been treated with doxycycline and a multivitamin injection three days previously. There had been some improvement in the bird's condition over the three days, but it had shown a marked yellow discoloration of the urate fraction.

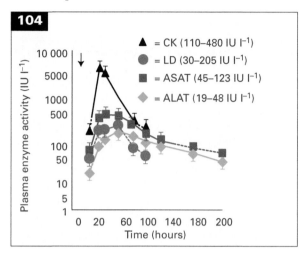

INVESTIGATION. A Kodak Surecell antigen capture test for chlamydophilosis was performed on a cloacal swab and found to be negative. Plasma chemistry to evaluate hepatic and renal function revealed the following enzyme activities: AST 400 u/l (normal = 57–194 u/l); CK 250 u/l (normal = 45–265 u/l); BUN concentration 5 mmol/l (14 mg/dl) (normal = 0.9–4.6 mmol/l [2.52–12.88 mg/dl]); uric acid concentration 300 mmol/l (5,070 mg/dl) (normal = 72–312 mmol/l [1,217–5,273 mg/dl]); TP 55 g/l (5.5 g/dl) (normal = 33–50 g/l [3.3–5.0 g/dl]) with an albumin:globulin ratio of 3:1.

DIAGNOSIS. The history and response to initial therapy are very suggestive of an infectious disease, possibly chlamydophilosis.

ETIOLOGY. The yellow discoloration of the urate fraction is probably caused by the multivitamin injection. The results of the Kodak Surecell test are misleading, since the test was performed three days after the doxycycline injection. The elevated AST is at least partly caused by the i/m injection of doxycycline. The absence of elevated CK activity three days after the injection can be explained by the relatively short half-life of CK compared with AST (**104**). Elevated BUN with normal uric acid concentrations and elevated TP are indicative of dehydration with prerenal azotemia.

MANAGEMENT. The most important action is to initiate fluid therapy: estimated fluid deficit (10% of body weight) plus maintenance (50 ml/kg per 24 hours) plus ongoing losses. One quarter of the calculated daily amount for the first day should be given slowly i/v by bolus; the rest can be given s/c q12h. Continuation of the doxycycline therapy (75 mg/kg i/m every 7 days for 6 weeks) might be considered, since this has shown a good response.

DISCUSSION. Examination of paired serum samples is recommended and the potential zoonotic risk must be discussed with the owner. PCR testing for antigen will be fruitless in light of the doxycycline injection already administered.

Case 105: **Anthracosis in an Amazon parrot**

CLINICAL PRESENTATION. A spectacled Amazon parrot presented for surgical sexing. During the procedure, black spots were observed on the lungs and air sacs (**105**). There were no signs of inflammation in the areas of the black spots.

DIAGNOSIS. Anthracosis.

MANAGEMENT. Anthracosis does not have to be treated. It is often observed on routine laparoscopic examination.

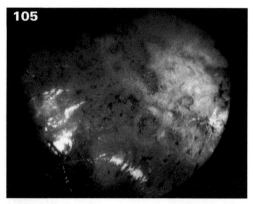

Case 106: **Mycobacteriosis in an Amazon parrot**

CLINICAL PRESENTATION. An adult, 370 g, female, blue-fronted Amazon parrot presented for necropsy. It had been housed in a pet shop for several years as the shop pet. It was found dead in its cage the morning that it was presented. The bird had exhibited no previous signs of illness and no other bird in the store appeared ill.

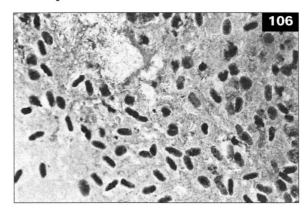

INVESTIGATION. Necropsy of the bird revealed multiple, raised lesions throughout the liver parenchyma. The lesions varied in size and were generally round. No other gross lesions were observed. A contact smear of one of the hepatic lesions was made for cytopathologic evaluation, and it was stained with Wright's stain.

DIAGNOSIS. The oil immersion field shown (**106**) is typical of the appearance of this lesion. The background of the smear demonstrates numerous bacterial rods that have failed to stain with Wright's. This finding is highly suggestive of a mycobacterial infection, because the waxy cell walls of *Mycobacterium* species fail to stain with Romanowsky stains. A macrophagic inflammation is also typical of mycobacterial lesions and macrophages are often found full of the rod-shaped bacteria. In this case a strong presumptive diagnosis of avian mycobacteriosis is made based on the cytologic findings. A definitive diagnosis for avian mycobacteriosis can be obtained by a positive culture for *Mycobacterium* species, usually *M. avium*.

Case 107: **Proventricular dilatation syndrome in an African grey parrot**

CLINICAL PRESENTATION. An African grey parrot presented because it had been chronically ill and losing weight, while passing whole seeds in the stool (**107**).

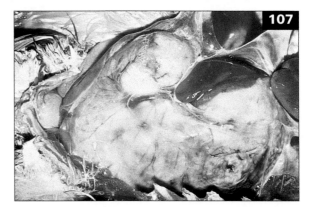

DIAGNOSIS. This bird has proventricular dilatation syndrome. A definitive diagnosis may be made on histologic examination of a crop biopsy. The bioposy should include a blood vessel and, usually, a nerve. Occasionally, lesions will also be found in peripheral nerves and the CNS.

ETIOLOGY. This disease is considered to be due to a virus, but the exact organism has not yet been confirmed. Macaws were the first species identified with this disease, but the condition is seen in many species of psittacine birds. Histologic lesions that are similar have been found rarely in nonpsittacines such as Canada geese, toucans, spoonbills, and finches. The nerves and nerve ganglia of the proventriculus and ventriculus have the highest incidence of lesion development, but histologic changes are occasionally found in other portions of the GI tract.

Case 108: **Liver disease in an African grey parrot**

CLINICAL PRESENTATION. An African grey parrot presented terminally ill and subsequently died.

INVESTIGATION. A necropsy was performed and the liver was markedly abnormal (**108**).

DIAGNOSIS. Chronic cholangiohepatitis, bile duct proliferation, fibrosis, and hepatic lipidosis (cirrhosis).

ETIOLOGY. Chronic infections, bile excreted toxins (particularly aflatoxins), endotoxemia, and nutritional/metabolic disorders have all been proved or suggested as causes of liver disease in psittacines. The cause in many cases may be multifactorial and the exact cause of chronic cases may not be determined. The highest incidence is in cockatiels, Amazon parrots, and macaws, but similar changes are also seen sporadically in other birds.

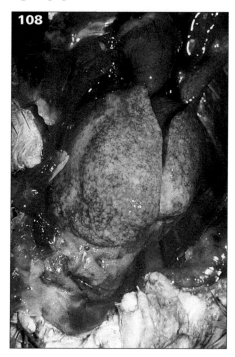

Case 109: **Crooked neck in an African grey parrot chick**

CLINICAL PRESENTATION. An African grey parrot chick presented with a crooked neck, which was present at hatching.

ETIOLOGY. This type of deformity may be associated with positioning of the chick in the egg or excessive incubation temperatures.

MANAGEMENT. This condition is frequently seen and many such deformities can be corrected by the application of a neck brace such as the one shown (**109**). The brace is constructed of a piece of towelling material and fastened with Velcro. The brace can be easily removed for feeding.

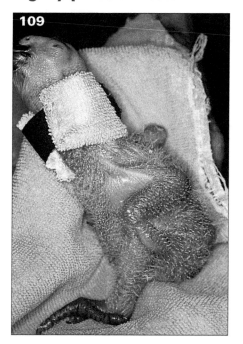

Case 110: **Atypical red feathers in an African grey parrot**

CLINICAL PRESENTATION. An African grey parrot presented with multiple red feathers (**110**).

DIFFERENTIAL DIAGNOSES. Malnutrition, especially deficiencies in certain essential amino acids, has been implicated as the cause of abnormal feather coloration. Liver disease is commonly blamed for the presence of abnormal red feathers on African grey parrots, but this is not well-documented. In poultry, hypothyroidism may cause normal black feathers to turn red. Abnormal feather colors is often associated with psittacine bird and feather disease (PBFD) infection.

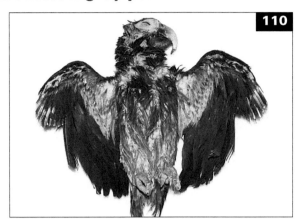

Case 111: **Crop fistula in an African grey parrot**

CLINICAL PRESENTATION. An eight-week-old African grey parrot presented as an emergency because the owner noticed food coming from its throat (**111**). The bird was still being syringe fed and weaning had not yet been started. The bird was bright, alert, and active.

DIAGNOSIS. This bird has a crop fistula, which is characterized by a fistula between the ingluvies (crop) and the skin, allowing ingested food to pass out of the ingluvies.

ETIOLOGY. The fistula is most likely the result of feeding inappropriately heated food to this baby bird. Most commonly, the food has been heated in a microwave oven but, unfortunately, microwaves do not heat food evenly. Though the temperature of the food is tested and apparently of appropriate temperature, pockets of overly heated food may be present. When the food is syringe or tube fed into the ingluvies, the overheated area remains in contact with the ingluvies and causes thermal burns. Once the burn has healed and the scab falls off, a fistula remains. In many cases the owner does not notice the original injury and only becomes aware of the problem when food spills from the crop. At this stage it is not an emergency, but it is very frightening to most owners.

MANAGEMENT. Surgical management is usually postponed until the patient is stable and the wound has matured. In some cases the demarcation between viable and nonviable tissue is readily apparent. In others it may be difficult to distinguish healthy tissue from devitalized tissue. It generally takes 3–5 days from the time of injury for the demarcation to mature. Once it is obvious, the eschar is removed along with any scar tissue uniting the wall of the ingluvies to the skin. The ingluvies is dissected away from the skin to allow the two structures to be closed as separate tissues. The ingluvies is closed in an inverting pattern, if possible, to allow serosa to serosa contact. The skin is closed over the crop as a separate layer. In cases with severe damage and necrosis of the ingluvies, every effort is made to maintain the longitudinal integrity of the esophagus. Resection and anastomosis of the esophagus and ingluvies is not recommended, as the incidence of stricture is much greater. An esophageal feeding tube may be placed in cases of extensive tissue loss to serve as a stent around which the esophagus may heal. This will also allow the patient to receive alimentation during the healing period without stressing the repair.

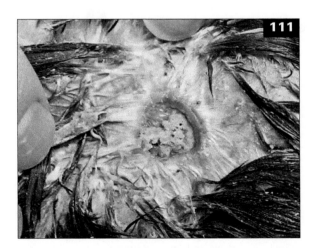

Case 112: Enucleation of the eye in an African grey parrot

CLINICAL PRESENTATION. A 12-year-old male African grey parrot (112a, b) presented for enucleation of the right eye in order to gain access to a retrobulbar mass that had been diagnosed using ultrasound.

MANAGEMENT. Compared with mammals, birds have a very short optic nerve, so excessive traction on the globe can result in damage to the optic chiasma and the contralateral optic nerve, rendering the contralateral eye blind. It is also possible that the brain could be adversely affected by excessive traction. Many birds have bone within the sclera (scleral ossicles), which can inhibit removal of the globe. In an effort to achieve better visualization of the muscles and blood vessels surrounding the globe, the cornea is incised and the lens and vitreous extruded to allow the globe to be collapsed. It is important to remove the lacrimal tissue as well as the eyelid margins to eliminate glandular tissue and provide a cut surface for the eyelids to heal to each other. The eyelids may be sutured together first and the skin along the lid margins incised a few millimeters from the edges circumferentially. Dissection is continued subcutaneously to remove all of the palpebral conjunctiva. Muscle attachments are transected until the optic nerve and associated vessels are all that remain attaching the globe to the orbit.

Hemostatic clips are applied to the stalk blindly without applying significant traction to the globe. The optic stalk is then transected distal to the clips. An angled clip applicator is preferred, as it allows the clips to be applied with minimal traction on the globe. Remaining hemorrhage is controlled with bipolar radiosurgical forceps. The eyelids are then closed routinely. An ocular prosthesis may be used to prevent the sunken appearance characteristic of avian enucleation.

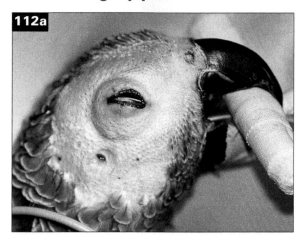

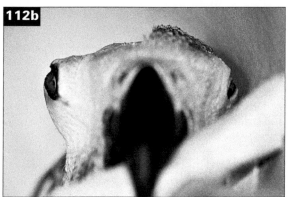

Case 113: Mycobacterium avium infection in an Amazon parrot

CLINICAL PRESENTATION. A Salvin's Amazon parrot presented with chemosis and granular conjunctivitis of the left eye (113a).

DIFFERENTIAL DIAGNOSES. Possible clinical differential diagnoses for this disease (which also occurs in other bird species, in particular pigeons, water fowl, and predatory birds) are infections with *Pasturella multocida*, *Yersinia pseudotuberculosis*, *Staphylococcus aureus*, *Mycoplasma* species, *Candida* species, *Cryptosporidium* species, *Cryptococcus* species, herpesvirus, and poxvirus (which may result in follicular conjunctivitis).

INVESTIGATION. The lower eyelid was everted and this revealed multiple subconjunctival granulomas (113b). Under combined isoflurane and topical local anesthetic, a conjunctival biopsy was taken for a crush preparation

for Ziehl–Neelsen staining. This specific stain directly identified the mycobacterial organisms as acid-fast red rods (113c).

DIAGNOSIS. Chemosis and granular conjunctivitis caused by a localized *M. avium* infection.

MANAGEMENT. There is no recommended treatment. Affected birds must always be euthanased.

DISCUSSION. In-contact birds must be examined serologically to demonstrate antibodies; hematology should be performed to look for a leukocytosis with a hypochromic microcytic anemia and hyperfibrinogenemia; and samples taken via coproscopy should be examined, using enrichment methods (Sputofluol), for the acid-fast bacilli of *Mycobacteria* (open tuberculosis). Birds may be

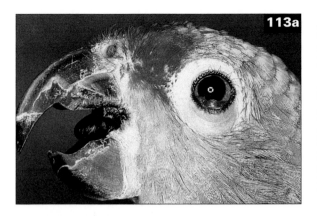

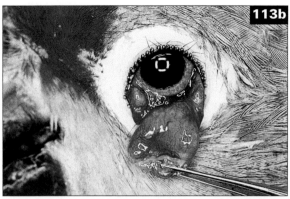

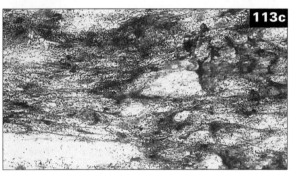

radiographed to demonstrate possible tuberculous granulomas of other organs, and hepatic endoscopy can be useful. PCR testing of swabs, aspirates, and feces is valuable if available. Aviaries must be decontaminated using special tuberculocidal disinfectants. When localized cutaneous tubercular lesions are found in birds, these are often caused by *M. tuberculosis* infections (i.e. human pathogenic organisms). Although *M. avium* is zoonotic, *M. tuberculosis* is a much more serious human pathogen. It can certainly be passed from man to bird and possibly bird to man. It is essential to warn owners and handlers of the zoonotic risk.

Case 114: **Psittacine proventricular dilatation syndrome in an African grey parrot**

CLINICAL PRESENTATION. An anorexic Amazon grey parrot presented because it was regurgitating its food and had undigested seeds in the feces. A radiograph showed the proventriculus to be severely distended, the wall very thin, and gas in the intestinal loops (**114**).

DIFFERENTIAL DIAGNOSES. Likely diseases that can lead to an enlarged proventriculus and undigested seed in the feces are PPDS, heavy metal poisoning, or any other cause of severe proventriculitis and physical or functional outflow obstruction. Proventriculitis may be caused by bacterial agents (e.g. *E. coli* or *Klebsiella* species) or by *Candida* species infection. Severe infestations of nematodes or cestodes, GI tract neoplasia, or radiolucent foreign bodies can also lead to an enlarged proventriculus.

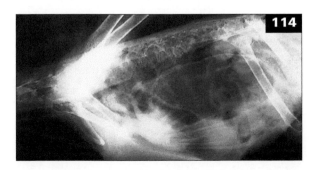

INVESTIGATION. Crop biopsy revealed a lymphoplasmocytic infiltrate of the nervous tissue, which is characteristic of psittacine proventricular dilatation syndrome.

DIAGNOSIS. Psittacine proventricular dilatation syndrome.

ETIOLOGY. The disease is thought to be of viral origin.

MANAGEMENT. Treatment involves administering the cox 2 NSAID celecoxib (10 mg/kg bid for at least 6 weeks), the use of a pelleted diet, and prokinetics. Due to delayed gut emptying, gut active antibiotics may be required periodically.

DISCUSSION. Clinical signs of psittacine proventricular dilatation syndrome often start with a change in the consistency, color, and composition of the feces, which becomes very thin, intense green in color, and may contain undigested seeds. The feces of pellet-eating, psittacine proventricular dilatation syndrome affected birds becomes voluminous and fetid and is usually pale brown. Most patients also exhibit signs of weakness, anorexia, and depression, and, sometimes, CNS signs such as ataxia.

The disease is segmental in nature. Because the nerves proximate to blood vessels, biopsy tissue should include a blood vessel. The pathologist is then more likely to examine a relevant section of tissue.

Case 115: **Chlamydophilosis in an Amazon parrot**

CLINICAL PRESENTATION. A six-month-old hand-reared, orange-winged Amazon parrot presented because it was depressed (**115**).

INVESTIGATION. Biochemistry showed a biliverdinuria, an elevated WBC count (44.5×10^9/l [44.5×10^3/µl]), and elevated AP, AST, and bile acids values. An indirect fluorescent antibody test titer and a DNA PCR fecal swab were both positive for chlamydophilosis.

DIAGNOSIS. Chlamydophilosis.

MANAGEMENT. Doxycycline is the drug of choice for the treatment of chlamydophilosis in a single pet bird. For treatment using doxycycline to be successful, blood levels should be kept at 1 mg/ml for most of the dosage interval. Several dosage regimes are published using a variety of doxycycline preparations, both oral and injectable.

Oral doses of doxycycline should be administered at 25–50 mg/kg daily. Recent work has shown that there is considerable interspecies variation in the dose rate required. Injectable preparations formulated for intravenous use are available in some countries and may be given intramuscularly. The dose for intramuscular weekly administration is 75–100 mg/kg. Some formulations can cause severe muscle necrosis and should not be used for intramuscular administration. An approved long-acting doxycycline injection is now available in the USA. Treatment should be continued for at least 45 days.

DISCUSSION. Members of the tetracycline family of drugs tend to chelate with calcium, and this reduces the bioavailability of the doxycycline; therefore, dietary calcium levels should be limited and items such as cuttlefish and mineral blocks removed during therapy. Many birds treated in this way will require some antifungal therapy within the course of the treatment to avoid the consequence of enteric yeast infections.

Owners of birds with confirmed chlamydophilial infection must be warned about the zoonotic potential of the infection and should be advised to consult their own physician. Owners should also be informed that there is no way of detecting whether their bird has been 'cured' of chlamydophilosis by the end of the therapy. Follow up testing is recommended.

Many birds with chlamydophilosis are immuno-suppressed and should be evaluated for secondary bacterial and fungal infections, which will require treatment. Supportive care should include heat and fluid therapy, hepatoprotective therapy, and paraimmunity inducers, as indicated.

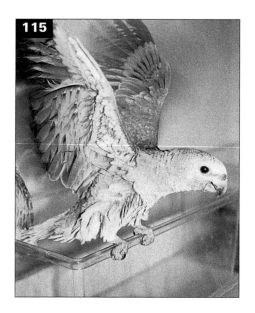

Case 116: **Mycotic granuloma (aspergillosis) in an Amazon parrot**

CLINICAL PRESENTATION. A festive Amazon parrot presented with tail bobbing and severe respiratory distress.

INVESTIGATION. Tracheoscopy and radiography were performed. The combination of these two techniques can yield much information. A structure (**116**) could be observed near the syrinx.

DIAGNOSIS. A mycotic granuloma within the trachea is suspected. It should be confirmed on cytology.

ETIOLOGY. Mycotic granulomas in the trachea are most often caused by *Aspergillus* species.

MANAGEMENT. Specific antimycotic treatment (e.g. amphotericin 1.5 mg/kg i/v q8h; itraconazole 10 mg/kg p/o q12h; voroconazole 14 mg/kg p/o q12h) should be instigated, as well as symptomatic treatment (fluids, vitamin A, tube feeding). Because of the severe respiratory distress, in many cases an abdominal air sac tube should be used. Surgical removal of the granuloma should be performed. This is often the only sign of systemic fungal infection. Nebulization with a suitable antifungal agent (e.g. enilconazole or F10, q8h for 30 minutes each time) is also indicated. The bird should be checked for the presence of granulomas in the lung and/or air sac, as this would have an influence on the prognosis.

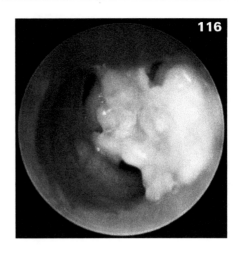

Case 117: **Sinusitis in a Solomon Island eclectus**

CLINICAL PRESENTATION. A female three-year-old Solomon Island eclectus presented with a swelling rostral to the eye (**117**). The bird was dyspneic and showed upper respiratory signs.

INVESTIGATION. Samples were taken for cytology and microbiology. A *Chlamydophila* titer was negative. Bacterial culture revealed a pure growth of *Escherichia coli* sensitive to several commonly used avian antibiotics, including amikacin and enrofloxacin. An acid-fast stain of the debris was negative. A CBC might have proved useful.

MANAGEMENT. The lesion should be lanced and a microbiology swab collected. It should then be curetted and flushed under isoflurane anesthesia, and left open to heal by second intention.

Based on the microbiology results, follow-up treatment should comprise systemic therapy with enrofloxacin (7 mg/kg p/o q12h). In addition, any debris from the convoluted avian sinus system can be removed mechanically by sinus flushing with sterile saline (plus antibiotics and hyaluronidase). In some cases, systemic antibiotics alone may not reach therapeutic levels in the sinuses and nasal cavities.

DISCUSSION. These cases can be frustrating and refractory to systemic therapy alone. Fortunately, in this case, response to therapy was excellent and after ten days of therapy the bird appeared normal. Nonresponsive cases may require nebulization therapy with sterile saline and antibiotics to treat the condition effectively, or sinus flushing with a combination of saline and antibiotics. The topical application of Tris-EDTA can be helpful in refractory cases.

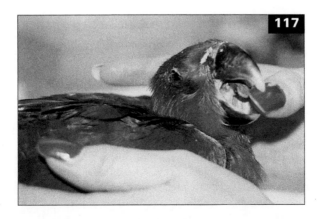

Case 118: **Splay leg in a blue and gold macaw chick**

CLINICAL PRESENTATION. A nine-week-old blue and gold macaw chick presented with a splay leg (valgus deformity) of its left limb, which was associated with trauma (**118**). The chick had two deformities: a rotational deformity of the femur and a premature closure of the lateral side of the growth plate in the cranial tibiotarsus. The chick was severely stunted.

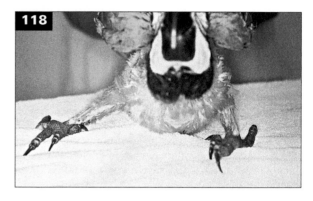

MANAGEMENT. The premature closure of the lateral side of the growth plate in the cranial tibiotarsus was corrected by immediate cauterization of the medial side of the growth plate, followed by derotational osteotomy of the femur three weeks later (delayed in order to allow calcification of the femur to occur prior to surgery).

DISCUSSION. If this problem is observed in a chick that is much younger than this one, it can be corrected by hobbling or packing the chick with its limbs pushed together in a small container. However, at nine weeks of age the bones are too well ossified for such manipulations to be successful.

Case 119: **Aspergillosis in a Meyer's parrot**

CLINICAL PRESENTATION. A Meyer's parrot presented with an exudative folliculitis with secondary feather dystrophy (**119**).

DIFFERENTIAL DIAGNOSES. Psittacine beak and feather disease (circovirus infection), polyomavirus infection (budgerigar fledgeling disease), adenovirus infection, and various bacterial and fungal infections should be considered, as all can cause similar pathologic changes in a follicle.

INVESTIGATION/DIAGNOSIS. The large amount of exudate and hyperkeratotic debris is suggestive of a bacterial or fungal infection. *Aspergillus* species was isolated by culture and easily identified on direct examination.

ETIOLOGY. The bird also had pssittacine beak and feather disease. This resulted in immune depression, which predisposed the bird to aspergillosis.

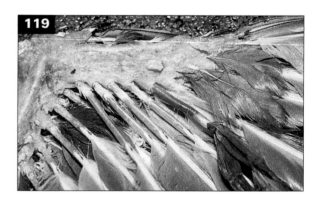

Case 120: **Annular toe deformity in an eclectus parrot**

CLINICAL PRESENTATION. A young hand-reared eclectus parrot presented with an annular toe deformity (**120**). The distal portion of the toe was warm but edematous.

MANAGEMENT. African grey parrots and macaws are most often afflicted by this condition. Some annular toe deformities (also called 'constricted toe syndrome'), if mild, may be managed medically by increasing the ambient humidity, massaging the toe, and providing hot compresses, as well as removing any obvious constricting bands. In cases where the constriction is deep and is causing severe edema or necrosis, surgery is indicated.

Isoflurane anesthesia should be used and additional care taken in relation to the risk of hypothermia (as neonates are at greater risk) during the procedure. A tourniquet is applied to the limb to control intraoperative bleeding and, with the aid of magnification, the constricting band is cut four times at 90 degrees. Having freshened up the tissues on either side of the constriction, a hydroactive dressing is applied after surgery to prevent scab formation, which could in itself cause a further constriction.

It is recommended that the chick is kept at a higher than normal humidity and not placed on substrate that might desiccate the feet. The ambient humidity should be maintained at at least 50%. Lotion-impregnated facial tissues work well as a container substrate to keep the feet moist and supple. Sutures should be removed after 7–10 days.

Serious constrictions (or cases where presentation has been delayed) may require digit amputation. Multiple annular toe deformities may occur, necessitating surgery on several toes at the same time. If surgery is performed aseptically, postoperative antibiotics should not be necessary. If the toe is necrotic, amputation alone is indicated.

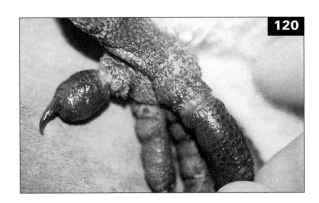

Case 121: **Cataract in a macaw**

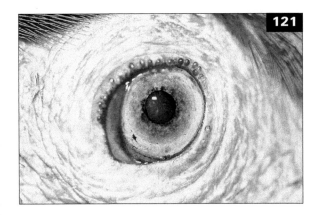

CLINICAL PRESENTATION. A macaw presented with an opacity in its eye (**121**).

DIAGNOSIS. The opacity is a cataract in the lens associated with ageing.

ETIOLOGY. Cataracts are common in aged macaws and often occur at 35–45 years old.

MANAGEMENT. The cataract can be surgically removed, preferably by phacoemulsification. Careful surgery will return sight to a blind eye as long as retinal function is normal. The eye will generally be aphacic (i.e. have no lens), therefore close focusing is not normal due to the lost accommodative function of the lens. After a few weeks' adjustment, sight returns close to functional normality. Hypermature cataracts may degenerate, resulting in phacolytic uveitis with secondary glaucoma and permanent loss of sight. In other cases, cataracts can arise secondary to trauma or systemic disease, or as a hereditary defect.

Case 122: **Convention on International Trade in Endangered Species (CITES)**

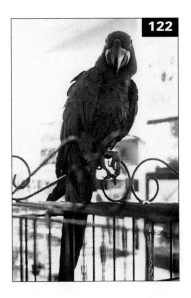

DISCUSSION. International trade in hyacinth (or hyacinthine) macaws (**122**) is restricted due to the species being listing in Appendix I of CITES, an international treaty with over 100 signatory countries. Such international trade requires an import as well as an export permit. The hyacinth macaw is not listed in Appendix II of CITES, nor on the US Endangered Species List or the Brazilian National List for Endangered Species.

Case 123: **Cloacal papilloma in a macaw**

CLINICAL PRESENTATION. A macaw presented with a history of choanal and cloacal papillomas that had been present for several years.

INVESTIGATION. Necropsy revealed a bile duct carcinoma (**123**).

ETIOLOGY. Herpesvirus has now been shown to be the causative agent for cloacal and choanal papillomas. Because it is an oncogenic virus, all birds affected with herpesvirus will eventually go on to develop hepatobillary, pancreatic, or renal neoplasia.

DISCUSSION. Papillomas and carcinomas may also be found in the pancreas and throughout the GI tract, therefore the whole of the abdomen should be examined for the presence of lesions.

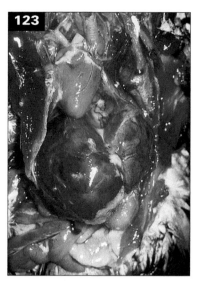

Case 124: **Laparoscopy on a blue and gold macaw**

CLINICAL PRESENTATION. A laparoscopy was performed on a blue and gold macaw using a left lateral approach from the caudolateral thoracic wall. One air sac had to be passed before the viewing field could be seen (**124**).

DISCUSSION. The tip of the endoscope is within the abdominal air sac. The visible organs are within the intestinal peritoneal cavity and are clearly visible from the abdominal air sac, even though they are covered by the air sac wall and the confluent peritoneum. Introduction of the endoscope in itself causes penetration of the caudal thoracic air sac. The visible structures are (1) the proventriculus; (2) the spleen; and (3) the ventriculus.

The spleen can be interpreted as slightly enlarged, although this is not an objective diagnosis. The ovaries of blue and gold macaws are melanistic, with translucent follicles; all the other organs appear normal. Depending on any other clinical signs, a test for *Chlamydophila* antigen is recommended because of the splenic enlargement.

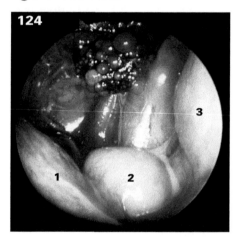

Case 125: **Cloacal papilloma in a macaw**

CLINICAL PRESENTATION. A nine-year-old female hybrid macaw presented for treatment of a mass protruding from its vent (**125**). The mass had been removed approximately a year earlier and the base cauterized with silver nitrate. The mass has recurred and the bird strained and vocalized when voiding urine and feces. On physical examination the mass appeared to arise from the cloaca and was circumferential.

DIAGNOSIS. Cloacal papilloma, though histology would be required to confirm the diagnosis.

ETIOLOGY. Cloacal papillomas are now shown to be caused by a herpesvirus. In some cases, autogenous vaccine has been thought to be efficacious in controlling disease. Surgical debulking may be advantageous.

Bile duct, pancreatic, and renal carcinoma have been associated with cloacal papillomas in Amazon parrots.

MANAGEMENT. Various methods for surgical removal of these masses have been employed, including cold blade excision, application of caustic substances, radiosurgical excision, cryosurgical removal, and laser surgery. None of these methods has been consistently successful and recurrence is common.

All such cases will go on to develop internal carcinomas given time. As it is now known that this is an infectious disease, Amazon parrots and macaws should always have their cloaca and choana inspected at all health checks.

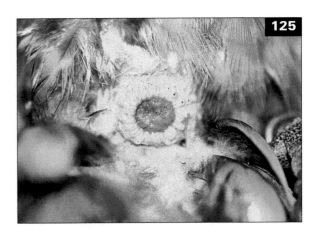

Case 126: 'New wire disease' in a hyacinth macaw

CLINICAL PRESENTATION. A two-year-old female hyacinth macaw presented because she had loose, voluminous, malodorous, brilliant lime green droppings. She was anorexic, had lost weight, and had developed polyuria/polydypsia. The bird was housed with a two-year-old male and they had recently been moved into a new cage made out of galvanized wire (**126**). The pair had been chewing on the cage, and had popped many welds.

INVESTIGATION. Radiographs were negative for wire densities. Blood lead levels were normal, but zinc levels were elevated.

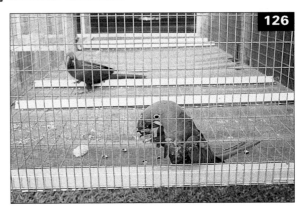

DIAGNOSIS. 'New wire disease'.

ETIOLOGY. 'New wire disease' can be seen when galvanized wire is used in the manufacture of cages and has not been treated properly (i.e. brushed with a wire brush and vinegar, cleaned with soapy water, and then set out to dry prior to the placement of birds in the cage). Traces of lead and considerable quantities of zinc are found in this type of wire.

The pancreas, liver, and kidneys and the reproductive and GI tracts are all affected by zinc. Necrotizing ventriculitis is a common sequela of zinc intoxication and may result in koilin exfoliation, intestinal obstruction, and death. Zinc may cause ileus, gastroenteritis, and dilated intestinal loops.

MANAGEMENT. Dimercaptosuccinic acid (DMSA) (30 mg/kg p/o q12h for 10 days or 5 days per week for 3–5 weeks) is the recommended treatment for lead and zinc poisoning in birds. DMSA is safe, is not nephrotoxic (which CaEDTA may be), and has been shown to

decrease serum zinc concentrations experimentally in pigeons. Laxatives should be given to help mechanically remove any remaining metallic particles in the gut. Supportive care including rehydration, antibiosis, antifungals, gavage feeding, and any other treatment based on additional diagnostic findings should be administered. If the patient is stable, surgery to remove radiographically visible metal densities can be attempted, or endoscopy or ventricular lavage may be used to remove metal particles. If particles still remain in the ventriculus, lavage is generally the easiest, quickest, and least traumatic method of removal. For ingested galvanized wire, a neodymium–ferro–barium alloy magnet attached to a small diameter catheter may be used to retrieve metal from the GI tract. The cage mate should also be checked for plumbism and zinc toxicosis.

Case 127: **Tunnel on the cranial aspect of the tarsometarsus in Falconiformes and Psittaciformes**

DISCUSSION. Falconiform birds (e.g. peregrine falcons) have a tunnel on the cranial aspect of their tarsometatarsus (**127a**). This bony tunnel is formed by the supratendinal bridge, which runs over the tendon of insertion of the long digital extensor (LDE) muscle and keeps the tendon close to the surface of the bone as it runs over the joint. There is a difference in parrots (e.g. red-fronted macaws) in that the supratendinal bridge is fibrous and not bony (**127b, c**).

If fractures in the distal tarsometatarsal region are repaired by immobilization of the intertarsal joint, the tendon's free running will be compromised and this joint, and those of the toes, will be prevented from extending.

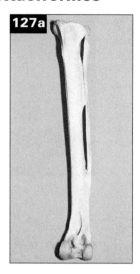 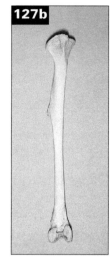 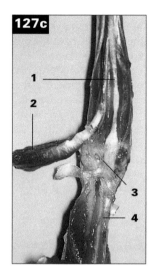

Key: 1 = LDE tendon; 2 = *M. tibialis cranialis*; 3 = supratendinal bridge; 4 = LDE muscle.

Case 128: **AST value elevations in a cockatiel**

CLINICAL PRESENTATION. A ten-week-old cockatiel that had been purchased from a pet shop presented for a general health examination.

INVESTIGATION. A blood sample was collected from a nail clip (rather than via venipuncture) and submitted for a screening blood panel. In addition to a monocytosis, the salient clinical findings included the following: AST 1,450 u/l (normal range 130–390 u/l).

DIAGNOSIS. As in mammals, elevated AST levels in birds are nonspecific. It is impossible to differentiate this elevation between hepatocellular leakage and damage from similar insults to cardiac, skeletal, or smooth muscle.

DISCUSSION. The enzyme CPK is of assistance in differentiating elevations. A patient presenting with an elevated CPK level as well as an elevated AST level is less likely to be affected by hepatocellular damage or leakage.

Case 129: **Oral candidiasis in a cockatiel**

CLINICAL PRESENTATION. A juvenile cockatiel presented with oral lesions (**129**).

DIFFERENTIAL DIAGNOSES. Trichomoniasis, candidiasis, poxvirus infection, an accumulation of hand-rearing food.

DIAGNOSIS. The lesions are those of oral candidiasis.

ETIOLOGY. Oral candidiasis is a common problem in cockatiel chicks, both in the nest and in chicks being hand raised. It is often associated with inappropriate temperature or consistency, or with frequency of feeding. It may also proliferate following antibiotic therapy.

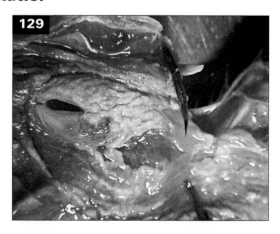

Case 130: **Egg binding in a cockatiel**

CLINICAL PRESENTATION. A three-year-old female pearl white-faced cockatiel presented because she was sitting on the bottom of the cage, feathers ruffled, and obviously depressed (130). The bird was of good weight (96g) with a distended lower abdominal region. A mass was palpable within the cloaca.

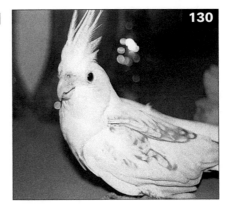

INVESTIGATION/DIAGNOSIS. Radiography was performed and this revealed the presence of an egg in the cloaca. Radiography will also reveal any additional eggs present in the oviduct.

MANAGEMENT. Initially, dystocias should be managed medically. Dystocic birds are often dehydrated and most have circulatory disturbances. Therefore, it is extremely important to stabilize the hen and correct any fluid deficits. Any calculated deficit should be replaced over a period of 36–48 hours, 50% being replaced in the first 24 hour period, in addition to maitenance fluids of 50 ml/kg per day. The maximum intravenous bolus for a cockatiel is 2 ml. The bird should also be given a parenteral multivitamin injection and parenteral calcium (0.5–1.0 ml/kg 5% calcium borogluconate s/c) and be maintained at 30–33°C (86–91.4°F) and increased humidity. Vitamin D_3 facilitates the uptake of calcium. Seed-eating, egg-laying females are often hypocalcemic and therefore benefit from parenteral calcium.

Mineral oil per cloaca is not an effective therapy and prevents subsequent incubation of the egg. Intracloacal application of prostaglandin E_2 vaginal gel is indicated, although it is important to be aware of Health and Safety issues related to this medication. This gel acts similarly to arginine vasotocin, the hormone responsible for normal uterine contractions and relaxation of the uterovaginal sphincter in birds. Birds do not use an oxytocic system for uterine contractions, so oxytocin should probably not be used . Prostaglandin gel should be applied directly to the vaginal opening using a sterile, cotton-tipped applicator inserted into the cloaca. Gloves should always be worn by humans handling this drug or treated birds in order to prevent contact with the skin or mucous membranes; this is particularly important in women. If the prostaglandin does not cause expulsion of the egg within two hours, surgical intervention is necessary. The egg contents should be aspirated and the shell imploded. If the crumpled egg shell is not expelled naturally by the hen with 12 hours, it should be removed via the cloaca. The oviduct may be removed to prevent future oviposition, although prevention of laying by removal of the nest material and nesting box, reducing the energy content of the diet, and behavioral modification training is indicated.

Case 131: **Growth and development differences in two cockatiels**

CLINICAL PRESENTATION. Two four-week-old cockatiels presented with differences in their growth and development. One bird (131a) received 20% protein on a dry weight basis and weighed almost three times the weight of the other bird (131b), which received only 5% protein on a dry matter basis.

DISCUSSION. The differences in these birds are due to different levels of protein in the diet. Protein levels varying from 5–20% resulted in intermediate growth rates. It is important to note, however, that relatively few nutrient deficiencies demonstrate characteristic signs of deficiency and the signs of deficiency of a specific nutrient differ between the species. Therefore, determination of the underlying nutrient deficiency is often impossible. In most cases of nutrient deficiency in which there is no response to vitamins or trace minerals, it is best to simply replace the suspect diet with one that is known to provide adequate nutrition.

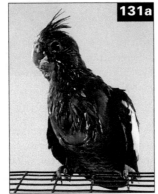

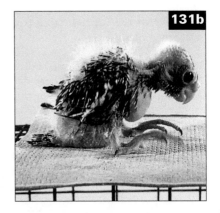

Case 132: **Smoke inhalation in a cockatiel**

CLINICAL PRESENTATION. A cockatiel presented after being immediately evacuated from a flat where the stove had caught fire and filled the room with smoke. The bird looked a little stressed and it had slightly labored breathing and occasional sneezes (**132a**).

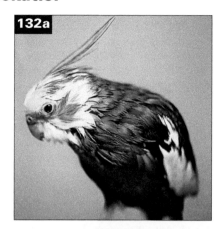

MANAGEMENT. Even though the bird does not appear very ill now, clinical disease caused by delayed, complicated pulmonary failure can occur up to three days post exposure. Treatment should include fresh air, humidified oxygen, and, if indicated, bronchodilator therapy, fluids, diuretics, and prophylactic antibiosis. Glucocorticosteroid use is controversial in smoke inhalation cases and may be detrimental.

DISCUSSION. The initial prognosis must be guarded due to the potential for delayed complicated pulmonary failure from irritant gases released from the fire (e.g. aldehydes, hydrochloric acid, and sulphur dioxide). In view of the potential for delayed reactions, as well as for residual odors in the apartment, it would be prudent to maintain the bird in the hospital for observation and oxygen therapy (**132b**).

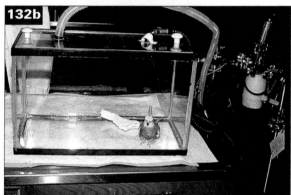

Case 133: **Abdominal mass in a cockatiel**

CLINICAL PRESENTATION. A female cockatiel presented with progressive respiratory distress. The bird was eating normally and the abdomen appeared thickened but soft on palpation.

INVESTIGATION. A barium contrast radiograph (**133**) showed an apparent large, soft tissue mass in the caudal abdomen.

DIFFERENTIAL DIAGNOSES. Ovarian cysts, renal neoplasia, a disease of the reproductive tract, or ectopic or malformed eggs.

DIAGNOSIS. Ultrasound can be used to differentiate fluid-filled cysts, which appear dark (hyperechoic). Abdominal paracentesis may be useful. Removal of fluid rapidly reduces the dyspnea. Exploratory surgery will provide a definitive diagnosis.

MANAGEMENT. Cystic paracentesis and, possibly, surgical removal of ovarian cysts will relieve the acute respiratory distress. Testosterone therapy has been used in an attempt to prevent recurrence of the cysts.

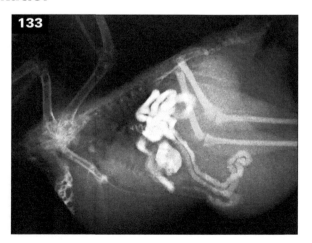

Surgery is the only possible therapy for neoplastic disease, and it may be efficacious for neoplasia of the reproductive tract. Renal neoplasia is generally untreatable.

Removal of ectopic eggs is usually successful, although the prognosis is guarded when complicated by peritonitis.

Case 134: *Serratospiculum* species infection in a Gyr falcon

CLINICAL PRESENTATION. A Gyr falcon presented with laborious breathing and poor flight performance.

DIFFERENTIAL DIAGNOSES. Aspergillosis, amyloidosis or other systemic illness, *Syngamus trachea* in the crop, *Capillaria contorta* in the esophagus, *Serratospiculum* species in the air sac.

INVESTIGATION/DIAGNOSIS. Endoscopy of the air sac revealed a large number of *Serratospiculum* species roundworms (**134**).

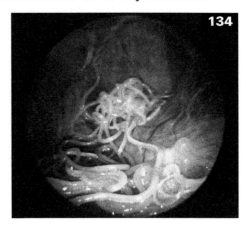

ETIOLOGY. *Serratospiculum* species is a large filarial worm found within the air sac walls, the visceral membranous serosa, and the connective tissue of the coelomic cavity of raptors. Studies in central Asia suggest that up to 10–15% of the wild saker falcon population are infected with *Serratospiculum* species. Wild prairie falcons are also commonly affected in the US.

The life cycle of *Serratospiculum* species is currently unknown. *S. tendo* is probably transmitted by the ingestion of locusts (*Locusta migratoria*) containing infected larvae. Other species are probably transmitted by blood-sucking arthropods.

MANAGEMENT. Current treatment for *Serratospiculum* species infection includes ivermectin (0.5–1.0 mg/kg i/m every week for 3 weeks) and mebendazole (25 mg/kg p/o q24h for 2 weeks). Following treatment of heavily infected birds, dead worms may need to be removed from the coelomic cavity using endoscopy.

PREVENTION. Although very little is known about the life cycle of *Serratospiculum* species, it is strongly recommended that all ectoparasites on birds and in their environment should be controlled. Quarantine of newly imported birds, and isolation and treatment of infected birds, coupled with ectoparasite treatment, is recommended.

Case 135: Fractured ulna and radius in a Harris' hawk

CLINICAL PRESENTATION. A Harris' hawk presented three weeks after repair of a compound fracture of the ulna and radius. The fracture was stable, but the healing was not normal and the flight capability was impaired.

INVESTIGATION. Radiography was performed.

DIAGNOSIS. The radiograph shows an active osteomyelitis with the presence of a bone sequestrum, as well as a synostosis between the radius and ulna (**135**). These two pathologic conditions might prevent a return to normal flight.

MANAGEMENT. The bird should be anesthetized, the pins and wire removed, and swabs taken for microbiology and sensitivity testing. The bird should receive systemic antibiotics. Antibiotic-impregnated methylmethacrylate beads, which are effective in releasing antibiotic for a prolonged period of time, may be implanted at the site of the infection. Once the infection is controlled and the bone callus has fined down, a compressed air drill should be used to remove the synostosis that is currently fixing the ulna and radius in relation to each other. Such fixation of these bones prevents normal wing action. A fat pad should be placed between the radius and ulna at the site of the surgery in an attempt to prevent a synostosis reforming. One weeks rest should be enforced to allow reduction of any post-surgical inflammation, after which the bird should be encouraged to keep the wing mobile.

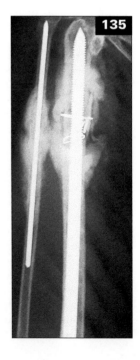

Case 136: *Mycobacterium avium* osteomyelitis in a goshawk

CLINICAL PRESENTATION. A three-year-old female Northern goshawk presented lame. The owner was concerned that she might have traumatized the leg while out hunting the previous week.

INVESTIGATION. Radiographs were taken, with two views at 90° to each other (**136**).

DIAGNOSIS. The radiograph shows a locular area of bone lysis in the tarsometatarsus. Such a lesion is most likely to be due to *Mycobacterium avium* osteomyelitis. Biopsy of the mass and staining with Ziehl–Neelsen stain for the presence of acid-fast bacilli is diagnostic. If required, the organism may also be cultured.

ETIOLOGY. Theoretically, infection can arise due to fecal contamination of open topped aviaries by infected feral birds or following the ingestion of infected quarry or food. In practice, the vast majority of cases arise after the ingestion of infected quarry or food.

MANAGEMENT. In view of the poor success rate of treating this infection, together with the zoonotic potential, therapy is not recommended. The bird should be euthanased, and any birds that have been kept in the same aviary or who may have access to ground on which this bird has defecated, should be screened for *M. avium*.

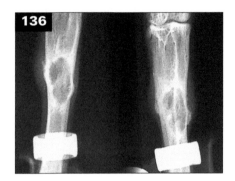

Case 137: Post-traumatic ocular hemorrhage in a sparrowhawk

CLINICAL PRESENTATION. A European sparrowhawk presented with severely impaired vision (**137a**).

INVESTIGATION. Ophthalmoscopic examination of the ocular fundus was carried out.

DIAGNOSIS. Post-traumatic epistaxis and subcutaneous hematoma at the supraorbital process.

MANAGEMENT. The patient should be immobilized immediately in a darkened box. Tissue plasminogen activator has been used (50 mg by intraocular injection at least 24 hours after the cessation of hemorrhage) with encouraging effects in an attempt to reduce the effects of, and increase the speed of, resolution following post-traumatic hemorrhage from the pecten. Euthanasia may be indicated in patients with extensive subretinal choroidal bleeding that leads to blindness resulting from retinal detachment.

DISCUSSION. As 85% of cases of post-traumatic hemorrhage affect only the posterior chamber, ophthalmoscopic examination of the ocular fundus is obligatory in trauma patients. The examination is conducted after inducing mydriasis by air sac perfusion anesthesia. Induction of mydriasis by the topical application of muscle relaxants (e.g. d-tubocurarine) is problematic and carries a number of inherent risks. Thirty two percent of trauma cases have intravitreal haemorrhage; 80% of the bleeding originates in

the pecten oculi (**137b**), a free, pleated projection of choroid into the vitreous body that provides nutrition to the retina.

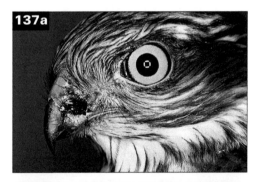

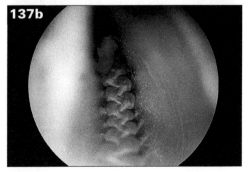

Case 138: **Cloacal prolapse in a hawk and a goshawk**

CLINICAL PRESENTATION. A red-tailed hawk (**138a**) and a Gabar goshawk (**138b**) both presented with a cloacal prolapse.

DIFFERENTIAL DIAGNOSES. Three structures can prolapse in these two species: the colon, the oviduct, and the cloaca (rare in raptors but relatively common in psittacines).

INVESTIGATION. Differentiation of which structure has prolapsed requires careful examination in an anesthetized patient. Visual examination will usually allow differentiation, the oviduct being a much larger, fleshier structure.

DIAGNOSIS. Prolapse of the colon as a consequence of an intersusception, as in the red-tailed hawk; prolapse of the oviduct in the Gabar goshawk.

MANAGEMENT. Cloacal prolapse is treated by a cloacopexi, typically to the caudal sternum or last rib as well as into the laparotomy closure. Both oviduct and colon prolapse must be treated via a coelotomy, with full retrieval of the affected organ, and pexi if the tissues appear healthy. If nonviable tissue is present, either a salpingohysterectomy or intestinal resection, followed by an anastomosis, should be performed.

DISCUSSION. Male ostriches and geese both have a phallus that can prolapse (e.g. with goose gonorrhoea caused by *Neisseria* species).

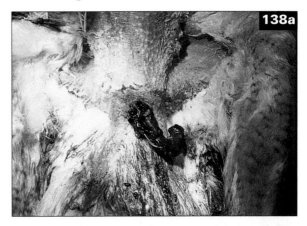
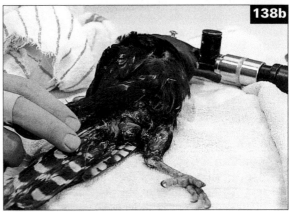

Case 139: **Cloacal urolith in a tawny owl**

CLINICAL PRESENTATION. A tawny owl presented apparently weakened, straining frequently, and passing only small volumes of feces and uric acid (**139**).

DIAGNOSIS. Cloacal urolith.

ETIOLOGY. Cloacal uroliths occur most often in breeding birds during or following incubation of their eggs. Some birds sit very tight, failing to get off the eggs, and they void their cloacal contents at irregular intervals. Precipitation of urates in the cloaca can, in time, lead to the formation of a uric acid concretion: a urolith.

Three other possible causes of abdominal straining are enteritis, which, if severe, can lead to intussusception followed by colonic prolapse; egg binding; and oviductitis, which can lead to a prolapsed oviduct.

MANAGEMENT. Once diagnosed, the urolith may be broken up inside the cloaca with a pair of forceps and removed piecemeal. A certain amount of local trauma is likely to be caused, therefore prophylactic antibiotics should be administered for 3–5 days following removal.

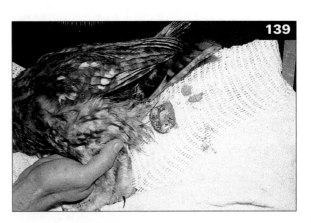

Case 140: 'Eagle owl and tawny owl keratitis'

CLINICAL PRESENTATION. A tawny owl presented with superficial keratitis characterized by superficial pale red dendritic vessels crossing the corneal limbus, and interstitial keratitis characterized by deep blue-red ciliary vessels of the epi- and intrascleral vascular system running dichotomously over the cornea, apparently cut off at the limbus of the cornea (140a).

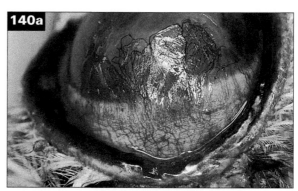

DIFFERENTIAL DIAGNOSES. Differential diagnoses in tawny owls should include owl herpesvirus infection as well as other mycotic and bacterial infections, but especially so-called 'eagle owl and tawny owl keratitis'.

INVESTIGATION. The extent of the corneal ulcer was demonstrated by staining the cornea with fluorescein. *Salmonella* species infection was diagnosed serologically by demonstrating antibodies and bacteriologically by examining conjunctival smears and faeces. The fundus oculi of the left eye was examined (140b).

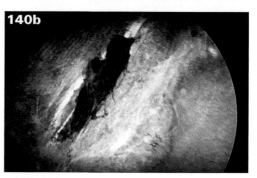

DIAGNOSIS. Superficial and chronic interstitial ulcerative keratitis caused by infection with *Salmonella typhimurium* (140a); chorioretinitis with marginal hyperpigmentation and severe atrophy of the pecten oculi (140b).

ETIOLOGY. The etiology of these conditions remains unclear. The reddening of the palpebral margins is physiological. The anterior chamber, which cannot be examined because of the massive keratitis, is usually found to have anterior uveitis, with secondary raised intraocular pressure (secondary glaucoma) attributable to destruction of the pecten oculi. A lateral view of the hemiresected bulb is shown (140c). The pecten oculi is also important for intraocular nutrition and pressure regulation.

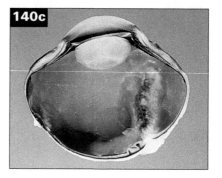

Case 141: Injury to the propatagium and elastic membrane

DISCUSSION. Any injury to the propatagium and elastic membrane of a bird will prevent it from flying. The two structures are shown in this dissection of the ventral aspect of the wing of a Harris' hawk (141). The triangular fold of skin (1) is the propatagium; it increases the surface area of the wing and forms the aerofoil shape. The leading edge of the propatagium (2) is supported by the tendon of the *m. tensor propatagialis longa*. This muscle has a small, fleshy belly mainly attaching to the clavicle. The distal fifth of the tendon is fibrous and unyielding, but the majority of the tendon is elastic and will maintain the tension of the leading edge of the wing even when it is not fully extended, thereby keeping the aerofoil shape while flying;

When the propatagium is repaired, the elastic tendon must be found and, if damaged, be repaired by suturing

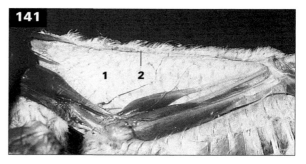

the ends together. Birds can fly well even when they have lost a significant part of the ligament, provided it is repaired correctly.

Case 142: **Bumblefoot in a Lanner falcon**

CLINICAL PRESENTATION. A Lanner falcon presented as a second opinion case, having been suffering from bumblefoot for several weeks.

INVESTIGATION. A radiograph was taken as part of the clinical assessment (**142**).

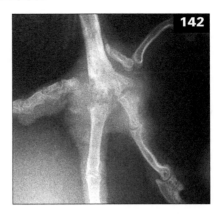

DIAGNOSIS. The radiograph shows marked osteomyelitis of the lateral and medial trochlea of the distal tarsometatarsus, as well as the proximal phalanges digits 2 and 3. The bird is therefore classified as suffering from class IV to class V bumblefoot (i.e. there is physical damage to bone or deeper structures of the foot, with possible loss of functional use of the foot).

It is important that the radiograph is considered concurrently with the clinical assessment.

MANAGEMENT. Success rates for treatment of bumblefoot of this severity are very poor. Treatment should comprise extensive surgery, supportive and weight redistributive dressings on both feet, and the implantation of antibiotic-impregnated polymethylmethacrylate beads, together with long-term (at least 30 days) parenteral antibiotics. However, the prognosis is grave and euthanasia should be advised prior to further therapy in this particular case.

Case 143: **Feeding of pigeons to raptors**

CLINICAL PROBLEM. Many diseases are associated with feeding freshly killed, wild pigeons to raptors, such as the Harris' hawk shown (**143**).

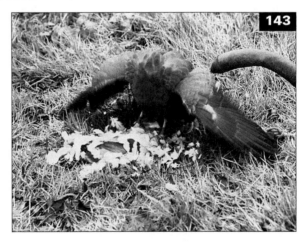

DISCUSSION. The feeding of pigeons to raptors may transmit or cause a number of diseases. The common infections or other disease risks are listed below:

- Infectious diseases: Newcastle disease (PMV1); paramyxovirus (PMV1 pigeon) and PMV3; falcon herpesvirus; avipox; *Mycobacterium avium*; salmonellosis; trichomoniasis.
- Poisonings: lead; alphachlorulose; mercury; pesticides (e.g. fenthion, DDT).

Although pigeon carcasses are nutritionally beneficial to raptors, their ingestion is associated with a number of disease risks. Therefore, ideally pigeons should never be fed to raptors. As trichomonads are temperature sensitive, the chilling or freezing of a carcass prior to thawing and feeding will greatly reduce the risk of this disease, although freezing has little effect on the risk of viral infections. Alternatively, where possible, one can medicate a pigeon population for trichomoniasis prior to killing them and feeding them to raptors.

Case 144: **Varus of the distal tibiotarsus in a Lugger falcon**

CLINICAL PRESENTATION. A 15-day-old Lugger falcon presented with an abnormality of the distal tibiotarsus.

INVESTIGATION/DIAGNOSIS. A radiograph (**144**) revealed varus of the distal tibiotarsus.

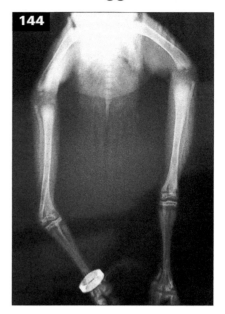

ETIOLOGY. Luxation of the calcaneal tendon often presents as a soft tissue complication with this varus of the distal tibiotarsus. In addition to varus, tibial dyschrondroplasia, bowing in the midsection of the tibiotarsus, and valgus or varus and rotation along the longitudinal axis of the tibiotarsus are often seen as part of the same clinical situation.

Varus of the tibiotarsus is secondary to trauma to the growth area, although there is often a dietary imbalance of calcium to phosphorus (i.e. insufficient calcium in relation to the level of phosphorus). Alternatively, the contents of the egg itself, when laid, may have been deficient in calcium. Clinical incidence can be reduced by supplementation with 1a,25-dihydroxycholecalciferol and avoided by the ingestion by both parents and young of a balanced 'whole carcass' diet. Excessive growth rates can lead to problems even when a normally adequate diet has been supplied.

MANAGEMENT. Surgery should be performed to remove a strip of periosteum and growth plate from the inner curvature. The limb may then be realigned in a straight position and a cast applied for 14 days. When the cast is removed, the limb should be straight and fully functional.

DISCUSSION. Generally, raptor chicks suffering from this condition are second or third clutch chicks, where the first clutches have been pulled and the female recycled in a short period. It is suggested that any female raptor that is likely to recycle should receive a good diet with a suitable Ca:P ratio, together with a Ca and vitamin D_3 supplement.

Case 145: **Endoscopy of the abdomen of a buzzard**

DISCUSSION. Endoscopic examination of a buzzard revealved the structures shown in **145**. The structures were identified as follows:

1 Cranial portion of the left kidney. The color, size, and structure appear normal.
2 Oviduct with the supporting ligament to the infundibulum. This structure is part of the dorsal ligament of the oviduct and is absent in juvenile males.
3 Inactive ovary. Note the distance to the oviduct in this bird. If the ovary was not visible because it was covered by intestinal loops, it would be easy to confuse the infundibulum with a testicle.
4 Adrenal gland, which is always close to the gonad. The triangle comprising kidney, gonad, and adrenal should always be identified to avoid confusion.
5 Intestinal loop.

All the structures visualized in this buzzard appear normal.

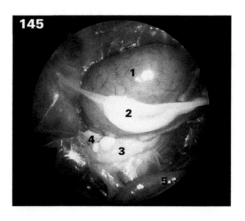

Case 146: *Leucocytozoon* species infection in a red-tailed hawk

CLINICAL PRESENTATION. A red-tailed hawk presented for a routine 'well-bird' examination.

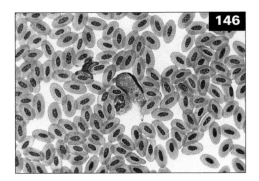

INVESTIGATION. Diagnostic assessment included a hematology and chemistry profile. A 'strange object' was found in a stained blood film (**146**).

DIAGNOSIS. Infection with *Leucocytozoon* species, a blood parasite affecting leucocytes and, probably, erythrocytes.

ETIOLOGY. Simulid (biting) flies are the common source of *Leucocytozoon* species. Leucocytozoan infection is common in a variety of raptor species, but clinical disease due to the parasite is uncommon.

MANAGEMENT. Pyrimethamine has been suggested as a treatment.

Case 147: Fractured digit/osteomyelitis of the digit of two raptors

CLINICAL PRESENTATION. Two raptors presented, both with acute onset swelling of a toe and an outwardly similar clinical appearance.

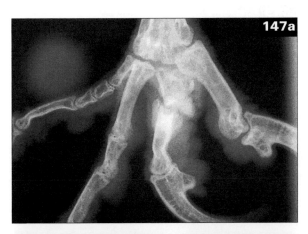

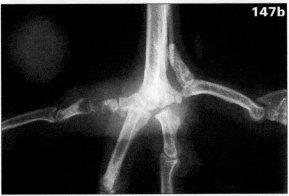

INVESTIGATION. Radiographs were taken of both birds (**147a, b**).

DIAGNOSIS. One bird (**147a**) has a fracture of digit 1, with minimal soft tissue swelling. The other bird (**147b**) has an acute, severe osteomyelitis affecting the lateral digit. The clinical history confirmed that this lesion had occurred following a cat bite to the toe seven days previously. There is significant soft tissue swelling that has extended to the metatarsophalangeal joint (the ball of the foot).

MANAGEMENT. The bird with the fractured toe should be rested in the dark (to keep it quiet). A ball bandage encompassing the whole foot may be applied, but it must not be left on for more than seven days. Any attempt to immobilize just the one toe will lead to disaster. If the whole foot is immobilized until the toe is fully healed, the flexor and extensor tendons may become involved in the bridging callus, preventing normal toe function in the future.

The osteomyelitis affecting the bird in **147b** is clearly very lytic. In view of the tremendous lysis that has occurred in as little as seven days, the future viability of the foot as a whole is at risk. In this situation a decision should be taken immediately to amputate the affected toe, effectively a damage limitation exercise. In this case the infection was subsequently controlled and the foot saved, even though it was believed that the toe was already well beyond help.

Case 148: **Multifocal follicular and feather pulp hemorrhage in a cockatoo**

CLINICAL PRESENTATION. A young umbrella cockatoo was presented after it had died following a short clinical illness. The gross appearance of the feathers is shown (**148**).

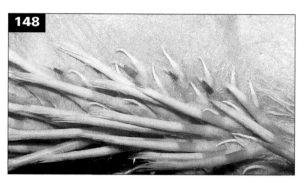

INVESTIGATION. Autopsy revealed hepatic enlargement and necrosis, and splenomegaly. The characteristic lesions and inclusion bodies of multifocal follicular and feather pulp hemorrhage were demonstrated on histology. Affected organs were swabbed and the swabs were submitted for DNA probe testing. This is a definitive test for multifocal follicular and feather pulp hemorrhage and, in cases with poorly developed lesions, may be the only way of making a positive diagnosis. Cloacal swabs were assessed by PCR testing for the presence of polyomavirus.

DIAGNOSIS. Multifocal follicular and feather pulp hemorrhage.

ETIOLOGY. These hemorrhages, which can vary in severity, are typical of polyomavirus infection in young psittacines.

DISCUSSION. The autopsy findings can vary depending on the species of psittacine. Generalized serosal hemorrhages may be present and, in a few cases, intestinal necrosis and hemorrhage are noted.

Case 149: **Psittacine beak and feather disease (PBFD) in a cockatoo**

CLINICAL PRESENTATION. A young lesser sulphur-crested cockatoo presented for a complete health check one week after arriving at its new home The bird had been recently purchased from a breeder with a PBFD-free, closed aviary and shipped by aeroplane to its new owner, who owned no other birds. The bird looked perfectly normal on physical examination (**149**) and had completely normal feathers. Its weight was perfect for its size and it was bright, active, and playful.

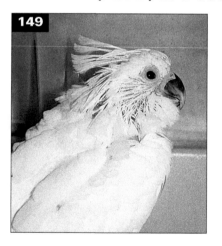

INVESTIGATION. Hematology revealed a somewhat depressed WBC count (4.5×10^9/l [4.5×10^3/ml], 58% heterophils, 42% lymphocytes). A PBFD DNA PCR test was positive. Blood for PBFD testing must be taken by clean venipuncture, and not a toe nail clip, as virus particles may otherwise contaminate the blood sample, leading to a false positive.

MANAGEMENT. A positive PBFD PCR test in a young bird with no feather abnormalities suggests that the bird has recently been exposed to the causative virus and is currently viremic, or that it is latently infected. The best advice that can be given to the owner is not to panic, as there is a good chance that the bird will be able to eliminate the virus on its own. If the bird was not shipped in a biosecure container, it may have been exposed to the virus en route in the cargo hold of the aircraft or at the airport, as Circoviridae can generally remain viable in the environment for quite some time.

Many young birds exposed to the virus will be transiently viremic but will eliminate the virus. These birds will only develop disease if the immune system is unable to clear the infection. A PBFD-positive young bird with normal feathers should be kept isolated and retested in 90 days. If it is still positive it should be considered to be latently infected or that it is being continually exposed to the virus. A negative test after 90 days indicates that the bird has eliminated the infection. However, if a young bird is PBFD positive and has feather abnormalities, then the bird has active PBFD infection.

Case 150: **Abdominal wall hernia in a cockatoo**

CLINICAL PRESENTATION. A 17-year-old female lesser sulphur-crested cockatoo presented with an abdominal swelling (**150a**) that had been getting larger over a period of approximately two months. The bird had recently begun straining to void feces and urine. On physical examination the translucent skin allowed visualization of urates within the cloaca directly below the skin (**150b**).

DIAGNOSIS. Abdominal wall hernia. Often the viscera are visible beneath the skin. Palpation or radiography may confirm the diagnosis.

MANAGEMENT. Many abdominal hernias are of little clinical significance. Most abdominal hernias in birds are very large and do not entrap viscera. However, the cloaca may herniate, affecting the bird's ability to void urine and feces. When this occurs, surgery is recommended. In female birds the risk of herniating an egg may warrant surgical treatment.

The major risk associated with abdominal herniorrhaphy in birds is respiratory compromise. With chronic hernias, reduction and replacement of the viscera within the coelom can compress the thoracic and abdominal air sac and compromise the bird's ability to breathe. If respiratory compromise is likely, it is better to use a polypropylene mesh to provide support for the abdominal viscera. Caution must be used when placing a mesh subcutaneously in birds, as they have very little subcutaneous tissue to support the mesh. Another problem frequently encountered with herniorrhaphies is failure accurately to identify the body wall. If the border of the body wall hernia is not identified and appropriately closed, herniation is likely to recur.

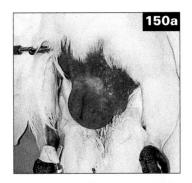

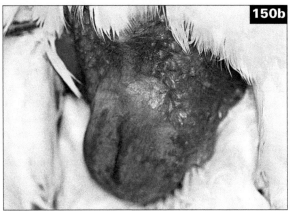

Hernia in psittacines is often linked to obesity and chronic hyperestroginism in females. All affected birds should be dieted to normal condition. If surgery is indicated, simultaneous salpingotomy/hysterectomy is advised.

Case 151: *Haemoproteus* **species infection in a cockatoo**

CLINICAL PRESENTATION. A nine-year-old captive-bred Moluccan cockatoo that had been purchased from a breeder presented for a health assessment.

INVESTIGATION. A hemogram was performed and abnormalities were observed within some of the erythrocytes (**151**).

DIAGNOSIS. *Haemoproteus* species infection.

ETIOLOGY. The bird was most likely a wild caught import, raising questions as to the bird's supposed history of being captive bred.

MANAGEMENT. Therapy is probably unnecessary, as this parasite is rarely, if ever, pathogenic in psittacine birds. However, chloroquine (250 mg/120 ml drinking water for 14 days) has been used successfully.

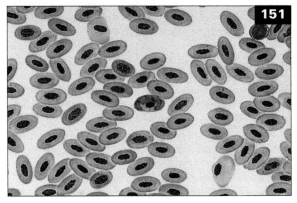

Case 152: **Chlamydophilosis in a cockatoo**

CLINICAL PRESENTATION. An umbrella cockatoo presented with symptoms suggestive of chlamydophilosis. A baby cockatiel from the same premises had died with postmortem signs consistent with chlamydophilosis.

INVESTIGATION. Samples from the bird tested strongly positive for chlamydophilosis. Cell culture is the 'gold standard' test for chlamydophilosis. Cell culture is sensitive and able to detect small numbers of chlamydophilial organisms within two or three passages. Unfortunately, it is only performed by specialized laboratories and takes about two weeks. Chlamydophilial organisms are often nonviable by the time they reach the laboratory. *Chlamydophila* antigen and serologic ELISA tests are commercially available and can be run in-house. False antigen positives may occur due to cross antigen reactions with certain bacteria. False antigen negatives arise due to intermittent shedding of the organism. Serology can be useful in identifying false antigen results, although they may give a negative result in acute cases. PCR testing is now commercially available in many countries. The test is very sensitive and specific, but takes one to two weeks. The prevalence of persistent, probably lifelong, infection within avian populations may require new concepts in control and differentiation between disease and infection.

DIAGNOSIS. Chlamydophilosis.

ETIOLOGY. The causative organism of chlamydophilosis is *Chlamydophila psittaci*. Other antigenically related species of *Chlamydophila* include *C. trachomatis* and *C. pneumonia*, which are restricted to humans. *C. psittaci* has a wide host spectrum among birds including most Psittaciformes and at least 130 non-Psittaciformes, mammals (horses, cattle, sheep, cats, guinea pigs, dogs) and humans. *C. psittaci* can be highly contagious and induces a disease called chlamydophilosis in parrots and ornithosis in all other animals and man.

DISCUSSION. Clinical signs of chlamydophilosis include conjunctivitis, greenish diarrhea, sinusitis, air sacculitis, hepatitis, and CNS signs including convulsions, tremors, and opisthotonus. Hematology may show severe leukocytosis, heterophilia, anemia, monocytosis (especially in Amazon parrots), and basophilia (especially in conures). Hepatic leakage enzymes such as AST, LDH, CPK, and bile acids may be elevated due to hepatocellular damage. No single sign is pathognomonic.

Case 153: **Cloacal prolapse in a cockatoo**

CLINICAL PRESENTATION. A 12-year-old male umbrella cockatoo presented with tissue protruding from the vent (**153**).

DIAGNOSIS. The most likely diagnosis is cloacal prolapse.

ETIOLOGY. The etiology for cloacal prolapse is unknown. Chronic bacterial infection and chronic hormonal influences have been proposed as potential etiologies.

MANAGEMENT. Rib cloacopexy, incisional cloacopexy, and body wall cloacopexy are the three most commonly used techniques to maintain the cloaca in the reduced position. Because of the high recurrence rate, these procedures are often used in combination. For all cloacopexy techniques it is important to remove the ventral fat pad on the surface of the cloaca, as fat will inhibit scar tissue formation, resulting in breakdown of adhesions and recurrence of the prolapse.

For the rib cloacopexy, a moist, cotton-tipped applicator is inserted into the cloaca to push the cloaca cranially as far as possible. Sutures are placed through the craniolateral extremity on each side of the urodeum of the cloaca and around the last rib on each side (usually two sutures are placed on each side).

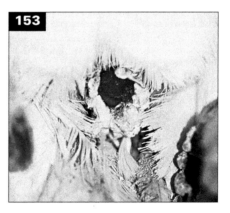

With an incisional cloacopexy, the ventral aspect of the cloaca is sutured into the body wall. A ventral midline incision is made and the fat removed from the ventral aspect of the cloaca. Sutures are passed from one side of the body wall, through the full thickness of the cloaca, and through the other side of the body wall in a simple interrupted pattern, sandwiching the cloaca between the sides of the body wall.

The body wall cloacopexy is performed by making two parallel incisions in the serosal surface of the coprodeum on each side of midline. Corresponding incisions are made in the peritoneal surface of the body wall at points that will maintain the cloaca in position, with slight inversion of the vent. Sutures are placed between each side of each incision so that the sub-serosal tissues are in contact, and the serosal surfaces of the cloaca and peritoneum are sutured in two rows on each side of the midline. The ventral midline incision is closed and the skin closed in a separate layer.

The three procedures described are used for definitive treatment. Often, a purse string or transvent suture is used temporarily to prevent recurrence following reduction of the prolapse; however, recurrence following suture removal is common.

Castration may be helpful in some cases where it appears that the prolapse is related to chronic masturbation or hormonal influences. Hormone injections may also prove to be beneficial in some cases. Behavioral modification training to gain dominance over the bird and reduce sexual behavior is indicated. Likewise, reducing the energy density of the diet is important because it will reduce the nutritional drive to breed.

Case 154: **Fracture of the maxillary tip in a cockatoo**

CLINICAL PRESENTATION. A Moluccan cockatoo chick presented with a fracture of the maxillary tip (**154**).

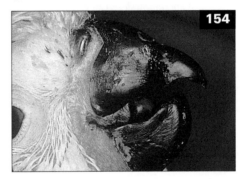

MANAGEMENT. A fracture such as this is so severe that successful repair is unlikely, particularly as the bird completely broke the tip off before it could be repaired. As the growth center in the tip of the maxilla was damaged, the tip did not regrow. Less severe fractures can be successfully repaired with pinning and/or cerclage wires and then strengthened by the application of dental acrylics.

Case 155: **Bradygnathism of the maxilla of a cockatoo**

CLINICAL PRESENTATION. A 14-day-old lesser sulphur-crested cockatoo chick presented with a problem affecting its beak (**155**).

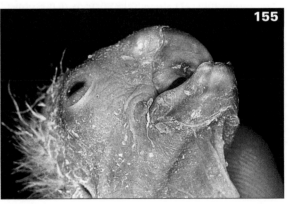

DIAGNOSIS. Severe bradygnathism of the maxilla.

MANAGEMENT. Due to the severe nature of the defect in this bird, it must be corrected in order to prevent the beak from growing into the mouth. In mild cases the bird can move the tip of the maxilla into the mandible and may hold it there at times. To correct this defect in a small chick, the inside of the tip (caudal surface) of the maxilla can be trimmed with cuticle clippers and the tip pulled cranially with each feeding, or as frequently as needed for correction.

The mandible should also be examined. If it is compressed laterally so that it is narrow and/or pointed in front, it should be manipulated so that it becomes flatter in front and more spread out at the sides. If the defect is not corrected before the beak becomes hardened it should be corrected by applying an acrylic extension to the tip of the maxilla.

Case 156: *Filaroides* species infection in a cockatoo

CLINICAL PRESENTATION. A Moluccan cockatoo that resided in a hotel display was found dead.

INVESTIGATION. A postmortem examination was performed. Samples taken included organ impression smears, which were stained with Gimenez for *Chlamydophila* inclusion bodies. The slide was examined under high power (**156**).

DIAGNOSIS. The preparation is negative for *Chlamydophila* inclusion bodies, but a microfilaria is visible.

ETIOLOGY. Blood-sucking insects are the source of the infection. Mostly, nonpathogenic adults reside in subcutaneous and serosal areas. Filarids rarely cause clinical disease, but occasional aberrant lesions can cause death.

MANAGEMENT. Repeated treatment with avermectins can be given; however, there is no proven effective therapy available that will clear microfilaria and adults.

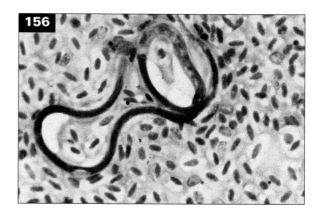

Case 157: Visceral urate deposition (gout) in a cockatoo

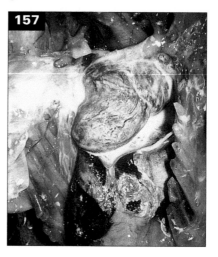

CLINICAL PRESENTATION. A lesser sulphur-crested cockatoo presented for necropsy. A lesion was found in the heart region (**157**).

DIFFERENTIAL DIAGNOSES. Infectious pericarditis and epicarditis, as well as severe myocardial mineralization.

DIAGNOSIS. This is a case of severe visceral urate deposition (gout). Histologically there is deposition of amorphous urates in the pericardial sac, the epicardium, and within the fluid found in the pericardial sac.

ETIOLOGY. Severe visceral gout is usually secondary to severe renal disease, but it may also occur due to metabolic disorders of protein metabolism or severe dehydration.

Case 158: Tracheal endoscopy in an umberella cockatoo

CLINICAL PRESENTATION. A 14-year-old female umbrella cockatoo presented with acute onset of dyspnea. The bird was initially recumbent on the bottom of the cage and gasping for breath, but it had been stabilized by placing an air sac cannula to allow the bird to ventilate through the caudal thoracic or abdominal air sac (**158**).

INVESTIGATION. Tracheal endoscopy was performed. A number of sunflower seeds were visible in the trachea at

the syrinx. However, it was not possible to retrieve them through the endoscope, so tracheotomy is indicated. In order to best visualize the trachea and syrinx, the bird is positioned with the shoulders elevated at 50–60°. A mid-ventral skin incision is made and the crop reflected to the right, allowing the surgeon to look down into the thoracic inlet. The trachea and associated sternotrachealis muscles are visualized. The syrinx cannot generally be retracted into the cervical region. The sternotrachealis muscles are transected using radiosurgery (to control hemorrhage). Stay sutures are placed through the trachea between rings and used to pull the syrinx into view. Alternatively, a hook can be inserted through the thoracic inlet to engage the syrinx and retract it into view. Access can be increased by elevating the proximal superficial and deep pectoral muscles on one side and transecting that clavicle.

MANAGEMENT. A transverse tracheotomy should be created several rings orad (towards the mouth) from the syrinx on the ventral aspect of the trachea and through half of its diameter. Following removal of the seeds, the tracheotomy is closed with fine absorbable, monofilament material, encompassing at least two rings on each side of the tracheotomy in a simple, interrupted pattern. It is important to suture the crop back over teh thoracic inlet, so as to achieve an air tight seal. Subcutaneous tissues and skin are closed routinely.

Potential postoperative complications include subcutaneous emphysema, stricture, and granuloma formation at the site of the suture material. It is best to place knots external to the lumen of the trachea and to limit the number of sutures so as to minimize the chances for intraluminal granuloma formation.

DISCUSSION. Placing an air sac cannula is primarily indicated to relieve respiratory distress associated with an upper airway obstruction; it does not generally help birds with primary lung disease. However, forced ventilation with oxygen through an air sac cannula may improve the arterial oxygen saturation.

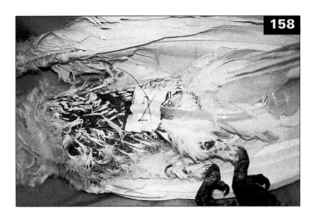

Case 159: **Candidiasis in a cockatoo**

CLINICAL PRESENTATION. A three-week-old hand-fed Moluccan cockatoo chick presented with a three-day history of delayed emptying of the crop. The chick weighed 186 g.

INVESTIGATION. An aspirate of the crop was performed for cytologic evaluation (**159**).

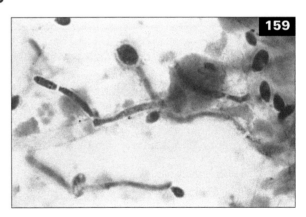

DIAGNOSIS. The Wright's-stained smear reveals many oval yeast and hyphae. There is no apparent inflammatory response. The yeast and hyphae are compatible with a severe yeast infection, most likely candidiasis, involving the ingluvies.

ETIOLOGY. Immunosuppressive conditions and trauma to the ingluvies lead to the development of candidiasis. Predisposing factors include hypothermia, feeding a formula that is too cold or too hot or of incorrect consistency, poor nutrition, antibiotic therapy, and systemic illness from other causes.

MANAGEMENT. An antifungal drug is indicated for the treatment of candidiasis. The presence of hyphae is suggestive of invasion of the mucosa by the yeast and the potential for a systemic infection. Therefore, a systemic antifungal drug should be used (e.g. itraconazole: 10 mg/kg p/o q12h for 7 days) along with a local or topical antifungal preparation (e.g. nystatin: 300,000 IU/kg p/o q12h or q8h for 7–10 days).

Case 160: **Lead and zinc poisoning in two cockatoos**

CLINICAL PRESENTATION. A pair of rose-breasted cockatoos (**160**) presented with a history of infertility during the last breeding season. The breeder reported that the birds had not seemed as active lately and on the day of presentation he had noticed some digested blood in one of the bird's droppings. Further questioning revealed that the birds had been moved into a new breeding cage that had been made out of galvanized wire.

INVESTIGATION. Based on the clinical signs and the potential exposure to galvanized wire, the following tests were performed: CBC/chemistry profile; fecal examination and culture; blood lead and zinc analysis (blood must not be collected in rubber-topped containers); radiographs; *Chlamydophila* titers.

DIAGNOSIS. The diagnostics revealed abnormally high blood zinc levels in both birds (>32 µmol/l (209.28 µg/dl). No metallic particles were seen on the radiographs. The melena reported in the history was most likely due to necrotizing ventriculitis, which is a common sequela to zinc toxicity.

MANAGEMENT. Treatment involves removal of the birds from their accommodation as well as administration of CaEDTA (35 mg/kg i/m q12h for 7 days). DMSA (30

mg/kg for 10 days or for 5 days per week for 3–5 weeks) is considered by some authors to be the preferred treatment of lead and zinc poisoning, as it is may be safer than CaEDTA, although the choice of therapeutic agent is governed primarily by availability, which varies between countries.

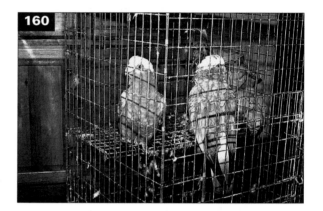

Case 161: *Cnemidocoptes* species infestation in a budgerigar

CLINICAL PRESENTATION. A male four-year-old budgerigar, living in a flight cage with five other clinically normal birds, presented with a powdery crust around the eyes, on the cere, in the intermandibular space, on the feet, and around the vent (**161**).

INVESTIGATION/DIAGNOSIS. Skin scrapings confirmed the presence of *Cnemidocoptes* mites.

MANAGEMENT. Treatment is simple and effective using ivermectin (0.2 mg/kg p/o on 2 or 3 occasions at 2-week intervals). Infestation may be refractory in immunosuppressed birds. All in-contact birds should be treated even if they are asymptomatic.

In some cases the beak is rigid and overgrown. If the beak is overgrown, it may be shaped with a hand-held file or mechanical burr. If the germinal epithelial layer is damaged, the beak may continue to grow abnormally, even after the mites have been eradicated.

DISCUSSION. Immunosuppressive diseases, such as hepatic lipidosis, diabetes mellitus, or neoplasia, must be considered in affected adult birds. Since it is thought that there is some genetic disposition to *Cnemidocoptes* mite infestation, affected birds should not be used for breeding. All in-contact birds should be treated in order to eradicate the parasite from the population as a whole.

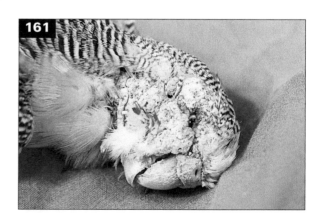

Case 162: **Candidiasis/trichomoniasis in some budgerigars**

CLINICAL PRESENTATION. Some budgerigars owned by a fancier presented because a number of them were vomiting. Because budgerigars flick their heads when vomiting, some of the vomitus landed on the top of the head and caused matting of the feathers (**162a**). Some of the affected birds were dying.

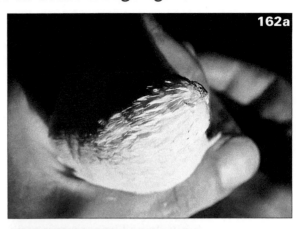

DIFFERENTIAL DIAGNOSES. Trichomoniasis or candidiasis; both diseases produce the same symptoms and lesions, though the former condition usually affects individual birds.

INVESTIGATION. Postmortem examination revealed an enlarged and inflamed cranial esophagus and proximal part of the crop (**162b**). There was an accumulation of yellow diphtheritic material on the crop mucosa (**162c**). A cytology sample can be collected from live birds by introducing a swab into the crop *per os*. The sample should be immediately examined in warm saline under a microscope. This will reveal motile trichomonads if present. Diff Quik-stained slides will demonstrate *Candida* species. Examination of necropsy lesions will reveal *Candida* organisms, but trichomonads are more difficult to visualize when they are dead and no longer motile.

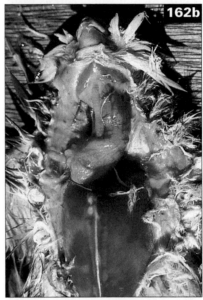

MANAGEMENT. Because asymptomatic carriers will be present where trichomoniasis has been diagnosed, all the birds on the premises should be treated. The usual treatment is dimetridazole in the drinking water. Care should be taken not to overdose, as the margin of safety is not great. Signs of overdose are 'drunkenness' and incoordination, followed by more severe signs of CNS disturbance, collapse, and death. Other drugs that can be used to treat trichomoniasis are ronidazole, carnidazole, and metronidazole; it is not usually necessary to treat the secondary bacteria in cases of trichomoniasis. The treatment of individual birds with candidiasis should include an antifungal agent such as nystatin (300,000 IU/kg p/o q12h for 10 days).

DISCUSSION. Occasional false negatives are found when examining crop washes from live birds. As trichomonads die and disintegrate a few hours after the death of the bird or after a crop wash is taken, only fresh samples are suitable for diagnosis of this disease. A wet film will show the highly motile trichomonads, and a Gram or Diff Quik stain of a mucosal scrape will reveal the yeast typical of *Candida* species. The lesions of both diseases are heavily infiltrated with a mixed population of secondary bacteria.

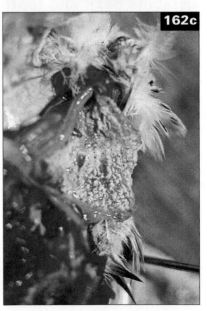

Case 163: **Egg related peritonitis in a budgerigar**

CLINICAL PRESENTATION. An approximately six-year-old female 38 g budgerigar presented with a history of labored breathing. The bird had exhibited a gradual onset of lethargy and weakness, with a recent development of dyspnea. The bird shared a cage with another female budgerigar, which appeared normal. The birds were fed a seed diet supplemented with fruits and vegetables. Physical examination revealed abdominal enlargement and dyspnea. Abdominal palpation suggested the presence of fluid in the abdominal cavity.

INVESTIGATION. Whole body radiographs revealed a fluid-filled abdomen with loss of detail and cranial displacement of the proventriculus and ventriculus, which contained grit. An abdominocentesis easily produced a yellow, slightly turbid fluid. The specific gravity of the fluid was 1032. A smear of the fluid was stained with Wright's stain (**163**).

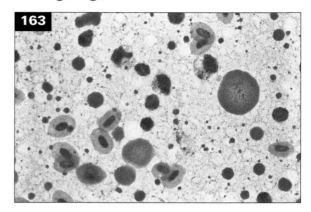

DIAGNOSIS. The smear is moderately cellular and contains erythrocytes, macrophages, and heterophils; the blue granules are either a staining or a photographic artefact. The slightly heavy background material contains round vacuoles or droplets suggestive of lipid material, and small to large basophilic globular material suggestive of protein aggregates. The cytology is compatible with a mixed cell inflammation as seen with egg related peritonitis.

ETIOLOGY. Egg related peritonitis can be associated with an ectopic ovulation (i.e. failure of the ovum to enter the infundibulum), rupture of the oviduct, or salpingitis. The condition may be either nonseptic or be septic in association with a septic salpingitis or secondary infection.

MANAGEMENT. Dyspneic birds should be provided with a warm, oxygen-rich environment. Abdominocentesis should be performed to remove a sufficient volume of fluid from the abdominal cavity to relieve the dyspnea. Parenteral fluids, broad-spectrum antibiotics and antiinflammatory drugs should be provided. Low doses of corticosteroids for 2–3 days will help to reduce the inflammation. In severe cases, or in cases that are unresponsive to medical treatment, it may be necessary to perform a laparotomy and abdominal lavage.

Case 164: **Psittacine beak and feather disease (PBFD) (circovirus infection) and polyomavirus infection (budgerigar fledgeling disease).**

CLINICAL PRESENTATION. Advice was sought because a small proportion of budgerigars in a collection showed poor plumage and areas of feather loss affecting the body, tail, and wings. Affected young birds failed to grow to full adult size (**164**). Apart from the feather abnormalities and small size, the birds appeared well and active.

DIFFERENTIAL DIAGNOSES. This is likely to be either PBFD (circovirus infection) or polyomavirus infection (budgerigar fledgeling disease).

INVESTIGATION. Commercially available PCR tests were performed using blood or feather pulp for PBFD and a cloacal swab for budgerigar fledgeling disease.

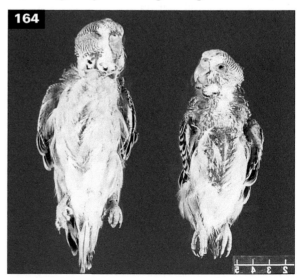

DIAGNOSIS. Birds showing clinical signs and testing positive for PBFD have the disease, which will persist for the rest of their lives, with progressive feather loss. Birds with no lesions but a positive test may be transient carriers and should be retested 90 days later.

Polyomavirus-positive birds may have the disease, may develop the disease, or may remain as infectious carriers for the rest of their lives.

Immunoperoxidase staining can be also be used to confirm the diagnosis.

ETIOLOGY. Unlike the larger members of the Order Psittaciformes, budgerigars with PBFD do not appear to develop beak and claw lesions. The disease is infectious, but appears to spread only slowly in a breeding colony.

Polyomavirus also causes an acute disease of neonatal budgerigars, characterized by a high mortality rate that can reach 100%.

MANAGEMENT. With larger parrots kept in pairs or small groups, it is suggested that affected and contact birds are culled, unless they are an endangered species. However, with the studs of exhibition budgerigars kept communally, this would involve culling the whole stud.

Psittacine birds should be tested for PBFD and polyomavirus before being introduced into a collection. As the PBFD virus has been found in pigeons and doves, new birds of these species should also be tested to see if they are infected.

Case 165: **Articular gout/bacterial arthritis in a budgerigar**

CLINICAL PRESENTATION. A five-year-old male budgerigar presented with lameness and articular swelling of the foot and intertarsal joint (**165**). Whitish material could be seen through the skin.

DIFFERENTIAL DIAGNOSES. Articular gout or bacterial arthritis.

INVESTIGATION. In order to confirm a diagnosis, material was collected for further examination.

In cases of articular gout, the whitish material looks macroscopically like toothpaste. The presence of urate crystals can be confirmed by performing a murexide test. A drop of nitric acid is mixed with a small amount of the suspected material on a slide and dried by evaporation in a Bunsen flame. After cooling, one drop of concentrated ammonia is added. In the presence of urate, a mauve color will develop. Alternatively, a polarizing microscope can be used to identify urate crystals.

In cases of bacterial arthritis, bacteria and white blood cells can be identified in a smear prepared for cytologic examination. The bacteria can be isolated and identified by culture.

MANAGEMENT. A chronic renal disorder or a high-protein diet should be suspected in cases of articular gout. Fluid balance and vitamin A status should be checked (history and physical examination) and corrected when necessary. A low-protein diet is recommended. Treatment with allopurinol and probenecid is controversial, but has been used

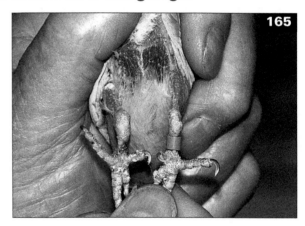

successfully by some clinicians. High doses of allopurinol have been shown to induce gout in red-tailed hawks. Probenecid is contraindicated in birds. In man the uricosuric action of probenicid is based on reduced absorption of uric acid in the tubuli, although glomerular secretion is also slightly inhibited. Since birds lack the resorptive mechanism for uric acid, and uric acid excretion is mainly based on active secretion by the tubuli, the net effect of the use of probenicid in birds might even be a reduced uric acid excretion.

Following antimicrobial sensitivity testing, bacterial pododermatitis should be treated with a combination of antibiotics and surgery.

Case 166: **Trichomoniasis in a group of budgerigars**

CLINICAL PRESENTATION. Five adult budgerigars of varying ages and three juveniles (fledgelings) from a large aviary presented with a history of regurgitation and weight loss. The aviary had been experiencing a disease outbreak characterized by a sudden onset high morbidity and low mortality. The eight birds were submitted for diagnostic evaluation of the flock problem. The affected birds exhibited evidence of regurgitation, with accumulation of regurgitated material on the feathers surrounding the mouth and on the head.

INVESTIGATION. A crop aspirate for cytologic evaluation was performed on all eight birds and the cytologic findings were identical (166).

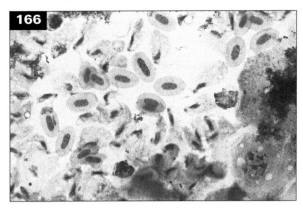

DIAGNOSIS. The smear is highly cellular and contains numerous pale blue-staining, piriform-shaped cells, each with a prominent nucleus, eosinophilic flagella, eosinophilic undulating membrane, and axostyle. The cells are indicative of trichomonad protozoa and a cytodiagnosis of trichomoniasis.

MANAGEMENT. Nitroimidazole drugs such as metronidazole (10–30 mg/kg p/o q12h for 10 days), dimetridazole (1 × 5 ml measure per 3.8 litres [1 teaspoon per gallon] of drinking water for 7 days), and carnidazole (100–200 mg/kg p/o once) are usually effective in the treatment of trichomoniasis. Treatment in the drinking water or food, which is a better route for budgerigars, is necessary for flock problems.

Case 167: **Megabacteria, otherwise known as avian gastric yeast or *Macrorhabdus ornithogaster*, in some budgerigars**

CLINICAL PRESENTATION. A budgerigar fancier reported that a small proportion of his birds had been losing weight and dying over the past two months. A few of the diseased birds had vomited and some had diarrhea.

INVESTIGATION. A postmortem examination of one bird showed enlargement and pallor of the proventriculus (167a, b).

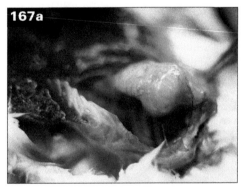

DIAGNOSIS. As a number of birds are affected, the condition is likely to be gastric yeast infection (167c). Other causes of proventricular dilatation are likely to affect only individual birds at any one time.

ETIOLOGY. Care must be taken in diagnosing flock problems from a single postmortem examination, as the bird examined may not be typical of the problem. Diagnosis in live birds depends on demonstration of the organism in crop washes or feces, but the number of organisms in these sites may be small. There is no way of distinguishing the carrier state from the clinical disease except on the basis of the clinical signs, but the bird could be ill due to another disease. After death, a postmortem examination will reveal proventricular dilatation and a degree of thickening at the proventricular–ventricular junction, often with

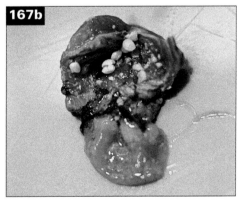

ulceration. There is an excess of mucus in the otherwise usually empty proventriculus. Gram-stained films of this mucus will reveal the organisms in large numbers. The contents of the proventriculus will be about pH neutral instead of the normal pH of 0.7–2, since affected birds do not produce hydrochloric acid.

MANAGEMENT. A 10-day course of a high dose (0.5 mg per budgerigar) of amphotericin B given orally at least twice a day will eliminate the organism; however, about half the birds will not recover clinically due to residual proventricular damage. Acidification of the drinking water with hydrochloric, citric, or acetic acid is effective in some flock situations, but often the birds, which originate from the desert, drink insufficient acidified water for it to to be therapeutic. Megabacteriosis is extremely common in exhibition budgerigars in the UK.

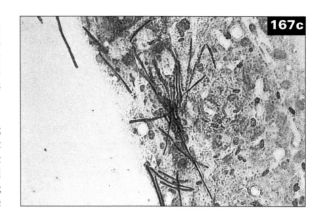

Case 168: **Atoxoplasmosis in a canary**

CLINICAL PRESENTATION. A young canary presented with an enlarged liver that could be seen as a blue spot at the right side of the abdomen caudal to the sternum (**168a**).

INVESTIGATION. Necropsy revealed an enlarged, spotted liver.

DIAGNOSIS. The most likely diagnosis is atoxoplasmosis, which is referred to by fanciers as 'thick liver disease'. The diagnosis can be confirmed with impression smears of the liver, spleen, and lungs. The parasites are found in the cytoplasm of the monocytes (**168b**). The nucleus of the host cell is crescent shaped. Coccidia are seldom found in the feces.

ETIOLOGY. Atoxoplasmosis is caused by *Isospora serini*, a coccidium with an asexual life cycle in the organs and a sexual cycle in the intestinal mucosa.

MANAGEMENT. The therapeutic agent of choice is sulfachlor–pyrazin (150 mg/l drinking water administered until after moulting for 5 days per week) or toltrazuril (2 mg/l for 2 consecutive days per week). This treatment affects only the production of oocysts and has no effect on the intracellular stages. Additional measures include feeding one part egg food and one part seed mixture to neonates until after moulting. Population control and improved hygiene are recommended.

DISCUSSION. This disease is found in young canaries, 2–9 months old. It is also a common problem in other captive European finches. In the acute phase of the disease, a huge, dark red spleen and, often, an edematous duodenum with vascularization are seen on necropsy.

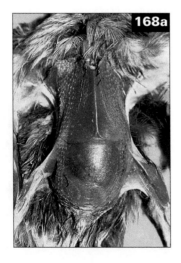

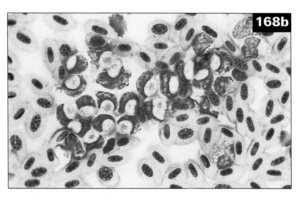

Case 169: **Feather cysts in a canary**

CLINICAL PRESENTATION. A canary presented with abnormal plumage (**169**).

DIAGNOSIS. Feather cysts.

ETIOLOGY. Cysts occurring in the body feathers of canaries often have a familial pattern and are thought to be inherited, although this is not well-documented. They may occur secondary to traumatic or infectious damage. Cysts occurring in the flight feathers of other birds, especially cockatiels, are usually the result of traumatic damage to the follicle.

In this case the cysts involve only body feathers. The lesion consists of a grossly swollen follicle containing a balled-up, ingrown feather that has curled around and not emerged. Such lesions often have large amounts of keratin debris in the follicle of the feather.

MANAGEMENT. In the case of a single cyst of a flight feather, the affected follicle may be carefully incised, the feather and debris removed, and the follicle left to heal by second intention. This treatment often results in recurrence of the cyst, in which case the whole follicle must be removed surgically.

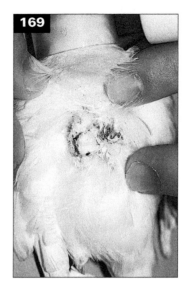

In canaries, there are often multiple cysts occurring in a single feather tract. In severe cases the whole affected feather tract may need to be removed.

Case 170: *Yersinia pseudotuberculosis* (or, less likely, *Salmonella typhimurium*) infection in a flock of canaries

CLINICAL PRESENTATION. A flock of canaries presented with ruffling of the feathers, debilitation, and high mortality.

INVESTIGATION. At necropsy, a dark, swollen, congested liver and spleen, with small, yellow, focal granulomas, was found (**170**). Impression smears were prepared from all the organs and these revealed the presence of many rod-shaped bacteria.

DIAGNOSIS. The most likely diagnosis is infection with *Y. pseudotuberculosis* (or, less likely, *Salmonella typhimurium*), which is regularly seen in canaries of all ages during the winter months. The clinical signs are not specific. In addition to those mentioned above, an acute catarrhal pneumonia and a typhlitis may be present. The diagnosis is confirmed after culturing the microorganisms.

MANAGEMENT. The mostly commonly effective antibiotics are trimethoprim (with or without sulfa), amoxycillin, or enrofloxacin via the drinking water or soft food. Once sensitivity test results are obtained, the antibiotic may need to be changed. Cleaning and disinfection are essential to prevent a relapse after therapy has been completed.

A connection has been suggested between contamination of food supplies by rodents and yersiniosis. Although serotypes are often similar between rodent and avian *Yersinia* species, no definite link has ever been proven. It is also likely that infection may occur through contact between infected feral birds and captive birds. In view of this contact and access by rodents to birds or their food supplies, control of these factors is necessary.

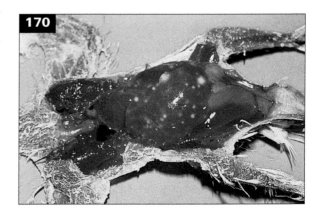

Case 171: **Air sacculitis and splenomegaly in a mynah bird**

CLINICAL PRESENTATION. A freshly imported mynah bird presented with a history of respiratory distress, vomiting, and weight loss.

INVESTIGATION. Laparoscopy was performed. The tip of the endoscope is within the abdominal air sac (**171**). The organ identified (1) is the spleen. The spleen of a mynah bird is bean shaped and more elongated, as in finches and pigeons. Its color should be purple to brownish-red (as in psittacines) and normally it is half the size of the spleen seen in this mynah bird.

Because air sacculitis was observed, a swab was taken from the air sac for Gram staining and culture. *Pseudomonas* species was isolated from the air sac and from a fecal swab.

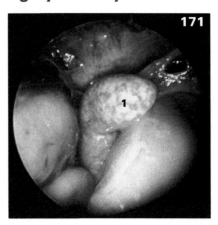

DIAGNOSIS. The symptomatic diagnosis is air sacculitis and splenomegaly. The etiological diagnosis is *Pseudomonas* species infection.

A diagnosis cannot be made by visualization of the organs alone. The discoloration and enlargement of the spleen is often seen in connection with septicemia. During the endoscopic examination, special attention should be given to the liver, air sacs, and kidneys. If the liver is enlarged, a biopsy would be a good choice to diagnose hemochromatosis.

MANAGEMENT. Enrofloxacin was administered i/m following the laparoscopic procedure. The bird recovered in three days.

DISCUSSION. Before undertaking laparoscopy, careful consideration must be given as to whether the patient's suspected problem might cause complications during the procedure. Ascites, for example, which is often seen in mynah birds due to hemochromatosis, greatly increases the potential risk of the procedure due to flooding of the air sacs and drowning.

Case 172: **Radiography of a mynah bird with severe dyspnea**

CLINICAL PRESENTATION. An anorexic mynhah bird presented with severe dyspnea (**172**).

INVESTIGATION. A dorsoventral radiograph was taken. It showed generalized abdominal enlargement and a piece of metal wire visible in the region of the left thoracic air sac, lung, and abdomen.

ETIOLOGY. The bird could have ingested the wire, which may then have caused peritonitis and ascites. Alternatively, the wire could be within the pectoral muscle and not within the abdomen. In the latter case the abdominal enlargement might indicate hepatomegaly and ascites due to hemochromatosis.

DISCUSSION. All cases should be radiographed from two views at a 90° angle to each other. A barium contrast (applied directly into the proventriculus p/o using a male dog urinary catheter in an anesthetized patient) and/or ultrasound would confirm the liver size.

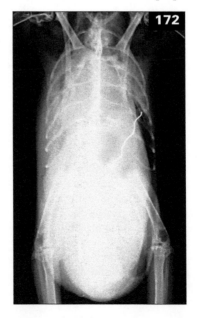

Case 173: **Paramyxovirus 1 infection in a loft of pigeons**

CLINICAL PRESENTATION. Profuse, watery diarrhea (**173**) was reported in a loft of pigeons. A high proportion of late-bred young birds were affected. In addition to the diarrhea, a few late-bred young birds exhibited nervous signs such as circling, incoordination, ataxia, and torticollis. The adult birds and young racing birds had been vaccinated against paramyxovirus 1 and had been treated for coccidiosis, worms, and trichomoniasis. The late-bred young birds had received no vaccination or other medication.

DIFFERENTIAL DIAGNOSES. Paramyxovirus 1 infection. Other conditions to be considered include *Salmonella typhimurium* infection, inclusion body hepatitis associated with a herpesvirus or adenovirus, the motile protozoal organisms *Hexamita columbae* and *Trichomonas gallinae*, and rotavirus and circovirus. Nematodes, cestodes, and trematodes may also cause diarrhea, and chlamydophilosis as a cause of diarrhea in young birds is not uncommon.

DIAGNOSIS. The most likely cause is paramyxovirus 1 infection. The diagnosis can be confirmed by combinations of isolating paramyxovirus 1 from tissues such as brain and intestine; demonstrating high antibody titres to paramyxovirus 1 in unvaccinated birds; and detecting histologic changes consistent with a viral encephalitis and interstitial nephritis.

ETIOLOGY. Paramyxovirus 1 infection can result in the sudden onset of watery diarrhea in a high proportion of susceptible birds. The feces consists of a clear pool of urine with a central core of green material originating from the digestive tract (**173**). When this becomes mixed by the movement of birds, a 'green diarrhea' results.

Also, affected birds are usually thirsty and a proportion develop a range of nervous signs including torticollis, inability to fly, circling, ataxia, and inability to pick up feed. When the birds are stressed, the severity of the nervous signs increases. Mortality is usually low except in young birds, but some do not fully recover from the nervous signs and must be culled.

DISCUSSION. Although pigeons must now be vaccinated prior to racing or showing, young late-bred pigeons, which are too young to race, may be left unvaccinated with the intention of vaccinating them along with adult birds later in the year. Should the racing teams of pigeons encounter paramyxovirus during transportation or racing, they may bring the organism back into the loft, resulting in infection and clinical disease in the in-contact, unvaccinated late-bred birds. An increased incidence of paramyxovirus from August to November has been observed in the UK over several years.

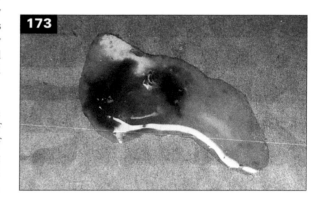

Case 174: **Trichomoniasis in a pigeon squab**

CLINICAL PRESENTATION. A pigeon squab presented with an umbilical infection (**174**).

DIAGNOSIS. Trichomoniasis.

ETIOLOGY. Trichomoniasis can also affect the upper GI tract, the liver, and the heart (endocarditis) of pigeons. The respiratory system (bifurcation of the trachea) has been reported to be affected in psittacines and raptors, in addition to the organ systems found in pigeons.

MANAGEMENT. The disease in squabs can be prevented by treatment of the parent birds with a nitroimidazole derivative (ronidazole, carnidazole, dimetridazole,

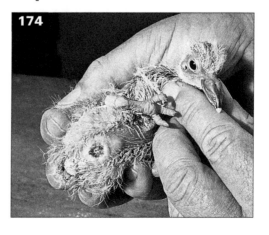

metronidazole) during incubation of the eggs, between days six and twelve. However, resistance problems have been reported in the Netherlands, possibly due to subtherapeutic drug dosages being given by pigeon fanciers during the racing season. *In vitro* studies have revealed that a fivefold dose of the recommended ronidazole dosage is effective in these cases; experimental pigeons have tolerated a tenfold dose. Other nitroimidazole drugs should not be given in dosages higher than those recommended by the manufacturer. Dimetridazole is well known for its toxic side-effects (neurologic signs). Overdosing occurs when pigeons drink more medicated water than usual (i.e. when feeding squabs or during warm weather).

Case 175: **Self-trauma of the breast feathers in a racing pigeon**

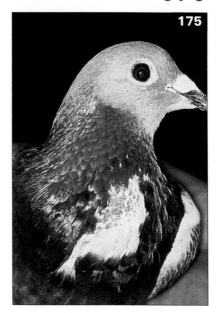

CLINICAL PRESENTATION. A racing pigeon presented with alopecia in the breast region due to a traumatic loss of feathers (**175**).

DIAGNOSIS. The fractures of the feather shaft are thought to be caused by rubbing the breast on the sharp edges of the drinking pan.

ETIOLOGY. This condition is seen especially in nervous male pigeons who show aggressiveness towards other males trying to approach the drinking pans. This 'nervous behaviour' causes repeated friction of the throat area over the sharp edges of the drinking pans.

MANAGEMENT. Treatment of the condition is by pulling out the broken shafts, after which the feathers will regrow in three weeks. At the same time, the number of drinking pans should be increased and the sharp edges covered with a plastic tube that has a longitudinal slit on one side. The level of the water in the pans should be raised.

Case 176: *Cnemidocoptes laevis* infestation in a racing pigeon

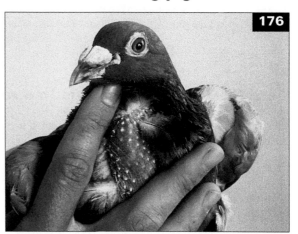

CLINICAL PRESENTATION. A racing pigeon presented with alopecia in the breast region due to a parasitic loss of feathers (**176**).

INVESTIGATION/DIAGNOSIS. The feather follicle and the thickened base of the feather shaft was brushed with a scalpel blade onto a microscopic slide. The parasite *Cnemidocoptes laevis* was found.

ETIOLOGY. Infection of other pigeons occurs through direct contact. The environment is not thought to be a reservoir for reinfestation.

MANAGEMENT. Treatment with ivermectin is unsuccessful. After degreasing the plumage in a warm detergent solution, affected pigeons can be bathed in a 0.15% trichlorfon solution and left to dry in a warm environment. Treatment can be repeated after 10 days.

Case 177: **Salmonellosis (paratyphoid) in a pigeon loft**

CLINICAL PRESENTATION. A pigeon loft owner reported multiple problems in his loft of racing pigeons including birds with swollen hock or wing joints, increased numbers of dead-in-shells and clear eggs, mortality in young squabs, and diarrhea with marked weight loss. An occasional bird exhibited nervous signs such as twisting of the neck (**177**) and difficulty feeding.

DIFFERENTIAL DIAGNOSES. Salmonellosis, poisoning, paramyxovirus 1 infection.

DIAGNOSIS. The history and clinical signs are typical of salmonellosis (i.e. paratyphoid, usually involving *Salmonella typhimurium* phage type 2 or 99).

MANAGEMENT. Treatment of all the birds in the loft with an antibacterial in the drinking water should be initiated. Suitable antibacterials include amoxycillin (1 g/l of water for 7 days), combined trimethoprim and sulfamethoxazole (20 mg trimethoprim and 100 mg sulfamethoxazole per litre of water for 10 days) or enrofloxacin (200 mg/l of water for 10 days).

The first course of antimicrobials may be unsuccessful in eliminating the organism from the flock; pooled feces from the birds should be screened for *Salmonella* species following treatment, with the possibility of repeat medication. Medication should be combined with effective disinfection of the loft, feeders, drinkers, nest bowls, etc. Severely affected birds should be culled if no signs of improvement are seen. Control measures should aim to reduce the risks of *Salmonella* species entering the loft, to reduce the effects of the *Salmonella* species should it gain entry to the loft, and should include loft monitoring for salmonellosis. The most likely source of *Salmonella* species is another pigeon, so steps should be taken to prevent stray or feral pigeons entering the loft. Good hygiene and avoiding overcrowding will reduce the subsequent spread of the organism. The use of an

inactivated *Salmonella* species vaccine has also been found to reduce spread in an infected loft. Strategic *Salmonella* species monitoring of pooled loft feces, prior to pairing up, should be part of the normal loft routine.

DISCUSSION. It is important to differentiate salmonellosis clinically from other causes of nervous disease in pigeons. Nervous signs may also be seen in pigeons that have been poisoned (e.g. by agricultural chemicals, alpha-chloralose, or the therapeutic agent dimetridazole). The history of access to such poisons would help in such a diagnosis. However, the most common condition to be considered in the differential diagnoses is paramyxovirus 1 infection. In lofts with this infection there is usually a higher proportion of birds with diarrhea and nervous signs than in lofts with salmonellosis, and the diarrhea with paramyxovirus is usually more watery. Loss of weight and appetite is more severe in cases of salmonellosis; swelling of the joints is a feature of salmonellosis, not paramyxovirus.

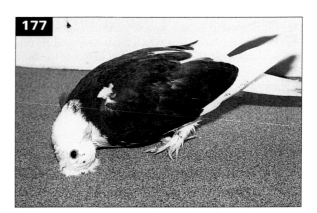

Case 178: **Bacterial arthritis in a racing pigeon**

CLINICAL PRESENTATION. A racing pigeon presented with a swelling in the region of the elbow joint (**178**).

DIFFERENTIAL DIAGNOSES. Bacterial arthritis, fracture, luxation, hematoma, tumor, and feather cyst. Clinical signs seen in other birds in the loft may include torticollis, diarrhea, skin abscesses, infertile eggs, and mortality.

INVESTIGATION/DIAGNOSIS. A tentative diagnosis of bacterial arthritis can be confirmed by culture of a

pooled fecal sample from the loft or by serologic examination if the pigeon has not been vaccinated against *Salmonella typhimurium*. Synovial culture of the elbow joint is often disappointing.

ETIOLOGY. The two most likely causes of bacterial arthritis are *Salmonella typhimurium* var. *kopenhagen* and *Streptococcus bovis* infection. Arthritis of the elbow joint is pathognomonic for salmonellosis in racing pigeons.

Streptococcus bovis is widespread in asymptomatic

pigeons (facultative pathogen), but may cause lameness of the wings (tenosynovitis of *M. supracoracoideus*) or limbs, emaciation, green slimy excreta, palpable areas of necrosis in the pectoral muscle, meningitis, and septicemia. Isolation of the organism requires special conditions (i.e. enrichment medium and Slanetz and Bartley agar).

MANAGEMENT. The whole flock should be treated with trimethoprim and sulfamethoxazole (50 mg/kg and 10 mg/kg q24h, respectively). Use of an inactivated vaccine should be considered for future prevention. The recommended treatment in cases with both clinical signs and isolation of *S. bovis* is ampicillin (175 mg/kg q24h [2 g/l drinking water] for 5 days).

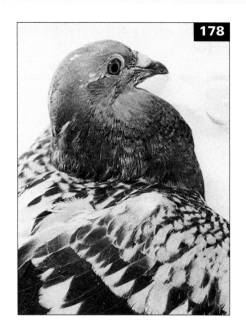

Case 179: **Human head louse infestation**

CLINICAL PRESENTATION. A pet dove presented because the owner was concerned that the bird might have been the cause of the 'bugs' on her own head. The dove was apparently healthy and free of obvious ectoparasites.

INVESTIGATION. One of the parasites from the owner's head was examined under the microscope (179).

DIAGNOSIS. The specimen examined is the human head louse (*Pediculus humanus* var. *capitis*).

MANAGEMENT. Treatment of the dove is not necessary as lice are generally species specific.

DISCUSSION. This can be a delicate situation. Although the dove is not the source of the infestation, it is not appropriate to advise the client as to how to control her own condition. The suggestion should be made diplomatically that she should seek advice from her own doctor. A variety of products have been used in humans including lindane and carbaryl.

Reinfestation will not be a problem for the dove. Human health workers can advise the owner on personal and environmental hygiene.

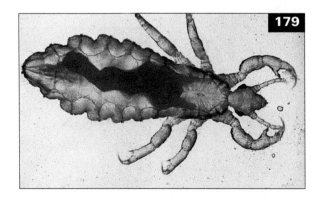

Case 180: **Duck virus enteritis (duck plague) in a group of Muscovy ducks**

CLINICAL PRESENTATION. During the spring breeding season, a Muscovy duck owned by a breeder presented with signs of neck weakness, drooped wings, and bloody diarrhea (**180a**). Some of the ducks in the group had died. The breeder reported that during the previous week she had observed some sick migratory waterfowl, which showed signs of ataxia, bloody nasal discharge, and acute death.

DIFFERENTIAL DIAGNOSES. Differentials include duck virus enteritis, duck virus hepatitis, pasteurellosis, necrotic enteritis, and toxicosis (e.g. lead poisoning).

INVESTIGATION. Initial diagnostic tests included necropsy and histopathology. At necropsy, petechiae and ecchymotic lesions were observed in the myocardium and visceral organs. Elevated white/yellow plaques were observed under the tongue and in the esophagus and intestinal lining (**180b**). Hemorrhagic annular bands were observed in the small intestine (**180c**).

DIAGNOSIS. The lesions are consistent with duck virus enteritis. The diagnosis can be confirmed on histopathology and viral isolation.

ETIOLOGY. Transmission of duck virus enteritis is direct or indirect, with an incubation period of 3–7 days. Muscovy ducks are very sensitive to this virus and call ducks (the smallest breed of domestic duck) are resistant. As the infection is caused by a herpesvirus, any surviving birds may become persistently infected and shed virus.

MANAGEMENT. Management should include removal of affected birds and all in-contact birds, and vaccination of adjacent captive populations. The collection should be vaccinated the following year two weeks prior to the disease outbreak as experienced in the current year.

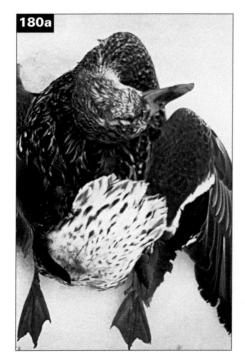

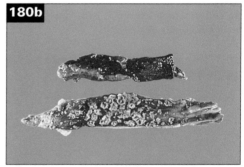

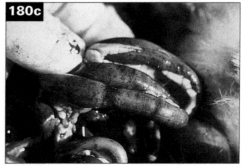

Case 181: **Brooder pneumonia in a duckling**

CLINICAL PRESENTATION. A two-week-old duckling presented because of increased open-mouthed breathing and lethargy (181a). The chick was very dyspneic and easily distressed.

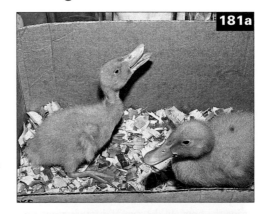

INVESTIGATION. Since the bird was easily stressed, oxygen was administered prior to slow induction with isoflurane anesthetic to enable a tracheal examination and radiography. An abdominal air sac tube was placed to help relieve the dyspnea. Enquiries were made as to how many other ducklings were affected and what sort of brooder and rearer equipment was being used.

DIAGNOSIS. The radiograph (181b) revealed pulmonary densities that were suggestive of aspergillosis lesions.

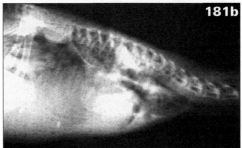

ETIOLOGY. Brooder pneumonia is caused by humid, cramped conditions with suboptimal ventilation.

MANAGEMENT. Treatment involves the setting of only clean eggs and the cleansing of egg shells prior to incubation (e.g. by UV light), together with improved brooder conditions and the administration of antifungal agents such as itraconazole to affected birds. The prognosis for affected young ducklings is poor.

Case 182: **Frostbite in a duck**

CLINICAL PRESENTATION. A duck presented with dry gangrene and loss of tissue from the extremity of its foot (182).

DIAGNOSIS. Frostbite.

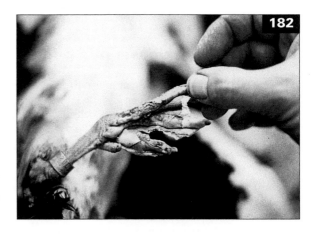

ETIOLOGY. Dry gangrene of the extremities, as seen in mammals, has not been recorded in birds. Ergot poisoning has not been reported in birds.

Waterfowl are most commonly affected by frostbite in this manner. Waterfowl lose heat by panting or heat exchange through their limbs. However, most waterfowl are remarkably tolerant of frost effects, particularly if they have open water to swim in. When sedentary, they tend to squat down, sitting on their feet in order to maintain temperature. Species endogenous to warm climates, but kept in temperate areas, are most susceptible.

Flamingos and other long-limbed birds, being unable to sit on their feet to maintain heat, simply reduce peripheral circulation. Although they often avoid frostbite, the long-term effect of poor pedal circulation is a marked deterioration in dermal quality, leading to cracking and low-grade bacterial infections.

MANAGEMENT. The condition can be avoided by either not keeping warm climate birds in cold areas, or by keeping them inside during extreme weather. Even in such circumstances, water temperature may have to be artificially raised, although water hygiene can be a problem if large numbers are housed together inside.

Case 183: **Duck virus enteritis ('duck plaque')**

CLINICAL PRESENTATION. The carcass of a duck that had died acutely, with a hemorrhagic cloacal discharge, was presented by the breeder (**183**). The same problem had occurred on this breeder's premises in three successive years, during April to June, with significant mortality in Muscovy ducks, Carolina (wood) ducks, blue-winged teal, and mallards, but cranes and call ducks had not been affected.

DIAGNOSIS. Duck virus enteritis ('duck plague').

ETIOLOGY. Duck virus enteritis is caused by a herpesvirus. Herpesviruses are enveloped, tending to be well-adapted to a particular species. The virus can survive for extended periods outside the body. In the case of duck virus enteritis, the virus can survive in water for up to one month. Individual birds that are not killed by the infection tend to develop lifelong latent infection with periodic recrudescence. The virus replicates in the cells lining the gut wall, forming characteristic intranuclear inclusion bodies. Spread may be vertical or horizontal. Infection can spread directly from cell to cell within the body, thereby avoiding circulating antibodies and leading to persistent infection.

MANAGEMENT. Herpesvirus vaccination will not currently prevent infection, but it will reduce the severity of infection. Also, vaccination will not prevent spread of the virus. Acyclovir can be used successfully in infected birds (10–40 mg/kg i/v or s/c q8h) or as prophylaxis in the face of an outbreak (80 mg/kg p/o q8h). If there are recurrent outbreaks of infection, all surviving in-contact birds should be euthanased or isolated to prevent subsequent recontamination of the environment (especially at times of stress).

DISCUSSION. Herpesviruses of the same family that cause duck virus enteritis are responsible for disease in other groups of birds such as psittacines, pigeons, poultry, and raptors (e.g. Pacheco's disease, as well as choanal and cloacal papillomas [caused by three separate serotypes of herpesvirus]; Amazon tracheitis virus; parakeet herpesvirus; herpesvirus-associated wart-like skin lesions [in cockatoos and macaws]; pigeon herpesvirus [causing inclusion body hepatitis]; Marek's disease [affecting poultry as well as other species]; falcon, eagle, and owl herpesvirus).

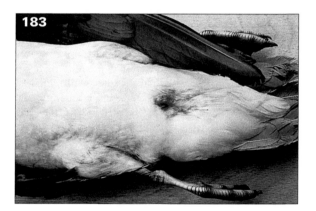

Case 184: **Oil toxicosis in a goose**

CLINICAL PRESENTATION. A goose presented that had been found on the shore of a local pond where oil had been dumped. Although the goose was weak, dehydrated, and covered in oil, it was alert and responsive (**184**).

DIAGNOSIS. Oil toxicosis.

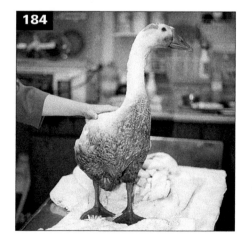

MANAGEMENT. The principal concernes of oil toxicosis are destruction of waterproofing and the insulatory properties of the plumage; diarrhea arising due to GI irritation following the ingestion of oil during preening; hemolytic anemia; hypothermia; and pneumonia (bacterial or fungal) due to immune suppression or inhalation of oil.

Treatment should include heat, supportive care, activated charcoal to inhibit the absorption of ingested oil, and, once stabilized, frequent high pressure (preferably 90 psi/620 kNm²), warm (40–45°C [104–113°F]) mild detergent baths and clean warm water rinses until the water coming off the feathers 'beads' freely. The birds should then be placed in a flow of warm air until dry. It is normal to maintain birds in captivity on self-skimming ponds for several days after washing to ensure that waterproofing is secure.

Case 185: **'Slipped' or 'angel' wing in a young goose**

CLINICAL PRESENTATION. A young goose presented with a problem involving the wings (**185**).

DIAGNOSIS. 'Slipped' or 'angel' wing. This condition involves an outward rotation of the carpal joint or the major metacarpal bone.

ETIOLOGY. Slipped wing is caused by the weight of the growing flight feathers placing an excessive force on the muscles and ligaments of the carpal area. The condition is most common in fast growing species such as geese, which would normally feed by grazing on grass and other vegetation. It is more common in males and is always seen during the blood feather growth phase. Manganese and vitamin D_3 deficiencies have been implicated, but genetics and in particular growth management have a greater role. Grazing birds typically eat grass having a crude protein content of 17–18%. If they are given a higher protein content grower pellet with a protein content greater than 18%, they will grow faster than they were designed to and slipped wing will occur.

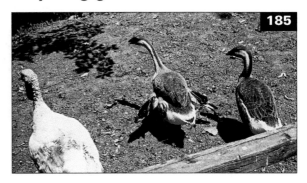

MANAGEMENT. Treatment involves the application, preferably within 24–48 hours of occurrence, of a figure-of-eight bandage to bring the primaries back against the wing itself. Such a dressing, if combined with nutritional restriction, will result in a correction in 3–4 days. If a mature bird is presented with this abnormality, it may be corrected by cutting the major metacarpal bone and introducing a pin into the medulla. The lateral rotation along the length of the metacarpal bone is corrected and the bone allowed to heal prior to pin removal.

Case 186: **Avian tuberculosis in a goose**

CLINICAL PRESENTATION. A Hawaiian (Nene) goose from a sizeable collection of mixed waterfowl presented for necropsy. Multiple white lesions were observed in the liver (**186**).

DIFFERENTIAL DIAGNOSES. The differentials in order of probability are avian tuberculosis (*Mycobacterium avium*), pseudotuberculosis (*Yersinia* species), and lymphosarcoma.

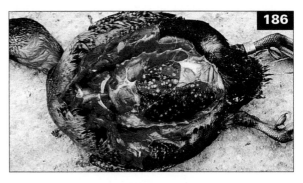

INVESTIGATION. The presence of acid-fast bacilli was confirmed by modified Ziehl–Neelsen stained impression smears of affected tissue, and by culture of the organism, though this took several weeks.

DIAGNOSIS. Avian tuberculosis caused by *M. avium*.

ETIOLOGY. Avian tuberculosis is highly contagious within a collection due to contamination of the ground by subclinical or preclinical cases, leading to subsequent ingestion of the *M. avium* organisms and potential infection of unaffected birds.

Because infection is generally by the oral route, the method of feeding affects the differential rates of infection in different species of waterfowl. Grazing, dabbling, or diving will affect the potential level of ingestion of infected material while feeding. Ducks that feed around the water margin (dabblers) will ingest the highest numbers of infective organisms. Furthermore, species being kept far from their climatic origin suffer stress as a consequence and hence show an increased incidence. Saltwater species kept on fresh water demonstrate an increased incidence. Certain species (e.g. the white-winged wood duck and Hawaiian goose) are more susceptible to infection, irrespective of the method of husbandry.

The rate of pathogenesis is variable between species. White-winged wood duck typically suffer rapid progress, dying within 2–4 months from the start of the infection, while some swans and geese will show no clinical signs of disease until 2–3 years from onset. However, during this period they may be continually shedding organisms in their feces, leading to high levels of environmental contamination.

Case 187: **Malpositioned flamingo embryos**

DISCUSSION. These two flamingo dead in shell illustrations (**187a, b**) show examples of malpositioned embryos, which are traditionally classified into seven types. Each type of malposition has a different effect on hatching viability:

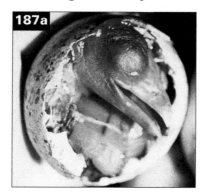
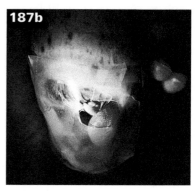

- Malposition 1 (**187a**). The embryo's head is found between the thighs; this is a normal position early in incubation. However, during the last third of incubation the embryo should move its head up and under the right wing. This malposition is always fatal; it can be associated with above normal incubation temperatures.
- Malposition 2. The embryo's head is located in the small end of the egg. The position is lethal in 50% of cases. Assistance in hatching improves the hatching success rate.
- Malposition 3. This occurs when the chick rotates its head under the left wing instead of the right wing. This malposition is nearly always fatal and is associated with malnutrition in laying females, high incubation temperatures, or improper positioning of the egg during incubation.
- Malposition 4. The body is rotated in the long axis of the egg; therefore, the head is away from the air cell and along the side of the egg. Without assistance, this malposition is often fatal, as the embryo never breaks through to breathe.

- Malposition 5. This occurs when the feet are located over the head. Because of this malposition, the limbs are not located properly to kick and cause the body to rotate as the chick is cutting out. Unless hatching is assisted, the results will often prove fatal.
- Malposition 6 (**187b**). The head is over rather than under the right wing. This can still result in a live hatch with few complications.
- Malposition 7. This occurs when the embryo is small or the egg is spherical. The embryo is found lying crosswise in the egg instead of in the normal orientation with the head up near the air cell. This malposition is often fatal.

Case 188: **Avian botulism in a group of waterfowl**

CLINICAL PRESENTATION. During the summer a number of waterfowl that resided on the lake of a city park were found dead on the shore or 'paralysed' (**188**). The lake was shallow and heavily overgrown with foliage.

DIAGNOSIS. Avian botulism (limber neck; alkali duck disease) based on identification of *Clostridium botulinum* type C toxin, which does not affect mammals. This toxin is most commonly found in maggots on carcasses. Serum toxin analysis or mouse inoculation neutralization tests confirm the diagnosis.

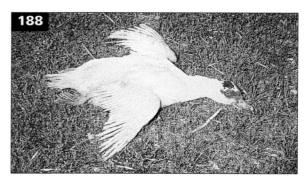

ETIOLOGY. Birds suffer an acute flaccid paralysis of the voluntary muscles, often occurring in mid swim and leading to death by drowning. Outbreaks occur in hot weather due to alkali and anaerobic conditions arising, often in stagnant water. As the water temperature rises, oxygen levels fall, the latter possibly being exacerbated by decaying organic matter in the water. Fish and invertebrate carcasses act as a substrate for clostridial spores and hence

toxin production. The toxin may then become concentrated in maggots that are feeding on the carcass.

MANAGEMENT. If the bird can still walk but not fly, good nursing and supportive care will often be effective. If the bird can swim but not walk, the prognosis is not so good, but it may recover. Therapy involves giving oral fluids with activated charcoal and bismuth. Antitoxins have not been proven to be effective and they are expensive. Control involves the removal of all carcasses from the water, as well as the removal of decaying vegetable material. The toxin is stable in water and the area of water will typically remain contaminated until the increased water flow caused by autumn storms, for example, washes the toxin away. Water flow and oxygenation should be improved if possible. Vaccination yearly with type C toxoid is helpful.

Case 189: **Hemochromatosis (iron storage disease) in a red-breasted toucan**

CLINICAL PRESENTATION. An eight-year-old red-breasted toucan (189) presented for postmortem examination. The bird had been in the collection for five years. It was an aviary bird whose mate appeared healthy. The bird was clinically normal the previous day. On external examination, no abnormalities were noted and the body weight was considered good at 435 g.

DIFFERENTIAL DIAGNOSES. The most likely diagnosis is iron storage disease (hemochromatosis).

INVESTIGATION. Autopsy revealed hepatomegaly. There is often a definite bronzed to bluish hue to the liver. The other abdominal organs were unremarkable, which is generally the case in cases of hemachromatosis.

ETIOLOGY. Cellular damage may or may not result from excessive iron deposition. Organ dysfunction and clinical illness or death may be the result. It is common for a bird to appear clinically healthy prior to acute death.

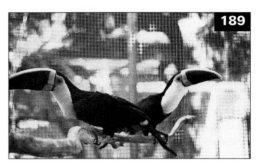

DISCUSSION. The liver is the predominant and frequently the only organ to be affected. Only rarely will iron pigment be identified in tissues other than the liver, but these could include kidney, pancreas, intestine, and lung, in that order of decreasing frequency of involvement. Iron deposition can also occasionally be noted in the spleen.

Case 190: **Hemochromatosis (iron storage disease) in a toco toucan**

CLINICAL PRESENTATION. A toco toucan (190) presented for a physical examination and advice regarding diet and potential medical problems. The client had never owned a toucan before but had owned three Amazon parrots for three years.

DISCUSSION. Diets recommended for toucans contain food elements that are all low in iron. Currently, advised diets are made up of a variety of diced fruits and a free-choice availability of dry, kibbled dog food or a commercially available soft bill diet. Recommended poultry dietary iron levels (40–60 ppm) are used as a guideline for ramphastides. It is recommended that a dry ration with an iron level less than 100 ppm is used. Fruit must be offered in bite size portions as ramphastides, unlike psittacines, do not chew or bite their food. Favorite fruits tend to be grapes, melon, papayas, and berries. Citrus fruits may enhance the bioavailability and subsequent uptake of dietary iron, so limiting the ascorbic acid-containing fruits in the diet is recommended. Toucans that are rearing young should also be offered pinkies, mice, or live foods such as mealworms, and crickets.

The most significant condition affecting many species of toucans is iron storage disease (hemochromatosis). Some species are particularly affected: channel-billed toucan, toco toucan, keel-billed toucan, red-billed toucan, ariel toucan, choco toucan, plate-billed mountain toucan, pale-mandibled aracari, chestnut-eared aracari, black-necked aracari, spot-billed toucanet, saffron toucanet, emerald toucanet.

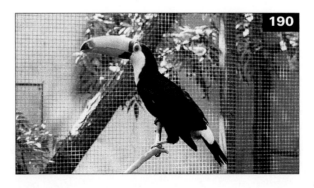

Case 191: **Syngamiasis in a group of pheasants**

CLINICAL PRESENTATION. An eight-week-old pheasant presented for postmortem examination. Affected birds in the group had been 'snicking' (a combination of a sneezing, coughing, and sideways flicking of the head). Some of the birds had been 'gaping' (extending their necks and gasping for breath through their opened beaks).

DIFFERENTIAL DIAGNOSES. Should include syngamiasis, mycoplasmosis, and aspergillosis. Mycoplasmosis is associated with swelling of the infraorbital sinus, between the eye and the nostril and around the eye. In gamebirds with aspergillosis there is usually silent gasping rather than the 'snicking' that occurs in birds with *Syngamus trachea* infection.

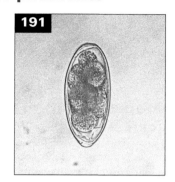

INVESTIGATION. Smears from the proventriculus, small intestine, and cecum showed large numbers of ova (**191**). No adult parasites were found in the digestive tract.

DIAGNOSIS. Syngamiasis (gapeworm) infection.

ETIOLOGY. *S. trachea* is a common nematode parasite found in the trachea of gamebirds. Syngamiasis is most likely to be a problem in gamebirds kept on ground that has carried birds in previous years. The parasite may use a direct life cycle, reinfecting the host species themselves, or use an indirect life-cycle, being taken up by earthworms, slugs, and snails, in which they survive from one year to the next. Wild birds also act as reservoirs of infection.

MANAGEMENT. Medications licensed and effective against *S. trachea* include benzimidazole group anthelmintics and nitroxynil. The benzimidazoles are best administered in the feed; nitroxynil is given in drinking water. Caution must be exercised in using nitroxynil, as it may result in toxicity, kidney damage, and egg production problems. It is not recommended for use in birds over 17 weeks old.

DISCUSSION. Mortality (especially among partridges), loss of weight, weakness, anemia, and reduced egg production may also be seen in syngamiasis.

Case 192: **Pheasant coronavirus infection**

CLINICAL PRESENTATION. High mortality was reported in a pen of adult pheasants that were just commencing egg production. Both sexes were affected, but especially the hens.

DIFFERENTIAL DIAGNOSES. High mortality rates in laying pens can result from coronavirus infection associated with nephritis, the viral condition marble spleen disease, bacterial conditions such as *Erysipelothrix rhusiopathiae* and *Pasteurella multocida* infection, septicemias, predator attacks, and poisoning incidents.

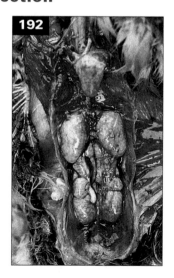

INVESTIGATION/DIAGNOSIS. Postmortem examination revealed a consistent finding of grossly swollen, pale kidneys (**192**), with urates distending the ureters of some birds. Visceral gout was also observed. Histopathology revealed an interstitial nephritis and kidney tubule necrosis, with infiltration by mononuclear inflammatory cells. Serology and virus isolation confirmed a diagnosis of pheasant coronavirus.

ETIOLOGY. This condition has been recognized in the UK since 1983. The disease most often affects adult pheasants in laying pens. Mortality may reach 50%; white diarrhea and reduced egg production may occur. It is believed that pheasants become infected early in life. Clinical disease is caused by the stress of catching and penning or the mobilization of calcium for eggshell formation by the hen pheasants.

MANAGEMENT. Currently there is no known method of control, so treatment can only be of a supportive nature. It is important to ensure easy access to adequate quantities of wholesome drinking water.

DISCUSSION. High mortality rates have been seen in pheasants that have been maliciously poisoned, and in adult pheasants treated with nitroxynil in drinking water to control *Syngamus trachea*. Nitroxynil should never be administered to pheasants over 17 weeks old, as it can result in kidney failure and death if wrongly administered (see *Case 191*).

Case 193: *Capillaria* species infection in a peacock

CLINICAL PRESENTATION. A wild neighborhood peacock presented for treatment of a leg fracture and a health assessment prior to release.

INVESTIGATION. A fecal flotation was performed and moderate numbers of ova were visualized (**193**).

DIAGNOSIS. *Capillaria* species infection.

MANAGEMENT. Treatment of this parasite can be challenging. The parasite often exhibits multiple drug resistance. Fenbendazole (25 mg/kg p/o q24h for 5 days), mebendazole, and ivermectin have been used. Repeat fecal flotations should always be carried out following the discovery of this parasite, to ensure that therapy has been effective.

DISCUSSION. If the peacock is released back into its habitual environment, reinfection is likely. Periodic testing and reworming is recommended.

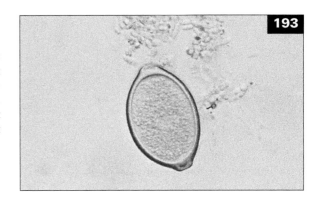

Case 194: **Blackhead in a peafowl**

CLINICAL PRESENTATION. An immature peafowl, which died acutely, presented for postmortem examination. The abdominal contents are shown (**194**).

DIAGNOSIS. Blackhead.

ETIOLOGY. Blackhead is particularly common in turkeys and peafowl. The disease is caused by the protozoan parasite *Histomonas meleagridis*. Young, nonimmune birds ingest *Heterakis gallinae* worms that are infected with *H. meleagridis*.

MANAGEMENT. If available, young birds may be fed a concentrate pellet containing dimetridazole. As most peafowl range freely, eating any garden morsels they can find, they often do not eat sufficient volumes of medicated feed to control the disease. The birds must be shut in daily for sufficient time to allow adequate medicine ingestion. Fecal samples should be screened for *Heterakis gallinae* and treated as required.

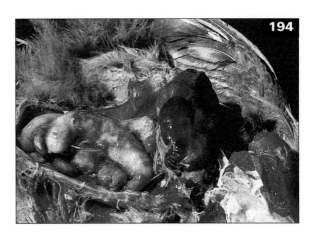

Case 195: **Polyfolliculitis in a lovebird**

CLINICAL PRESENTATION. A lovebird presented with a lesion of the skin between the shoulders (**195**).

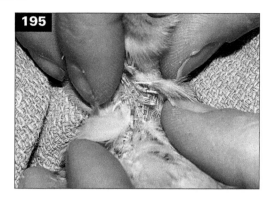

DIAGNOSIS. Polyfolliculitis. There is more than one feather emerging from a single follicle.

ETIOLOGY. This condition is relatively common in lovebirds. They generally present with intense pruritus and self-mutilation. The areas most frequently affected are the axillary and interscapular regions. A viral etiology is suspected but is, as yet, unproven.

MANAGEMENT. The lesions are often secondarily infected, therefore systemic antibiotics are usually indicated. Corticosteroids or NSAIDs may ease the pruritus. A collar can be applied to prevent further self-mutilation until the lesion has healed. However, these measures are only palliative, as the condition often recurs. The surgical removal of affected follicles may reduce the incidence of recurrence. Isolation of affected birds from other lovebirds is recommended.

Case 196: **Ostrich pox**

CLINICAL PRESENTATION. A three-month-old ostrich presented with a lesion involving the proximal dorsal lid of the right eye (**196**).

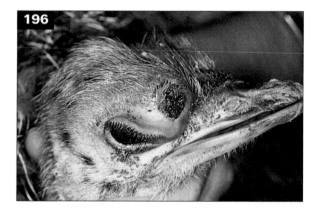

INVESTIGATION/DIAGNOSIS. A histopathologic examination of a biopsy sample of one of the lesions revealed the definitive intracytoplasmic inclusions (called Bollinger bodies) of ostrich pox (cutaneous form).

ETIOLOGY. The condition can be transmitted through blood-borne trauma (e.g. pecking at necrotic bloody lesions) or via arthropod vectors, commonly mosquitoes.

MANAGEMENT. The treatment for this condition can be divided into management and medical:
• Management. Unaffected birds should be removed from the clinical cases and exposure to arthropod vectors reduced. Affected birds should be cared for in an environmentally stable area with easy access to feed and water. If the birds have trouble drinking or eating, supportive fluid and nutritional measures must be taken. In most cases the birds will survive if they are managed properly.
• Medical. Since the patients are in a viremic state and immunosuppressed, antibiotic treatment is recommended, both parenterally and topically to the lesions.

Although most avian pox infections are species specific, there are fowl pox cutaneous vaccines available. Cutaneous application of the vaccine in the wing web of unaffected birds may provide some protection. The vaccine can be administered at 10–14 days of age.

Case 197: **Avian malaria**

CLINICAL PRESENTATION. An adult skua that had been placed in an outdoor aviary after being housed in an indoor aviary for several years presented with severe weakness and lethargy.

INVESTIGATION. Hematology showed a PCV of 0.18 l/l (18%) (normal = 0.35–0.55 l/l [35–55%]). A blood film was prepared (**197**).

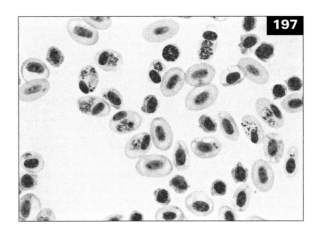

DIAGNOSIS. The blood film demonstrates a large number of immature erythrocytes suggestive of a marked regenerative response. Many of the erythrocytes contain intracytoplasmic inclusions that contain iron pigment and dramatically alter the position of the host cell nucleus. These inclusions are compatible with *Plasmodium* species gametocytes. Some strains of plasmodium are highly pathogenic, resulting in a severe hemolytic anemia (avian malaria).

MANAGEMENT. Chloroquine phosphate (10 mg/kg p/o once then 5 mg/kg at 6, 18, and 24 hours) and primaquine phosphate (0.03 mg/kg p/o q24h for 3 days) are used in combination to treat avian malaria. Treatment with these and other antimalarial drugs is often unrewarding and reinfection is common. Therefore, prevention by controlling the contact between birds and mosquito vectors is the best approach.

Case 198: *Ornithonyssus sylviarum* infestation in a barred rock rooster

CLINICAL PRESENTATION. A backyard poultry fancier presented a barred rock rooster for a shipping health certificate. During the examination it was noticed that there were some small parasites moving quickly through the skin and feathers of the fowl.

INVESTIGATION. One of the parasites was examined under the microscope (**198**).

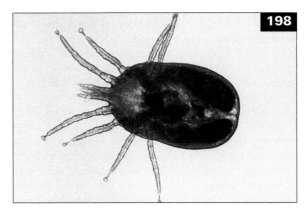

DIAGNOSIS. *Ornithonyssus sylviarum* (the northern poultry [fowl] mite) infestation.

MANAGEMENT. The birds should be treated with pyrethrin or carbamate powders, and the environment sprayed. This must be repeated at three week intervals. New arrivals must be isolated and examined and treated before being added to the flock.

Case 199: **Early embryonic mortality**

CLINICAL PRESENTATION. A suspected infertile or dead egg was presented for examination.

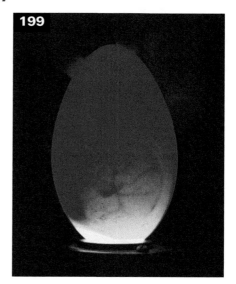

INVESTIGATION. The egg was opened and it showed a blood ring stage (**199**). This occurs when there is extravasation of blood into a partial or complete ring surrounding the remnants of a dead embryo.

DIAGNOSIS. Mortality during early incubation.

ETIOLOGY. Mortality during the first third of incubation can result from an improper incubation temperature, genetic abnormality, infection, rough handling or movement, or poor ventilation in the incubator leading to a build up of CO_2.

DISCUSSION. In both psittacines and domestic fowl eggs, approximately 33% of embryonic mortality occurs during the first third of incubation. The great majority (60%) of embryonic deaths occur during the last third. The smallest percentage of mortality occurs during the middle third.

Case 200: **Weighing incubating eggs**

DISCUSSION. It is important periodically to weigh eggs during the incubation process because the developing embryo's metabolism, combined with evaporation, will result in egg weight loss due to water loss. This is true of eggs under both natural (i.e. parental) and artificial incubation. Weighing eggs periodically and charting weight loss is an important technique used in monitoring the development and health of an embryo.

Acceptable weight loss from the start of incubation to piping is 13%, and 16% by the time of hatching; however, there is a range of 11–16%. Weight loss is not constant; the greater losses occur during early and late incubation. Charting weight loss is helpful to determine if the egg weight is on target for the time of elapsed incubation. The size of the air cell increases in proportion to the weight loss.

Weight loss greater than expected may be an indication of low humidity levels in the incubator. To increase humidity, a tray of water can be placed in the incubator, or the environment can be misted. If further control is required, a non-toxic white glue may be placed on part of the eggshell over the air cell, thereby reducing the area from which water vapour may be lost. Once applied, such glue is difficult to remove, therefore only a small application should be made.

Weight loss less than expected may result when an egg is incubated at too high a humidity level; it may also indicate an abnormal or dead embryo. Inadequate weight loss can be increased by desiccating the incubator (i.e. reducing the humidity using silica gel). If necessary, emery paper may be used to gently sand the eggshell over the air cell, or a small hole may be made in the shell over the air cell, without rupturing the membrane, in order to permit increased water loss. The egg should be candled for viability.

Case 201: **Chlamydophilosis**

CLINICAL PRESENTATION. A bird, one of a collection of six, presented with ocular and nasal discharge and watery green diarrhea (**201**).

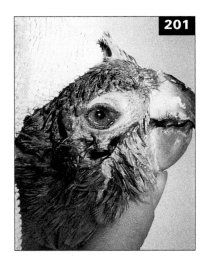

DIFFERENTIAL DIAGNOSES. The first and most important differential diagnosis is chlamydophilosis.

INVESTIGATION/DIAGNOSIS. The diagnosis of chlamydophilosis can be confirmed by PCR testing on blood or feces, or serology (ELISA). Paired samples are often required for serology. Blood and fecal PCR can give false negatives, as the organism is often latent and only shed intermittedly. During this stage, shedding may only occur once every 10 days; therefore, the tests yield a false negative.

MANAGEMENT. Treatment with doxycyline must be continued for 45 days. Doxycycline may be given as a long-acting injection (Vibravenous) every 5–7 days, although there is a risk of associated myositis; as twice daily medication in food if the birds will take a soft mix; or as impregnated pellets. Doxycycline hyclate in water has been shown to achieve and maintain MIC in cockatiels.

Consideration must be given by the clinician and the owner of the likelihood of complete eradication of the organism, especially in a collection of birds, as well as the potential for recurrence and the inability to prove eradication of the organism.

Following effective treatment, serologic titres should halve every 3–4 months. There is no way of ever proving a bird is cleared of latent infection. However, the clinician may advise periodic serologic testing, a gradually falling titer being indicative of effective therapy and the absence of recrudescence.

DISCUSSION. If therapy is carried out, the owner must be warned of the zoonotic potential and the health of his family and staff should be verified. The risk to other birds in the collection must be considered. They should be screened and treated if positive, or treated anyway if, for example, they share the same air space.

Summary questions and answers

Q1. How would one approach the diagnosis and treatment of a sick psittacine bird?

Q2. What is the fluid requirement for a bird, and how may this be provided to a sick bird?

Q3. Why is a sunflower or peanut based diet generally considered to be inappropriate for a psittacine bird?

Q4. What advice would you give to a client regarding the correct dietary options for a pet Amazon parrot?

Q5. What can a prospective bird owner do to minimize the risk of purchasing a new bird that is infected with PBFD?

Q6. A young hand-reared Amazon parrot, now 18 months of age, has recently started plucking its limbs and inguinal area. When presented at the clinic, the owner is reluctant to handle the bird. When the owner does get the bird out of its carrying box, it runs straight up her arm and onto her shoulder. What is the most likely cause for this bird to be plucking?

Q7. A cockatoo is presented. On radiography it is shown to have a dilated proventriculus. What are the differential diagnoses?

Q8. What is the most readily accepted 'safest anesthetic technique' for use in birds?

Q9. It is often suggested that clinical pathology samples should be collected with the patient anesthetized. How would you monitor isoflorane anesthesia in practice?

Q10. From which veins might one safely and usefully collect blood in a bird?

Q11. What clinical signs might be observed in a sick bird?

Q12. How would you treat a 'shocked' bird?

Q13. When is anemia a problem, and how would you treat it?

Q14. How would you triage an ex 'free-living raptor' in order to determine whether it will eventually be fit for release?

Q15. A five-year-old African grey parrot is presented to you with a three-month history of feather plucking. The bird is owned by a couple, who now both work (as of three months ago). You conduct a medical screen and no abnormalities are detected. What management options can be recommended?

A1. Birds hide signs of illness and, as a consequence of their higher metabolic rate, demonstrate rapid pathogenesis; therefore, veterinarians presented with a sick bird should take a comprehensive history and observe the bird carefully. Diagnostic samples should be collected (typically under isoflorane anesthesia, as this minimizes the stress for the bird), radiographs taken, and endoscopy undertaken if indicated. Blood should be collected for a CBC and *Chlamydophila* serology, and swabs and aspirates collected from any areas of clinical interest for culture and cytology.

Diagnostic samples should be processed in-house where possible in order to expedite the availability of results.

Symptomatic treatment and nutritional and fluid support must be provided, as must suitable nursing care and support. A sick bird should be weighed daily and fed sufficient food (by gavage if necessary) to maintain body weight. The bird should be considered to be potentially infected with *Chlamydophila* species until proven to the contrary.

A2. Although there will be great variation between species, the standard requirement is taken as 50 ml/kg/day. In addition, any sick or injured bird should be considered to be 10% dehydrated. Fluids may be provided orally (in particular with food when given by gavage), intravenously (preferred option), intraosseously, or subcutaneously.

A3. Birds eat to satisfy their energy requirements. Sunflower and peanut are 45% pure oil and have seven times the energy content of chocolate snack bars. Being fed on a high energy diet means that birds do not need to eat as much to meet their energy needs; however, they will then take in lower trace element requirements than are necessary to meet their long-term needs. Birds fed on a sunflower or peanut based diet tend long term to suffer from vitamin A and calcium deficiencies.

A high energy diet will act as a nutritional drive to breed. So, while such a diet might stimulate more breeding in a pair of birds (despite the deficiency aspects of the diet), they will also tend to stimulate excessive breeding drive in single pet birds.

A4. The two accepted options are (1) a wet mix diet comprising 1/3 cooked brown rice, 1/3 fresh fruit and vegetables, 1/3 sprouted (for 36 hours, washed at 12, 24, and 36 hours) beans and pulses, plus a suitable vitamin and mineral supplement; or (2) a good quality pelleted diet plus a small volume of fresh fruit or vegetables daily.

The latter is generally easier to manage for the average pet bird owner. In contrast, many parrot breeders and 'multiple bird' keepers do have the time available and so are able to make the effort to prepare a fresh wet mix diet each day.

A5. The prospective owner should be advised to go direct to a good quality breeder with birds of good health status. Any new bird should be purchased direct from the breeder and submitted for a 'new bird check' with an experienced avian veterinarian, who should maintain high standards of practice biosecurity so that the risk of infecting one patient with pathogens left previously by another patient is minimized.

A6. The bird is obviously dominant to the owner. Taking into account the fact that the bird was hand reared, is 18 months old, and is plucking its limbs and inguinal area, the most likely explanation is that the bird desires to breed with the owner. It is plucking because it is sexually frustrated. This problem is best controlled by: separating the amorous couple; reducing the amount of daylight; reducing the energy content of the diet; injecting leuprolide acetate injections every two weeks on three occasions.

Avoiding recurrence is achieved by gaining dominance over the bird and maintaining a low energy diet.

A7. Any cause that results in physical or functional GI tract stasis: psittacine proventricular dilarion syndrome; heavy metal (lead, zinc, copper, iron) toxicity; any cause of GI tract inflammation (bacterial, fungal, or parasitic infection); neoplasia, torsion, adhesions, endoparasites; foreign bodies (e.g. wood or plastic).

A8. There is no such thing as a 'safe anesthetic'; there are only safe anesthetists. If you do not have access to an experienced avian anesthetist, the safest anesthetic may be considered to be a systemic agent; for example, medetomidine (150–300 µg/kg) and ketamine (3–5 mg/kg) given mixed together intravenously, and reversed with a same volume of atipamezole as the volume of medetomidine used. This mixture will give 30 minutes surgical anesthesia (if the lower dose is used, it can be repeated once). While the bird should still be entubated and maintained on oxygen, provided the bird has been weighed and the dose correctly calculated, overdosage cannot occur and careful monitoring of anesthesia is less important.

If an experienced/trained anesthetist is available, either isoflorane or sevoflorane are considered to produce the safest anesthetic.

A9. Because of the bony ossicles in the sclera, the eye position in birds does not change in relation to the depth of anesthetic. Palpebral and digital responses will have been lost before surgical anesthesia is achieved. Heart rate can be monitored for response to noxious stimuli. Pulse oximetry can be used; changes in readings are relevant, although the absolute reading may not be. Respiratory rate and depth should be monitored. The most useful reflex is the corneal reflex. When the cornea is touched with a sterile cotton bud, the third eyelid should come across the cornea at a steady rate. If the rate is faster, the depth of anesthesia is light; if slower, it may be too deep. In addition, in the author's opinion the most useful monitoring aid is a capnograph, with a respiratory monitor included. The monitoring of expired CO_2 levels gives a very useful and efficient indication of cardiorespiratory function.

A10. The options are:
- The medial tarsal vein (particularly useful in waterfowl).
- The superficial ulna vein (otherwise known as the basilic vein). This is useful in any birds over 100 g in weight. Although some authors suggest hematoma is a risk, at least the haematoma can be seen and the hemorrhage controlled.
- The jugular vein (typically larger and easier to use on the right side, although this varies with individuals). The apteria (featherless tract) on the bird's neck overlying the jugular furrow is parted and and wetted away with spirit. The apteria is moved to the left or right so that it overlies the jugular vein. Effective pressure must be applied to the vein after the needle is removed, otherwise significant and at times dangerous hemorrhage can occur.

A11. Loss of weight or condition (note that a bird can lose condition without necessarily losing weight); decreased food conversion efficiency (i.e. a bird needing more food to maintain its weight than usual); increase or decrease in appetite; change in normal behavior or activity (e.g. less active, less vocal, more demanding); not as bright, alert, or responsive as usual; perching – using a different perch (higher/lower), perching on two limbs not one, perching with two limbs and holding onto the bars with the beak; sleeping more (slit-like/lemon-shaped eyes rather than big round shiny eyes) or lethargic; lame – limbs or wings, wings hanging down, paresis; exercise intolerance; abnormal bodily discharges (mouth, nares, eyes, ear, cloaca, preen gland) or cloacal prolapse, cloacal straining; respiratory effort, noise or tail bobbing, coughing (may be mimicry), sneezing, gaping; swellings, bleeding from any site; change in feces (note the fecal, urate and aqueous fractions); plumage – damage, no recent moult, plumage color abnormalities, bleeding into shafts, brittle feathers, feather loss, loss of waterproofing; skin changes – self-trauma, pruritus, erythema, swellings etc, loss of feather dust on beak and feet; CNS signs – fits, seizures, blindness.

A12. Warmth, darkness, oxygen therapy if indicated, fluid therapy (preferably 10 ml/kg i/v) and minimize stimulation.

A13. Any bird with a PCV less than the normal range (typically 0.45–0.53 l/l [45–53%]) for the species, should be thoroughly investigated. The cause of the anemia should be identified where possible and addressed. In the interim, any patient with a low PCV should receive fluid therapy, preferably a plasma colloid expander rather than crystalloids. Any bird with a PCV of <0.20 l/l (20%) should receive a transfusion. An homologous transfusion (i.e. same species or at least genera) as opposed to a heterologous transfusion (i.e. different genera) should be used wherever possible, as erythrocyte survival time is significantly longer (11 days compared with 2–3 days). Bovine hemoglobin glutamer 200 (Oxyglobin) can be safely and effectively used in anemic birds.

A14. The bird must be able to see well enough, fly well enough, hunt and kill well enough, and be able to eat and digest food in sufficient quantity to be able to maintain its body weight. The bird must also be able to relate safely with others of its own species and not present a risk to humans.

Therefore, a sight defect, flight impairment, digit 1 or 2 nonfunctional in either foot, beak damage, GI tract disorders, or imprinting would preclude release.

A15. Rehome the bird; one of the owners to take the bird to work with them; build an outside aviary at home into which the bird can be placed while the owners are at work, preferably with a second parrot.

An analogy is often drawn between a parrot and a four-year-old child, in particular a four-year-old child who is accustomed to living with many others in a large noisy gregarious group. If you were to take that four-year-old child and place it in solitary isolation in a cot in an empty room for 8–10 hours each day, you would not expect it to grow up normally; no more can you expect a solitary abandoned parrot to do any better.

Bibliography

Textbooks

Abramson J, Speer B, Thomsen J (1995) *The Large Macaws. Their Care, Breeding, and Conservation.* Raintree Publications, Fort Bragg.

Altman RB, Clubb S, Dorrestein GM, Quesenberry K (1997) (eds) *Avian Medicine and Surgery.* WB Saunders, Philadelphia.

Anderson Brown AF, Robbins GES (2002) *The New Incubation Book* (Millennium Edition). World Pheasant Association, Fordingbridge.

Baumel JJ, King AS, Breazile JE, Evans HE, Vanden Berge JC (1993) (eds) *Handbook of Avian Anatomy: Nomina Anatomica Avium* (2nd edn). Nuttal Ornithological Club, Cambridge, Mass.

Beynon PH, Forbes NA, Harcourt-Brown N (1996) (eds) *Manual of Raptors, Pigeons and Waterfowl.* British Small Animal Veterinary Association, Cheltenham.

Campbell TW (1995) *Avian Hematology and Cytology* (2nd edn). Iowa State University Press, Ames.

Campbell TW, Ellis CK (2007) (eds) *Avian and Exotic Animal Hematology and Cytology* (3rd edn). Blackwell Publishing, Ames

Coles BH (1997) *Avian Medicine and Surgery* (2nd edn). Blackwell Science, Oxford.

Coles BH, Krautwald-Junghanns ME, Herman TJ (1998) *Avian Medicine.* Mosby, St Louis.

Cooper, JE (2002) *Birds of Prey: Health and Disease* (3rd edn). Blackwell Science, Oxford.

del Hoyo J, Elliott A, Sargatal J (1994 and 1997) *Handbook of the Birds of the World.* Volumes 2 & 4. Lynx Edicions, Barcelona.

Forbes NA, Altman RB (1998) *Self-Assessment Colour Review of Avian Medicine.* Manson Publishing, London.

Fowler ME, Miller RE (1999) Special medicine: birds. In: *Zoo and Wild Animal Medicine, Current Therapy 4.* (eds ME Fowler, RE Miller) WB Saunders, Philadelphia, pp. 259–314.

Fudge AM (2000) (ed) *Laboratory Medicine: Avian and Exotic Pets.* WB Saunders, Philadelphia.

Harcourt-Brown NH, Chitty J (2005) *Manual of Psittacine Birds* (2nd edn). British Small Animal Veterinary Association, Gloucester.

Howard R, Moore A (2002) *A Complete Checklist of the Birds of the World* (3rd edn). Academic Press. Oxford.

Jordan FTW (1990) *Poultry Diseases.* Baillière-Tindall, London.

Kern JT (2000) Exotic animal ophthalmology. In: *Veterinary Ophthalmology* (3rd edn). (ed KN Gelatt) Lippincott/Williams & Wilkins, Philadelphia, pp. 1177–1208.

King AS, McLelland J (1989) *Form and Function in Birds.* Volumes 1 to 4. Academic Press, Oxford.

King AS, McLelland J (1975) *Outlines of Avian Anatomy.* WB Saunders, Philadelphia.

Krautwald ME, Tellhelm B, Hummel G, Kostka V, Kaleta EF (1991) *Atlas of Radiographic Anatomy and Diagnosis of Cage Birds.* Verlag Paul Parey, Berlin.

Lumeij JT (1997) Avian clinical biochemistry. In *Clinical Biochemistry of Domestic Animals* (5th edn). (eds JJ Kaneko, JW Harvey, ML Bruss) Academic Press, London, pp. 857–883.

Lumeij JT, Remple JD, Redig PT, Lierz M, Cooper JE (2000) (eds) *Raptor Biomedicine III.* Zoological Education Network, Lake Worth.

McLelland J (1991) *A Color Atlas of Avian Anatomy.* WB Saunders, Philadelphia.

Olsen GH, Orosz SE (2000) (eds) *Manual of Avian Medicine.* Mosby, St Louis.

Orosz SE, Ensley PK, Haynes CJ (1992) *Avian Surgical Anatomy.* WB Saunders, Philadelphia.

Petrak ML (1982) (ed) *Diseases of Cage and Aviary Birds* (2nd edn). Lea & Febiger, Philadelphia.

Redig, PT, Cooper JE, Remple JD, Hunter DB (1993) (eds) *Raptor Biomedicine.* University of Minnesota Press, Minneapolis.

Ritchie, B (1995) *Avian Viruses: Function and Control.* Wingers Publishing, Lake Worth.

Ritchie BW, Harrison GJ, Harrison LR (2000) (eds) *Avian Medicine: Principles and Application* (2nd edn). Wingers Publishing, Fort Worth.

Samour J (2000) (ed) *Avian Medicine.* Mosby, St Louis.

Schmidt RE, Reavill DR, Phalen, DN (2003) *Pathology of Pet and Aviary Birds.* Iowa State Press, Ames. (also as CD ROM)

Schubot R, Clubb S, Clubb K (1992) *Psittacine Aviculture.* Avicultural Breeding and Research Center, Loxahatchee.

Sturkie PD (2000) (ed) *Avian Physiology* (5th edn). Academic Press, San Diego.

Tudor D (1991) *Pigeon Health and Disease.* Iowa State University Press, Ames.

Tully TN, Lawton MPC, Dorrestein GM (2000) (eds) *Avian Medicine.* Butterworth Heinmann, Oxford.

Tully TN, Shane SM (1996) (eds) *Ratite Management, Medicine, and Surgery.* Krieger Publishing Company, Malabar.

Wobeser GA (2003) *Diseases of Wild Waterfowl.* Plenum Press, London.

Refereed journals

Avian Diseases
Avian Pathology
Journal of Avian Medicine and Surgery
Journal of Small Animal Practice
Journal of Exotic Pet Medicine (Elsevier) (Formerly Seminars in Avian and Exotic Pet Medicine [WB Saunders])

Proceedings

Association of Avian Veterinarians
European Conferences on Avian Medicine and Surgery
European College of Avian Medicine and Surgery

CD ROMS

Harcourt-Brown NH (2000) *Birds of Prey: Anatomy, Radiology, and Clinical Conditions of the Pelvic Limb.* Zoological Education Network Multimedia Series, Lake Worth.

Taylor M, Harrison GJ (2000) *Diagnostic Application of Avian Endoscopy.* Zoological Education Network Multimedia Series, Lake Worth.

Section 3
REPTILES & AMPHIBIANS

Fredric L Frye

Classification of cases by species

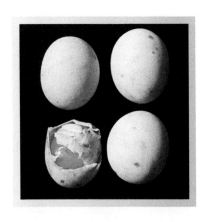
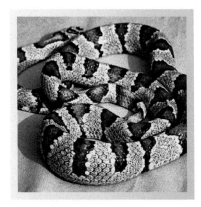
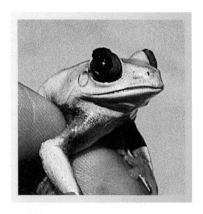

Introduction

Many people desire to have some form of animal companionship in their homes. If, however, they live in multifamily rental accommodation that prohibits noisy barking dogs, yowling cats, or squawking caged psittacine birds, there are alternative quiet animals that might be permissible. Keeping fish in an attractively planted aquarium is a possibility, as are a wide variety of relatively small lizards, snakes, chelonians (turtles, tortoises, terrapins), amphibian larvae, completely metamorphosed frogs, toads, salamanders, newts, and caecilians.

Many of us fondly remember our own childhood experiences keeping common small reptiles and amphibians for brief periods in glass jars, coffee tins, and terraria. These nascent experiences were often our first introduction to what developed into a lifelong interest in biology and animal husbandry. In reality, these ectothermic vertebrates, which have changed little since millions of years ago, are fascinating to observe. Many are relatively inexpensive to acquire, easy to keep as terrarium animals, simple to feed, not demanding of their owners' time, make no loud noises to disturb neighbors, and don't require regular exercise. When provided with appropriate diet and care, many reptiles and amphibians will live longer than they would under wild, natural conditions. This is largely attributable to lack of predation and other naturally occurring environmental stresses.

This section of the book focuses on those reptiles and amphibians that are most likely to be seen as patients by veterinarians with an interest in clinical herpetologic medicine and surgery. Today, many pet owners expect their veterinarian to have some degree of expertise in how to care for and treat a variety of exotic (nondomestic and wild) companion animal species. In accordance with the nondomestic pet-owning public's steadily increasing interest in this kind of pet, veterinary colleges and local, regional, national, and international veterinary conferences and seminars have moved proactively to meet the demand for formal training and dissemination of information on 'exotic' animal medicine. At least one institution (the Royal Veterinary College in the UK, in collaboration with the Institute of Zoology at the Zoological Society of London) has established a postgraduate course in Wild Animal Medicine in which successful students earn an MSc degree. In addition, several veterinary colleges in North America offer postdoctoral residencies in wildlife medicine. The has resulted in the subdiscipline of exotic animal veterinary medicine expanding and being enthusiastically supported by the veterinary profession, the veterinary educational establishment, and the companion pet owners.

Approximately a decade ago, the Association of Reptilian and Amphibian Veterinarians (ARAV), following the path blazed by the Association of Avian Veterinarians (AAV), was formed by a relatively few committed veterinary clinicians. Their desire was to share their expertise and efforts, and to foster a better understanding of the correct methods of husbandry, treatment, and surgery for the medical conditions affecting reptiles and amphibians. A similar interest in nondomestic animal veterinary medicine and surgery provided the stimulus for establishing the British Veterinary Zoological Society (BVZS), the European Association of Zoo Veterinarians (EAZV), and the World Association of Zoo Veterinarians (WAZV).

These specialty groups within traditional veterinary medicine are providing the knowledge required to improve the health of exotic animals. This information is now being transferred to the veterinary profession in general and to the owners of exotic pets. In addition to the abundance of textbooks devoted to exotic animal medicine, several scholarly, peer reviewed journals are now thriving, thereby facilitating the dissemination of sound knowledge. Slowly but steadily, veterinary colleges are including exotic animal medicine courses in their curricula and, therefore, students can often begin pursuing their special interests while still in their matriculating years.

As a visiting professor in the USA, the UK, Italy, Nicaragua, and Japan, I have had the privilege and pleasure of teaching in-depth courses regarding my specialty. Everywhere, the enthusiastic students want to learn more about these intriguing animals.

Concomitant with this nearly exponential expansion of the knowledge base of husbandry, medicine, and surgery is the rise in numbers of veterinary comparative pathologists who are competent to render diagnosis of disease in ectothermic animals. Like 'higher' vertebrates, reptiles and amphibians fall victim to a wide variety of traumatic injuries and metabolic, infectious/ inflammatory, and neoplastic disorders. Only within the last four decades has the veterinary profession taken a serious interest in the illnesses of these creatures and the methods by which many of them can be effectively diagnosed and treated. Interestingly, we now know that many immunohistologic staining reagents originally developed for diagnosing human conditions are fully applicable to reptiles and amphibians (Frye, 1991; Frye and Kass, 1991; Frye et al., 1994a; Frye et al., 1994b). An additional benefit of this research, in which immunohistologic reagents originally produced for human disease are applied to reptilian and amphibian tissues, is the fostering of cooperation between veterinarians and physicians. Furthermore, these products are relatively expensive, and the collaboration between veterinarians and physicians is essential from that aspect alone.

Regional and international restrictions concerning the capture (or even the possession) and trade in threatened or endangered species of reptiles and amphibians are being enforced, and excellent captive breeding programs that adhere to the rules and regulations have been established for many taxa. Numerous breeders specializing in one or more species of chelonians, lizards, snakes, frogs, toads, or salamanders are now thriving in market-driven pet animal enterprises. These enlightened captive-breeding efforts have reduced the incidence of both ecto- and endoparasitism, particularly pertaining to those parasites that utilize multiple hosts in order to complete their indirect life cycles. This is not to suggest that adequate quarantine of all new arrivals into an animal collection is no longer essential; to the contrary, quarantine is still mandatory because it facilitates impeding or totally preventing the risk of infection or infestation of some pathogens that require multiple hosts.

The goal of this section is to provide the interested veterinarian and/or veterinary student with instructive cases. It is not designed to be a stand alone textbook with a complete bibliography. Rather, it is a compilation of diverse clinically oriented cases, and the format reflects the manner in which clinical veterinary medicine is practiced.

The reader will notice that some reptiles are overrepresented in these 100 cases. This is not to imply that species such as green iguanas, California desert tortoises, boa constrictors, or tegu lizards have a greater incidence of diseases. Rather, it is a reflection of the popularity of these reptiles as pets. Over the many years that I was in practice, these animals were the reptiles most commonly brought to me as patients. Some extraordinary, rare cases are included in this chapter because they represent valuable instructive material. Furthermore, what might seem unique today might very well become nearly ordinary in years to come.

When the owner of a reptile or amphibian seeks veterinary care for a pet because it displays a particular condition or malady, the clinician obtains a history and observes the patient's symptoms (or signs of disease). Animals cannot speak to us and so provide some clues regarding their health; therefore, the clinician must be a keen observer. We now know that reptiles and amphibians can feel pain; therefore, they should be handled in a gentle fashion – the same way we prefer to be handled when we are not feeling well. Following observation, the clinician investigates and evaluates the signs or symptoms of disease in order to deduce the diagnosis. Sometimes, these signs and symptoms suggest differential diagnoses. However, radiography, hematology, cytology, and/or histopathology and, in some cases, necropsy contribute to the final diagnosis.

Questions invariably arise once a diagnosis is established. How should this patient be managed? What are the treatment options? Which husbandry techniques will prevent a problem from recurring?

The veterinarian or veterinary student with a developing interest in herpetologic medicine is encouraged to investigate the growing body of authoritative information covering morphology, physiology, nutrition, ophthalmology, infectious diseases, surgery, reproductive physiology, hematology, radiology, pathology, diagnosis and treatment, special techniques, practice tips, and other clinical aspects of

dealing with these fascinating animals. Fortunately, there are superb books that detail the captive care, nutrition, diagnosis, and treatment of exotic small wild animals; therefore, veterinarians now have relevant sources for reference that were unavailable only a few decades ago.

Special instruments are not required to diagnose and effectively to treat reptiles and amphibians; essentially, all of them are 'off-the-shelf' and, therefore, readily available. In some instances items that were designed for other uses are very useful for the veterinary surgeon with an interest in herpetologic medicine and surgery. An example of such dual usage is the employment of various size spoons (in assorted sizes from small espresso coffee to long-handled iced-tea spoons) for evacuating the contents of hollow viscus organs (e.g. shelled ova from oviducts, feces from intestines, urates and calculi from urinary bladders) and the purulent, necrotic contents of abscesses and pyogranulomata. In practice, these inexpensive common utensils are as effective as substantially more expensive surgical gallbladder spoons. Similarly, cerumen loops, originally designed to remove ear wax from humans, are invaluable in a myriad of clinical circumstances ranging from the atraumatic removal of premoistened retained tertiary spectacle shields of snakes and some lizards to the enucleation of small accumulations of necrotic debris in pyogranulomata. Common objects, from upended foam coffee cups to large buckets, are used to support chelonian patients and prevent them from scuttling off the examination table. Guitar picks facilitate opening the mouth of many reptiles without inflicting trauma.

The processing of specimens destined to be sent for pathology should utilize several specific, but simple, procedures, so that the maximum amount of information is yielded. These techniques, in addition to many other practical tips, stem from decades of clinical practice as well as trial and error.

Like any intellectual endeavor, herpetologic medicine and surgery will only grow and flourish as long as those who are involved in practice and research continue to disseminate their expertise. Fortunately, today there are many avenues open for clinicians to contribute their observations and techniques; therefore, I urge those who are in the field to share their discoveries so that all of us may continue to learn.

Many of the cases that I have chosen to include in this chapter are straightforward; others are far more complex. Because I am a comparative pathologist, as well as a former clinician, some of the cases came to me either as cadavers for dissection or as bits and pieces of tissue selected by those who submitted them for histopathologic diagnosis. For this reason, vital antemortem laboratory details may be either scanty or lacking altogether. Dermatologic cases may be interspersed with ophthalmological disorders, infectious diseases, nutritional deficiencies, traumatic injuries, reproductive problems, and/or cases demanding a working knowledge of comparative hematology, parasitology, cardiology, radiology, anesthesiology, surgery, pathology, etc. However, it is just this sort of variety that makes herpetologic medicine and surgery such a challenging and intellectually rewarding subdiscipline within our profession.

Whenever possible, the information regarding these cases is written using the present tense of grammar. This is a dynamic process – I am conversing with you and mentoring you.

The student is the most important person on the campus.
Without students there would be no need for the Institution.
Not a cold enrollment statistic but a flesh and blood human being with feelings and emotions like our own.
Not someone to be tolerated so that we can do our own thing.
Not dependent on us. Rather, we are dependent on them.
Not an interruption of our work but the purpose of it.
We are not doing them a favor by seeing them; they are doing us a favor by giving us the opportunity to do so.

Anonymous
On the office wall of one of my faculty colleagues.

Together, we shall contemplate these cases, and I hope that you enjoy reading about them as much as I enjoyed writing about them.

Acknowledgements

To my wife, Brucye, who read the manuscript and employed her editorial skills to ensure that the information in this section would be 'user-friendly' for the clinician just commencing his or her professional career and for the more seasoned colleague who has just begun to see exotic animals as patients.

To my veterinary colleagues, friends, and former students who, throughout my forty years of practice and biomedical research, referred cases to me and graciously contributed data and images for my textbooks.

Without their generous support, my career would have been less productive. I thank you one and all.

English and Latin names

African bullfrog	*Pyxicephalus adspersus*
African clawed frog	*Xenopus laevis*
African rock python	*Python sebae*
African spurred tortoise	*Geochelone sulcata*
American bullfrog	*Rana catesbiana*
Argentine horned frog	*Ceratophrys ornata*
Asiatic box turtle	*Cuora amboinensis*
Australasian bearded dragon lizard	*Pogona vitticeps*
Australasian blood python	*Python curtus*
Australasian skink	*Tiliqua* species
Box turtle	*Terrapene carolina*
Burmese python	*Python molurus bivittatus*
California mountain kingsnake	*Lampropeltis zonata*

Central American boa constrictor	*Boa constrictor imperator*
Children's python	*Antaresia* (formerly *Liasis*) *childreni*
Collared lizard	*Crotaphytus collaris*
Desert tortoise	*Xerobates (Gopherus) agassizii*
Emydid turtle	*Chryemys picta picta*
European green lacerta lizard	*Lacerta viridis*
False water cobra	*Hydrodynastes bicinctus*
Galapagos tortoise	*Geochelone elephantopus*
Garter snake	*Thamnophis sirtalis*
Gila monster lizard	*Heloderma suspectum*
Green iguana	*Iguana iguana*
Hermann's tortoise	*Testudo hermanni*
Indigo snake	*Drymarchon corais*
Jackson's chameleon	*Chamaeleo jacksoni*
Kingsnake	*Lampropeltis mexicana alterna*
Madagascar panther chameleon	*Furcifer pardalis*
Meller's chameleon	*Chamaeleo melleri*
Mexican beaded lizard	*Heloderma horridum*
Monitor lizard	*Varanus species*
Ornate box turtle	*Terrapene ornata*
Pacific pond turtle	*Clemmys m. marmorata*
Pacific tree frog	*Hyla regila*
Painted turtle	*Chrysemys picta*
Panther chameleon	*Furcifer pardalis*
Red-eyed tree frog	*Agalychnis callidryas*
Red-tailed boa constrictor	*Boa c. constrictor*
Rock iguana	*Cyclura nubila*
Royal (ball) python	*Python regius*
Savanna monitor lizard	*Varanus exanthematicus*
Snake-necked turtle	*Chelodina expansa*
Soft-shelled turtle	*Apalone* (formerly *Trionyx*) species
Solomon Island prehensile-tail skink	*Corucia zebrata*
South American red-legged tortoise	*Geochelone carbonaria*
Tegu lizard	*Tupinambis teguixin*
Texas tortoise	*Gopherus berlandieri*
Tree frog	*Hyla chrysoselus*
Veiled chameleon	*Chamaeleo calyptratus*
Water snake	*Nerodia species*
Western toad	*Bufo boreas*

Case 202: **Bowel obstruction in a green iguana**

CLINICAL PRESENTATION. An adult green iguana presents with an acute history of vomiting and general distress. A sausage-shaped mass is palpated in the caudal coelomic cavity.

DIFFERENTIAL DIAGNOSES. Constipation; obstruction from a gastrointestinal foreign body; obstruction from a mass of worms; intussusception of one or more segments of intestine; intestinal volvulus; intestinal ileus; gastric or intestinal neoplasia; an ingested toxic substance.

INVESTIGATION. Plain radiographs disclose a soft tissue density mass in the mid body with a gas-filled intestine proximal to the mass. Routine hematology and biochemistry studies reveal hemoconcentration, mild leukocytosis, lymphopenia, and mild hyperuricemia.

DIAGNOSIS. Intussusception.

ETIOLOGY. Intussusception is the telescoping of one segment of a hollow viscus organ, usually a length of intestine, into either a proximal or adjoining distal length or segment. Its prevalence is sporadic. Many instances of intussusception can be traced to chronic constipation and gastrointestinal parasitism, which often involves metazoan helminth parasites, predominantly nematodes. It can also be caused by intestinal protozoan infections. It is thought that these organisms induce local inflammation and accompanying repeated tenesmus. Continued straining, as if to produce stools, can induce one or more segments of intestine (duodenum) to invaginate either into the stomach proximally or distally into the jejunum (**202a, b**). Similarly, the jejunum can telescope proximally into the duodenum (histological section stained with H&E and photographed [**202c**] at ×27 magnification), distally into the ileum, cranially into the jejunum, or caudally into the colon (**202d, e**).

The clinical signs of intussusception are those associated with complete or partial intestinal obstruction. Vomiting, bloating, distress, fluid and electrolyte shifts and, finally, shock, are commonly observed. Often, one or more sausage shaped masses can be palpated in the coelom. Plain or contrast radiography reveals one or more fluid density masses with or without entrapped gas proximal to the obstruction. Intussusception is an emergency that demands immediate attention.

MANAGEMENT. The intussuscepted segment(s) are reduced surgically, which will restore the mesenteric blood circulation that has been compromised. The tissues must be handled gently. If the telescoped segment(s) can be reduced, and are found to be vital, they are sutured to the body wall by creating an enteropexy to prevent subsequent intussusception.

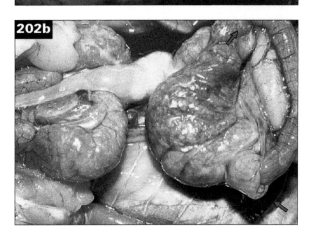

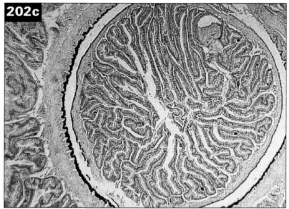

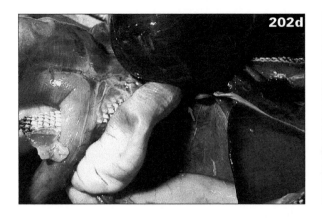

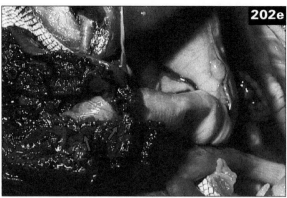

It is essential that any underlying (inducing) etiology is treated effectively as well. Routine fecal analysis is advised. Gastroenteric parasitism must be treated with appropriate parasiticidal therapy.

PROGNOSIS. Guarded because intestinal intussusception is often discovered only after irreparable ischemic necrosis has occurred.

Case 203: **Parasitic ovum identification in an Gila monster lizard**

INVESTIGATION. After appropriate dilution and mixing, the wet preparation of a fecal sample is ready for microscopic examination and interpretation. Spherical to slightly elliptical thick-walled embryonated ova are identified. The embryos are characterized by having tiny refractile hooklets (**203**).

DIAGNOSIS. Cestode ovum.

MANAGEMENT. The lizard is treated with praziquantel (5–8 mg/kg, repeated in 2 weeks). Gila monster lizards and Mexican beaded lizards are venomous, and extreme

caution must be taken when medicating them. Therefore, the medication is placed into a dead rodent before feeding it to these lizards, thus avoiding having to handle the patient.

PROGNOSIS. Favorable.

HUSBANDRY. Many, if not most, cestodes utilize an indirect life cycle. Therefore, limiting the prey to healthy, laboratory-raised rodents will facilitate reducing a reptile colony's incidence of endoparasitism.

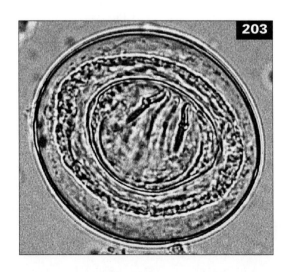

Case 204: **Anorexia and severe lethargy in an adult male green iguana**

CLINICAL PRESENTATION. A 1.4 kg adult male green iguana that was previously thriving presents with a history of anorexia that began approximately two weeks before the owners found the iguana upside down in its cage, apparently dead. However, when they prodded him, he responded by moving his limbs feebly. The iguana's diet consists primarily of mustard, collard, turnip, and dandelion greens and, occasionally, soft ripe fruit. The iguana is severely depressed. Its integument and oral mucosae are icteric and its oral mucus is viscid and sticky. The eyes are deeply sunken. No grossly visible lesions or palpable swellings are detected.

INVESTIGATION. Ultrasonic Doppler blood flow investigations detect loud bilateral atrioventricular and aortic valvular murmurs. A pretreatment whole blood specimen is withdrawn from the ventral caudal vein for hematology and biochemistry tests (below). The blood, which is very dark red, flows into the syringe substantially slower than normal and it clots almost immediately.

Based on the history, brief period of illness, and laboratory findings, various factors should be considered when attempting to arrive at a diagnosis. The diet is ideal. The blood sample is severely hemoconcentrated. Although the total WBC count is only mildly elevated, there is a substantial heterophilia. The monocytes are not increased; therefore, chronic disease is less likely to be a factor. There is a significant glycosemia; the glucose is markedly elevated, which suggests (but does not confirm) diabetes mellitus. The CPK is elevated, which suggests increased myocardial exertion due to the greatly elevated PCV, muscle necrosis, muscle wasting and/or muscle injury. The LDH is elevated, which suggests a liver dysfunction or hepatocellular insult. However, the ALT, AST, and AP are not significantly elevated; this tends to help rule out hepatic necrosis. The serum cholesterol is moderately elevated, which suggests that the iguana is mobilizing fat stores as an energy source. The calcium is just slightly above normal. The phosphorus is markedly elevated. The TP is markedly elevated. This reflects the hemoconcentration noted above in the PCV value. The globulin fraction of the plasma proteins is significantly elevated. This reflects the A:G ratio of 0.4, which suggests either an infectious or an inflammatory response to an antigenic stimulus, or a neoplasm involving plasmacytes (B lymphocytes). However, the hemogram does not reflect the lymphocytosis or plasmacytosis that would be expected to be found with a B-cell leukemia or multiple myelosis. The sodium is slightly lower than normal. The potassium is extremely elevated to a level that would be clearly cardiotoxic and, therefore, fatal, in most mammals. The uric acid is markedly elevated to several times normal value and represents severe hyperuricemia. Both the BUN and creatinine are within normal limits.

Hematology			Biochemistry		
PCV	0.62 l/l	(62%)	Glucose	32.8 mmol/l	(590.4 mg/dl)
WBCs	13×10^9/l	(13×10^3/μl)	ALT (SGPT)	30 u/l	
Heterophils	83%		AST (SGOT)	114 u/l	
Lymphocytes	13%		CPK (CK)	1,731 u/l	
Monocytes	2%		LDH	1,110 u/l	
Azurophils	2%		AP (SAP)	0 u/l	
Thrombocytes	adequate		Cholesterol	9.2 mmol/l	(355.2 mg/dl)
			Calcium	3.7 mmol/l	(14.8 mg/dl)
			Phosphorus	6.1 mmol/l	(18.9 mg/dl)
			TP	93 g/l	(9.3 g/dl)
			Albumin	24 g/l	(2.4 g/dl)
			Globulin	69 g/l	(6.9 g/dl)
			A:G ratio	0.4:1	
			Sodium	123 mmol/l	(123 mEq/l)
			Potassium	15.3 mmol/l	(15.3 mEq/l)
			Uric acid	4.1 mmol/l	(69.3 mg/dl)
			BUN	2.14 mmol/l	(5.9 mg/dl)
			Creatinine	53 μmol/l	(0.59 mg/dl)

DIAGNOSIS. The most likely tentative diagnosis, particularly when evaluating the hematology and biochemistry results, is acute or subacute renal failure. This could be due to any of the following etiologies:

- Interstitial nephritis, glomerulonephritis, or pyelonephritis. Interstitial is the most likely.
- Ingestion of or iatrogenic injection of a nephrotoxic substance or agent.
- A neoplasm of the kidneys, while possible, is less likely because it almost certainly would have to be bilateral. If unilateral, the ipsilateral kidney should be able to provide adequate renal function.

MANAGEMENT. Based on the tentative diagnosis of acute or subacute renal failure, and because of the markedly elevated hemoconcentration, elevated PCV, hyperkalemia, and hyponatremia, physiological saline was infused (35 ml i/v and 65 ml i/c). **NB:** Ringer's solution *must not* be used because it contains potassium. Within five minutes of receiving the saline infusion, the iguana became much more animated and within an hour the hemotocrit had been lowered to 42%. By the next morning the PCV had returned to normal (34%) and the blood flow murmurs were no longer detected with the Doppler device. Less than 24 hours after being presented in a moribund state, the iguana was actively trying to defend himself by lashing his tail and threatening to bite. Due to the hyperphosphatemia, the iguana should be placed on a regimen of saline diuresis, maintained at 45 ml/kg daily in two divided doses, plus as much orally provided fluid as it will tolerate without developing pulmonary edema or ascites. A course of enrofloxacin therapy was begun, and the iguana had an uneventful recovery.

The source of the hyperglycemia was not determined because the blood glucose level spontaneously returned to normal within a few days. The BUN and creatinine determinations in this iguana point to the fact that while these values are important in mammals, they are unreliable in reptiles because reptiles are uricotelic in their renal excretory functions. Therefore, the measurement of uric acid is the most accurate means for assessing urinary waste clearance of catabolyzed proteins in reptiles. Although the plasma calcium is essentially normal, the plasma phosphorus is approximately triple normal; this suggests that there is substantial renal retention of phosphorus. Had the loss of kidney function been more severe or more chronic, it is likely that the plasma calcium would have been significantly lower because hyperphosphatemia stimulates the secretion of parathyroid hormone (PTH) which, in turn, stimulates the mobilization of calcium stores from bone and eventually induces osteomalacia and (renal-associated) fibrous osteodystrophy ('renal rickets'). In this instance, skeletal disease was not observed because the course of the nephropathy was relatively brief and it resolved before it was manifested. Enzymatic diuresis was not employed because the iguana tolerated the saline diuresis well and voided abundant urates and fluid urine.

PROGNOSIS. Usually, severe renal failure and uremia proves fatal. However, this case illustrates that when the condition is diagnosed sufficiently early and is treated aggressively, acute renal failure can be resolved satisfactorily.

Case 205: **Parasitic ovum identification in a green iguana**

INVESTIGATION. After appropriate dilution, mixing, and centrifugation, the wet preparation of a fecal sample from a green iguana is ready for microscopic examination and interpretation. Elongated, 'D'-shaped embryonated ova are identified. The near-term embryos are characterized by having a very thin, curved, tail-like 'pin' structure at one end (**205**).

DIAGNOSIS. Oxyurid (pinworm) ovum.

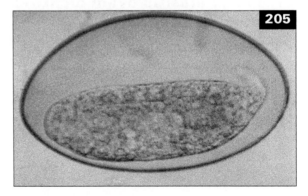

MANAGEMENT. The iguana is treated with pyrantel pamoate (5 mg/kg p/o, repeated in 2 weeks) or fenbendazole (50–100 mg/kg p/o, repeated in 2 weeks) or ivermectin (200 µg/kg i/m, repeated in 2 weeks).

PROGNOSIS. Favorable.

Case 206: Inky black, raised integumentary lesions in a European green lacerta lizard

CLINICAL PRESENTATION. A European green lacerta lizard is examined because its owner notices the relatively rapid appearance of multiple, raised, inky black integumentary masses on its rostrum, right thoracic wall, dorsum of pelvis, left forelimb, and tail (206a – photo courtesy Dr DR Mader). The masses are freely movable and, when touched, do not appear to elicit pain. The lizard is eating with a normal appetite, and its growth is normal.

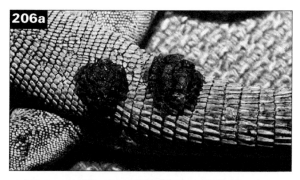

DIFFERENTIAL DIAGNOSES. Pigmented epidermal papillomata; malignant melanoma; benign pigmented nevi; eschar-covered healing traumatic wounds; mycotic dermatopathy; bacterial dermatopathy.

DIAGNOSIS. Transmissible epidermal papillomatosis.

ETIOLOGY. Transmissible epidermal papillomatosism is caused by a papillomavirus that is specific to lacertid lizards, especially *Lacerta viridis*.

PREVALENCE. Common, especially in naïve, usually young, lacertid lizards, which are most susceptible to this viral-associated, benign integumentary tumor.

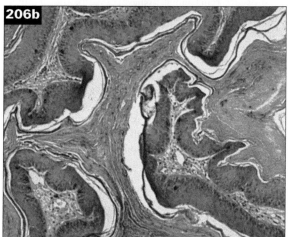

MANAGEMENT. The lizard is anesthetized and one or all of the masses prepared for surgical excisional biopsy. The surgical specimens are preserved in a tissue fixative and processed for histopathology (206b).

PROGNOSIS. After a variable period, most lizards mount an immune response to the etiologic viral agent and, as a result, these benign neoplasms usually will regress spontaneously.

Case 207: Parasitic ovum identification of a fecal sample from a savanna monitor lizard

INVESTIGATION. After appropriate dilution, mixing, and centrifugation, a wet preparation is ready for microscopic examination and interpretation. Elliptical, thin-walled embryonated ova are identified. The embryos are characterized by having four pairs of tiny appendages (207). These appendages are lost soon after the parasites emerge from their eggs.

DIAGNOSIS. Pentastomid ova.

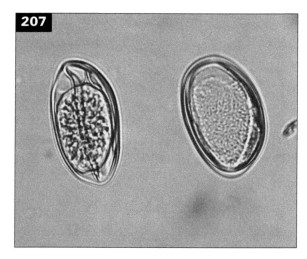

MANAGEMENT. The lizard is treated with ivermectin (200 µg/kg i/m, repeated after 2 weeks). **Warning:** Pentastomids have a potential zoonotic for human infection. Therefore, contamination when handling feces from reptiles known to be harboring these parasites must be prevented.

Case 208: **Dermatitis, irritability, hyperesthesia, and nonspecific electrocardiologic alterations in a Mexican beaded lizard**

CLINICAL PRESENTATION. A mature Mexican beaded lizard is suddenly exhibiting nonspecific signs consisting of dermatitis, irritability, and hyperesthesia. The lizard's diet consists of hen's eggs. After approximately three months of eating hen eggs, the lizard developed a moist dermatitis; it also twitched occasionally, as if it was being touched.

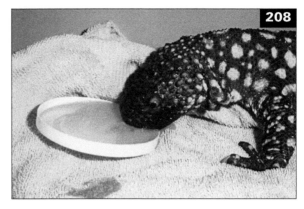

DIAGNOSIS. Biotin deficiency.

ETIOLOGY. Biotin is an essential water-soluble vitamin that is present in animal tissues, grains, and some other foodstuffs. It is only when the antibiotin antagonist, avidin, which comprises part of avian egg albumin, is present in significant quantity that biotin deficiency is induced. Avidin-induced biotin deficiency probably does not occur under wild, natural conditions because egg-eating animals usually consume embryonated bird (or reptile) eggs. Avian eggs in which embryos are developing contain much less avidin that nonfertile or unincubated fertile avian eggs. Moreover, the embryo also contains biotin, thus lessening the degradation of stored biotin in the egg predator.

PREVALENCE. Sporadic, depending upon the captive diet eaten.

MANAGEMENT. The egg yolks should be separated from the albumin portion of the eggs (**208**).

Case 209: **Identification of a mite found in a lizard cage**

CLINICAL PRESENTATION. Tiny arthropods are collected from a cage in which lizards are housed. It is necessary to identify them and determine if they are parasitic.

INVESTIGATION. These organisms can be identified by placing several of the organisms onto a glass microscopic slide, adding a drop of Hoyer's mounting medium (Frye, 1994), cover slipping, warming the slide gently until the mounted organisms have cleared and any bubbles have dissipated, and examining under low magnification.

DIAGNOSIS. Immature (nymphal) trombiculid grain mites.

ETIOLOGY. Pseudoparasitic mites, especially trombiculid grain mites, infest reptilian cages, especially those in which wood chips or similar particulate litter materials are used. During their immature nymphal stages, these mites can be truly parasitic. Nymphal mites are readily recognized by their three pairs of walking limbs (**209a**). Adults possess four pair of walking limbs (**209b**).

PREVALENCE. Frequently observed in reptile collections.

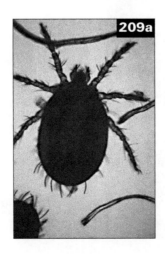

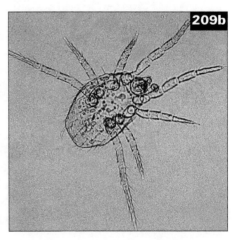

Case 210: **Bright red scleral coloration in a rock iguana**

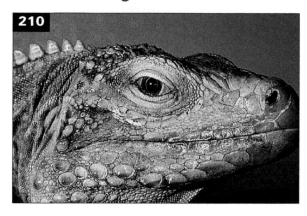

CLINICAL PRESENTATION. A male rock iguana is presented for evaluation because, as it has grown, it has gradually developed bright red sclerae (**210**). The iguana does not manifest any signs of illness or distress.

INVESTIGATION. When it is observed, care must be taken to differentiate the bright red-colored sclerae in males of this species from inflammatory ophthalmic disease such as keratoconjunctivitis.

ETIOLOGY. The males of this species (and some other species of *Cyclura*) possess bright red sclerae; this is a normal, sexually dimorphic characteristic.

PREVALENCE. Common.

Case 211: **Crusty circumnasal accumulation in a green iguana**

CLINICAL PRESENTATION. A mature green iguana has an accumulation of crusted white material around each nostril (**211a**). The iguana is healthy, and does not have any other medical problems.

DIFFERENTIAL DIAGNOSIS. Dried salt(s) of NaCl and KCl secreted from the nasal salt glands; an exudate arising from inflammation of the nasal mucosae.

DIAGNOSIS. Dried electrolytes secreted from the nasal salt glands.

ETIOLOGY. Some reptiles, particularly, but not limited to, those that have evolved to live in desert habitats, have behavioral and physiologic adaptations by which they conserve water. They are able to excrete electrolytes, especially sodium, potassium, and chloride ions, as NaCl and KCl salts in either their nasal (**211b, c**) or oral secretions. Some lizards, such as green iguanas, also employ extrarenal electrolyte secretion as a means of water conservation and electrolyte excretion.

Some plants, such as celery and many halogen sequestering plants native to deserts and some volcanic islands, contain very high levels of sodium and potassium.

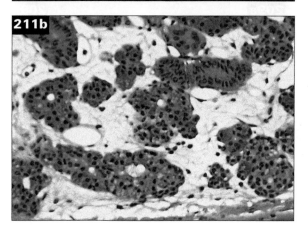

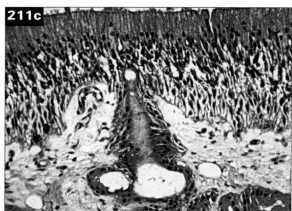

It is normal behavior for these lizards to sneeze out their electrolyte-rich secretions; therefore, it should not be interpreted as evidence of an upper respiratory tract disorder. Often, these dried deposits can be seen on the interior walls of a terrarium in the area where a lizard has sneezed.

PREVALENCE. Very common.

MANAGEMENT. These dried electrolytes are normal; therefore, unless there is evidence of inflammation, no treatment is required.

Case 212: **Swelling and lameness of all four limbs in a green iguana**

CLINICAL PRESENTATION. An adult male green iguana has become progressively reluctant to bear weight on its limbs. It can walk but only with great difficulty. The iguana is eating but, because of its reluctance to walk, the owner has to hand feed it. All four limbs are swollen, firm to the touch, and very tender to even the most gentle digital palpation. Bilateral, slightly raised longitudinal ridges are seen on the lateral thorax. These ridges are especially apparent when the iguana takes a deep breath (these ridges are analogous to the 'heave lines' observed in horses with pulmonary emphysema and other chronic respiratory conditions). The iguana is permitted to roam the owners' home, and has learned to use the tray filled with silica-containing diatomaceous earth cat litter that is provided for the household cats' toilet needs. The diet of the iguana consists of green leafy vegetables and small amounts of canned cat food and primate biscuits.

DIFFERENTIAL DIAGNOSES. Metabolic bone disease (secondary nutritional hyperparathyroidism); primary hyperparathyroidism due to one or more functional parathyroid adenomatous tumors; HPOA; multiple appendicular fractures; osteomyelitis; osteoarthritis; rheumatoid arthritis; multiple myeloma; osteoma or another benign musculoskeletal neoplasm; osteogenic sarcoma or another malignant musculoskeletal neoplasm; secondary bone metastasis from a distant primary site; osteopetrosis.

INVESTIGATION. Results of hematology and biochemistry investigations are shown (below).

The most significant laboratory findings are mild to moderate hypoproteinemia, hyperuricemia, and azurophilia. However, azurophilia might have been a laboratory misinterpretation of the granulocytic cell type; it is possible that what are identified as azurophils are actually heterophils.

	Immediate result		One month later		Normal value(s)	
Hematology						
WBCs	$16.3 \times 10^9/l$	$(16.3 \times 10^3/\mu l)$	$8.2 \times 10^9/l$	$(8.2 \times 10^3/\mu l)$	1.2–22.5	(1.2–22.5)
PCV	0.2 l/l	(20%)	0.35 l/l	(35%)	0.16–0.3	(16–30)
Metamyelocytes	$4 \times 10^9/l$	$(4 \times 10^3/\mu l)$	$0 \times 10^9/l$	$(0 \times 10^3/\mu l)$	n/a	
Bands	$4 \times 10^9/l$	$(4 \times 10^3/\mu l)$	$0 \times 10^9/l$	$(0 \times 10^3/\mu l)$	n/a	
Azurophils	$61 \times 10^9/l$	$(61 \times 10^3/\mu l)$	$28 \times 10^9/l$	$(28 \times 10^3/\mu l)$	n/a	
Lymphycotyes	$31 \times 10^9/l$	$(31 \times 10^3/\mu l)$	$71 \times 10^9/l$	$(71 \times 10^3/\mu l)$	21–91	(21–91)
Monocytes	0		0		0–10	
Eosinophils	0		0		0–3	
Basophils	0		0		0–3	
Thrombocytes	Adequate		Adequate			
Biochemistry						
AST (SGOT)	213 u/l		253 u/l		200–300	
Glucose	7.4 mmol/l	(133.2 mg/dl)	nd		<8.6	(<154.8)
Calcium	2.4 mmol/l	(9.6 mg/dl)	nd		2.9–3.5	(11.6–14)
TP	40 g/l	(4.0 g/dl)	28 g/l	(2.8 g/dl)	45	(4.5)
Uric acid	0.48 mmol/l	(8.1 mg/dl)	0.4 mmol/l	(6.8 mg/dl)	<0.3	(<5.1)

A whole body radiograph of the thorax (**212a**) is unremarkable. However, radiographs of the appendicular skeleton reveal severe osseous changes. The cross-sectional diameters of the long bones are grossly enlarged and they are very sclerotic with radiodense lines radiating outward from the periosteum (**212b, c**).

When informed that the radiographic findings are consistent with hypertrophic pulmonary osteoarthropathy (HPOA), and because of the progressive lameness and obvious pain that their pet is experiencing, the owners request euthanasia and grant permission for a complete necropsy. Significant gross pathologic conditions are identified in the skeleton, lungs, liver, myocardium, kidneys, and great vessels. The long bones are extremely dense and flinty; they are difficult to cut even with a new hacksaw blade. When defleshed and dried thoroughly, the left distal humerus, together with the radius and ulna, weigh an astonishing 39 grams. The marrow cavities of these altered long bones are normal in diameter; the mass of osseous tissue is composed of dense compact diaphyseal bone (**212d**). Small mucoid lesions that fill some of the airways in the incised lungs contain gritty gray material. The incised liver has a distinctly 'nutmeg' appearance and is firmer than normal (**212e**). The heart and great vessels are difficult to cut and are white and gritty on their incised surfaces.

Histopathology reveals massively dense compact bone, with numerous variably wide and irregular cement lines. The hepatic tissue is markedly fibrotic, with multiple seams of fibrocollagenous connective tissue that isolate cords of hepatocytes into islands that are often widely separated from each other (**212f**). The most interesting pathologic findings are in the lungs. Scattered throughout the pulmonary parenchyma are aggregates of amorphous microcrystalline material that are mixed with mucus (**212g, h**). When viewed with cross-polarized illumination, these aggregations are found to contain refringent glass-like material (**212i, j**).

Once these glass-like mineral crystals are identified as silica, the owners of the iguana are contacted and asked if their cats or any persons in the house are displaying respiratory distress. The answer is negative. The owners are provided with gauze surgical sponges saturated with distilled water, and are requested to secure the moistened sponges to the end of their vacuum cleaner wand, vacuum the areas around each of their cat-litter trays, and return the sponges in the sealed plastic bags that are provided. The returned sponges are rinsed in distilled water to dislodge any particles that have adhered to them. The water is centrifuged and the button that is spun down is examined microscopically. The recovered crystalline material is indistinguishable from the crystals that are identified within the pulmonary aggregates. A sample of cat litter is crushed, suspended in distilled water, and examined microscopically. This material is identical to the previous two sources.

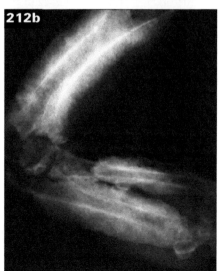

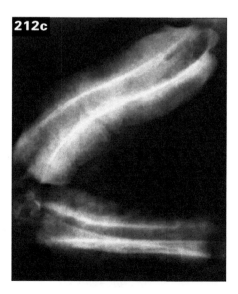

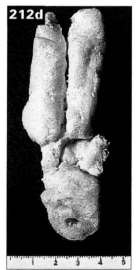

DIAGNOSIS. HPOA.

ETIOLOGY. Classically, HPOA is associated with any of the following disorders: pulmonary neoplasia or other chronic pathology (parasitism; inflammatory/infectious diseases affecting the lungs or mediastinal organs, including the esophagus); chronic cardiac dysfunction; chronic hepatocellular disease; chronic renal disease; chronic enteric disease.

Therefore, although HPOA is often associated with chronic pulmonary diseases, it also can be induced by several other disorders involving visceral parenchymatous organ systems (e.g. pulmonary silicosis; hepatic fibrosis; myocardial, aortic, or renal mineralization).

PREVALENCE. Sporadic.

MANAGEMENT. Captive reptiles must not be exposed to silica-containing diatomaceous earth cat litter.

PROGNOSIS. Guarded because HPOA is usually related to severe chronic disease in at least one vital organ system.

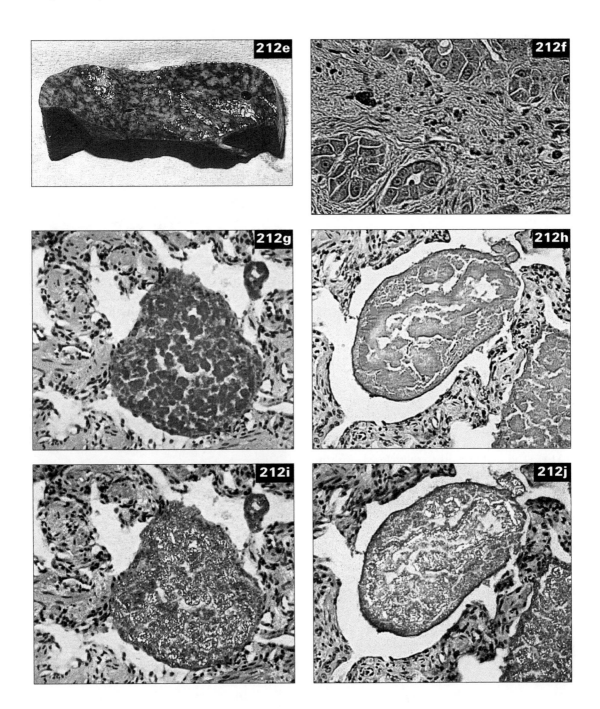

Case 213: **Parietal eye of a green iguana**

ETIOLOGY. Many lizards of the family Iguanidae possess a parietal, or 'third', eye that is located between the two lateral eyes (**213a**). The photomicrograph (**213b**) of a histological section of the parietal eye shows the relatively clear and hypocellular cornea at the top. The cellular lens, formed from parallel pink-staining columnar epithelial cells with basal or sub-basal nuclei, is seen immediately beneath the cornea. There is a slightly compressed, clear, fluid-filled central chamber that occupies the space immediately above the cup-shaped pigmented parietal retina, which is served by the parietal nerve and which exits through the parietal foramen. This interesting secondary sense organ serves as a physiologic dosimeter that helps regulate voluntary exposure to solar radiation. Experimental studies show that the parietal eye participates in hypothalamic, thyroidal, and gonadal functions.

When the parietal eye is either covered or ablated surgically, test lizards fail to bask or do not remove themselves from basking after what would be a normal period. Furthermore, when the eye is occluded or ablated, the lizard's thyroidal and gonadal functions are impeded.

The parietal eye might be misinterpreted either as an abnormal or anomalous integumentary scale or a pathologic item that requires excision.

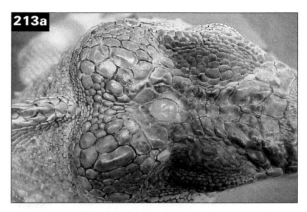

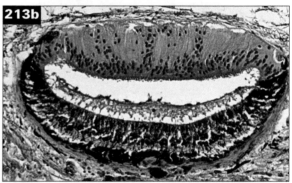

Case 214: **Sudden death in a neonate Solomon Island prehensile-tail skink**

CLINICAL PRESENTATION. The fresh cadaver of a 24-hour-old, fully formed skink is presented for necropsy. The neonate appeared to be normal when it was born.

INVESTIGATION. Necropsy reveals multifocal accumulations of chalky-white material that fill the pericardial sac, cover the epicardium, and are around both scapulohumeral articulations and between several ribs (**214**). The umbilicus is freshly closed, with no evidence of inflammation. The gastrointestinal tract is empty except for a very small amount of mucus. Histopathology confirms that the chalky-white accumulations are urate microcrystals.

DIAGNOSIS. Visceral and periarticular gout.

ETIOLOGY. In this instance the hyperuricemia with deposition of microcrystalline urates in soft tissues must have been referred from the maternal circulation to the developing fetus while it was *in utero*.

PREVALENCE. Sporadic.

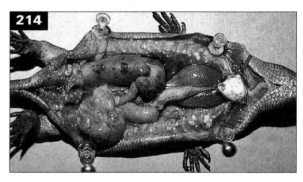

MANAGEMENT. In nature, Solomon Island prehensile-tail skinks almost exclusively eat the vine-like pothos plant, *Epipremnum* species, which is closely related to *Philodendron* species. It is estimated that their natural diet consists of approximately 95% *Epipremnum*, and the balance comprises small amounts of tropical figs, mango, papaya, and bananas. Fresh water must always be available.

Case 215: **Fecal parasitic ovum identification in a tegu lizard**

INVESTIGATION. After appropriate dilution, mixing, and centrifugation, the wet preparation of a fecal sample from a tegu lizard is ready for microscopic examination and interpretation. Elongated, thick, multiwalled embryonated ova with a plug-like operculum at each end are identified (**215**).

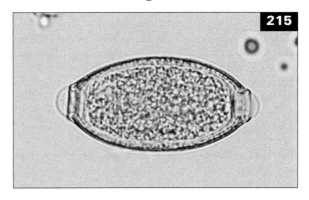

DIAGNOSIS. *Capillaria* species.

MANAGEMENT. The lizard is treated with pyrantel pamoate (5 mg/kg p/o repeated in 2 weeks) or with mebendazole (20 mg/kg p/o repeated in 2 weeks).

Case 216: **Chronic cholehepatic disease in a savannah monitor lizard**

CLINICAL PRESENTATION. The cadaver of a freshly dead, obese, mature female savannah monitor lizard that was depressed and anorectic for approximately two weeks prior to being found dead in her cage is presented.

INVESTIGATION. Necropsy examination reveals a massively enlarged, grossly thickened, and distended pale tan-colored gallbladder that bulges outward from the ventral incision that provides access to the coelomic cavity (**216a**). On incising the gallbladder, gallstones are not identified, but the bile is thick and viscid and it contains abundant coarse, dark green biliary 'sand'. Specimens are obtained of all organ tissues for histologic processing and microscopic examination (**216b**).

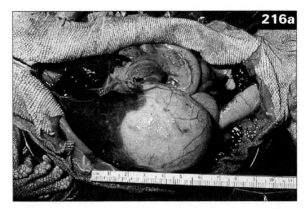

DIFFERENTIAL DIAGNOSES. The large, pale tan mass bulging from the coelom could be any of the following: a severely inflamed and thickened gallbladder; a primary hepatoma; secondary tumor metastasis from another site; pyogranuloma; mycetoma, (mycotic granuloma).

DIAGNOSIS. Suppurative cholecystitis and macro- and microvacuolar hepatocellular lipidosis.

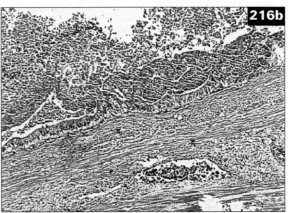

ETIOLOGY. Two of the most common disorders observed in captive savannah monitor lizards are gross obesity and chronic active pancreatitis. Both are related to overfeeding these robust animals. Once the lizards cannot sequester excess energy in the form of large intracoelomic adipose (fat) bodies and as subcutaneous and intermuscular fat, they tend to first develop hepatocellular lipidosis and, then, cholecystolithiasis and cholecystitis. Cholecystolithiasis (biliary 'sand' and formed gallstones) is believed to be promoted by a diet that is overly rich in lipids.

Cholecystitis is related to inflammatory disease induced by a variety of pathogenic microorganisms, or to the physical presence of gallstones, either within the body, the gallbladder, or in the biliary system, where they cause obstruction of bile flow to the duodenum.

PREVALENCE. Sporadic.

HUSBANDRY. It is vital not to overfeed captive savannah monitor lizards.

Case 217: **Facial dermatitis in an immature green iguana**

CLINICAL PRESENTATION. A half-grown common green iguana has a history of chronic anorexia and depression despite eating a nutritious diet of fresh salad greens, mulberry leaves, and occasional fresh tropical fruit. There are several small, discolored integumentary lesions on the head and neck as well as several raised lesions within the oral cavity (**217a**). The iguana is thin, depressed, and moves only when provoked to do so.

INVESTIGATION. Ultrasonic Doppler blood flow detection discloses very loud but muffled heart sounds that are transmitted to the aorta, brachycephalic trunk, carotid arteries, and as far as the internal iliac arteries. A blood sample reveals a leukocytosis of $32 \times 10^9/l$ ($32 \times 10^3/\mu l$), with a heterophilia of 84%.

Permission is granted for a complete necropsy. The individual lesions in the oral cavity (**217b**) and on the skin of the face and shoulders are filled with caseated exudate. The pericardial sac contains a large, wedge-shaped fibrin clot. The heart is grossly enlarged and misshapen due to the presence of several large, pale lesions that bulge from the surface of the myocardium. Additional lesions are scattered throughout the liver and lungs. When the pericardial sac is opened and the heart is incised in sagittal section, the normal myocardial tissue is revealed as being largely replaced with pale yellow, caseated exudate (**217c–f**).

Representative samples of all the parenchytmatous organs are gathered for histopathologic examination. Microscopic examination of stained histologic sections discloses massive replacement of the myocardium by pyogranulomatous inflammatory tissue. The lungs, liver, spleen, pancreas, kidneys, and thyroid also contain pyogranulomata, each characterized by multinucleated giant cells at their periphery.

DIAGNOSIS. Vegetative valvular endocarditis. The major lesions are in the myocardium and valvular endocardium, but other parenchymatous organs and tissues are also involved. In addition, there is evidence of possible multi-organ failure.

ETIOLOGY. The finding of multifocal pyogranulomatous inflammatory lesions in a reptilian patient is important with regard to the pathogenesis, as well as the prognosis, because it suggests that a septicemic process has occurred and that the vascular system has been 'showered' with infected emboli. Often, the cusps of the heart valves are infected and develop vegetations on their surfaces. These foci can shed emboli of infective exudate into the blood flowing over them. Once these emboli lodge in ever-smaller-diameter blood vessels that serve parenchymatous organs, they establish satellite inflammatory foci. The physical signs displayed by the patient clearly reflect the infected organs that are involved. If it is the heart and its valves, then adventitious valvular sounds are detected

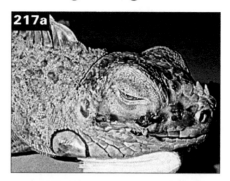

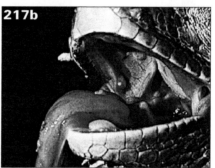

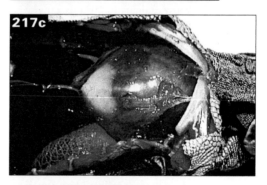

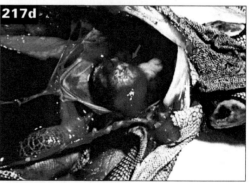

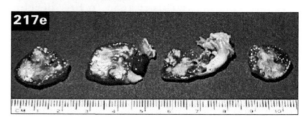

with an ultrasonic Doppler device. If it is the brain, CNS signs are to be expected. If it is the kidneys, then there will be renal insufficiency or, at least, urine that contains inflammatory leukocytes and tubular casts. If it is the liver, icterus, hypoproteinemia, and liver failure may ensue, depending on how much hepatic tissue is compromised.

PREVALENCE. Common.

PROGNOSIS. Guarded. Euthanasia is recommended because of the multiplicity of the inflammatory lesions (mouth, skin) and the very abnormal heart sounds.

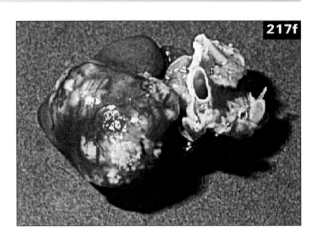

Case 218: **Bilateral firm post-cloacal vent swellings in a Jackson's chameleon**

CLINICAL PRESENTATION. An adult male Jackson's chameleon has bilateral swellings caudal to the base of its tail (**218a**). The chameleon was healthy and eating well until a few days prior to being presented for evaluation. The chameleon is housed by itself in a screened enclosure, which is kept outdoors in warm weather. The enclosure also contains a small mulberry tree on which mulberry silk-moth larvae feed. The chameleon has free access to these larvae and consumes them *ad libitum*. The chameleon's sole source of water is provided by the continuous slow drip that is directed onto the mulberry tree's foliage.

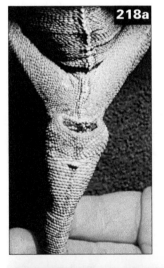

INVESTIGATION. Except for the bilateral enlargements, the physical examination is unremarkable. On gentle digital palpation, these bulges are quite firm and unyielding.

ETIOLOGY. Overly dry captive environment and solitary celibacy resulting in the accumulation of inspissated smegma plugs.

PREVALENCE. Common.

MANAGEMENT. The chameleon is restrained manually and a small volume of oily antibiotic ointment instilled into each hemipenial sulcus. This lubricant is massaged gently until it is evenly distributed and the perihemipenial soft tissues move freely over the twin bulges. Gentle pressure is directed cranially toward the anal opening to express the pair of dessicated smegma plugs (**218b**).

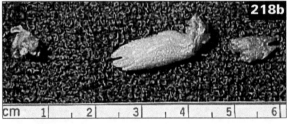

A moderately moist, humid environment that resembles the chameleon's native habitat should be provided. Additional moisture facilitates tropical reptiles in their periodic ecdysis (molting) and helps to moisturize secretions such as smegma and mucus. If the chameleon had a conspecific mate, hemipenial erections would help mobilize and eliminate surplus smegma, thus preventing its dessication and accumulation.

PROGNOSIS. Favorable.

Case 219: **Morbid obesity in a Bengal monitor lizard**

CLINICAL PRESENTATION. A mature male Bengal monitor lizard was gradually but progressively becoming obese, and it was lethargic. Previously, it was eating well but now it eats only occasionally. However, because the lizard was obese, the client was advised to feed his pet less often and to exercise it by encouraging it to swim in a bath-tub of tepid water at least twice weekly. Three months after it was first presented and examined, the monitor lizard, which is even more obese than before, is found dead in its cage. The owner admits that he continued to feed his lizard more meals and more frequently than recommended. Moreover, he did not exercise his pet even once since his last visit. The owner requests a necropsy.

INVESTIGATION. Necropsy examination reveals a pale tan, swollen liver that has rounded edges. When a piece of fresh liver is placed in a jar of formalin solution, it floats (**219a**). The pancreas has white foci that have the consistency of soap. The kidneys are slightly swollen and bulge cranially from their normal intrapelvic location. The heart is enlarged, and it has stopped in diastole; the single ventricle is distended with clotted blood. H&E staining of a histologic section shows that the liver is markedly altered by the presence of both large single and small multiple, clear lipid-like vacuoles within the hepatocytes (**219b**). Oil-Red-O staining confirms that these intracytoplasmic vacuoles are lipid (**219c**). The pancreas contains multifocal areas of chronic active pancreatitis, characterized by fibrosis and saponification of the peripancreatic fat.

DIAGNOSIS. Both chronic active pancreatitis and chronic macro- and microvacuolar hepatocellular lipidosis.

ETIOLOGY. Lipidosis is the abnormal deposition of intracytoplasmic lipid droplets in organs, most usually the liver, although it can also occur in kidney, spleen, and large arteries. Often, lipidosis is induced by chronic dietary intake of nutrients that far exceed what is essential for normal physical activity and metabolism.

Most monitor lizards are relatively sedentary in captivity, expending little energy in exploring their enclosures except when they are hungry and foraging. Many owners of these lizards tend to overfeed them; therefore, lacking exercise and being chronically overfed, these lizards soon become grossly obese. Chronic obesity tends to induce both hepatocellular lipidosis and chronic active pancreatitis. If the pancreatic disease is sufficiently severe, or if it continues unabated, diabetes mellitus may ensue due to the loss of insulin-secreting islet tissue.

PREVALENCE. Frequent in captive reptiles, especially monitor lizards.

PROGNOSIS. Favorable if the obesity can be significantly reversed and if the pancreatitis has not progressed too far. The hepatocellular lipidosis is reversible.

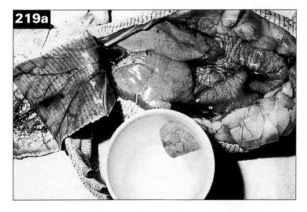

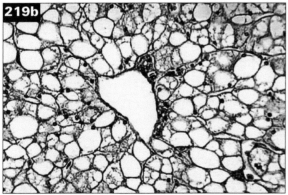

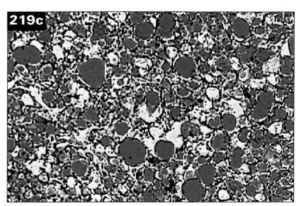

Case 220: **Sudden hemiparesis in a Meller's chameleon**

CLINICAL PRESENTATION. A recently acquired adult male Meller's chameleon presents with sudden left-sided hemiparesis. Both of the chameleon's left limbs are totally paralyzed (**220a**). However, the right forelimb and right hindlimb are mobile and the lizard can control them. There is a swelling immediately caudal to the anal vent (**220b**). The chameleon is able to move both of its turret-like eyes independently. Because the lizard was acquired very recently from a dealer, it is under a warranty of good health. The dealer elects to have the chameleon euthanatized and necropsied, with a promise to replace the sick lizard with a healthy one.

DIFFERENTIAL DIAGNOSES. Brain abscess; space-occupying parasitic cystic lesion in the brain; space-occupying neoplastic lesion in the brain; helminth parasites migrating through the brain (visceral larval migrans); traumatic injury to the brain; vascular insufficiency to the brain; ischemia, stroke.

INVESTIGATION. Parenchymatous tissues are collected aseptically, and selected tissues are submitted for microbiological culture. Microbiological culture of the brain and the postcloacal vent lesion yield *Peptostreptococcus* species in pure culture. Histopathology reveals at least two discrete abscesses within the right side of the cerebellum (**220c**).

DIAGNOSIS. Bacterial abscesses in the right cerebellum.

ETIOLOGY. The microbiological cultures of both the brain and subcutaneous postcloacal abscesses are identical; therefore, it is likely that the brain abscesses originated via hematogenous spread from the postcloacal lesion.

PREVALENCE. Sporadic. Depends on husbandry practices.

MANAGEMENT. Medical management of this case is difficult and problematical because a definitive diagnosis probably cannot be confirmed antemortem without employing highly sophisticated imaging studies. Once the diagnosis is made, an effective antibiotic drug that can cross the blood–brain barrier is employed. It is questionable whether the damaged brain in the area of the abscesses will heal sufficiently so that this chameleon can return to full neurologic function.

Frequent observation and cage hygiene are essential in keeping captive reptiles healthy. If this chameleon's postcloacal abscess was identified and treated early in the course of its abscessation, it is likely that it would not have become a nidus for septicemic dissemination and spread to the brain.

PROGNOSIS. Unfavorable.

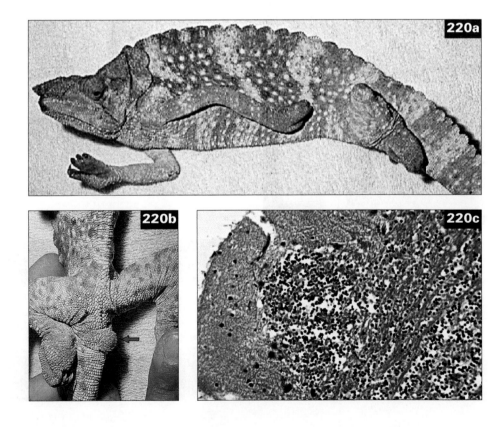

Case 221: **Multifocal skin lesions in a veiled chameleon**

CLINICAL PRESENTATION. An adult male veiled chameleon presents with multifocal integumentary lesions that developed over a period of three weeks. The chameleon is housed by itself in an indoor cage furnished with living plants.

INVESTIGATION. Several crusted lesions located on the caudal surface of the bony casque that rises from the back of the skull, along the dorsal spine, and on the right thoracic wall are identified (**221a**). The technique for examining samples of these crusted lesions is as follows: direct microscopy after macerating in 10% potassium hydroxide solution; direct microscopy as lactophenol cotton blue wet mounts; visualization with ultraviolet illumination (Wood's lamp) in a dark room; inoculation on dermatophyte test medium (DTM) slant, incubated at room temperature; direct microscopy of fungal growth gathered from DTM after approximately 10 days as a lactophenol cotton blue wet mount.

The crusts are examined with ultraviolet light display fluorescence (**221b**). The KOH wet-mounted specimen of crusted lesion is negative, as is the preliminary lactophenol cotton blue wet mount. However, fungal elements grow in the DTM culture and, after 10 days, exhibit significant numbers of conidia arising from mycelial hyphae (**221c, d**).

DIAGNOSIS. Mycotic dermatitis from *Microsporum* species.

PREVALENCE. Sporadic.

MANAGEMENT. The integumentary crusts are gently lifted and removed leaving a bed of inflamed granulation tissue (**221e**). Once every crust is removed, the underlying skin is gently cleansed with dilute (0.75%) povidone–iodine solution and air dried. Ketoconizole antifungal cream is applied twice daily. Ketoconizole is also administered orally (15 mg/kg q24h for 4 weeks). In order to administer oral medication, the chameleon's jaws are opened gently using a guitar pick as a lever and being careful not to injure the teeth or gingival tissue.

The source of the *Microsporum* infection is not established. The chameleon's owner has a cat that lives indoors and often sleeps on top of the chameleon's screened cage. Therefore, it is possible that the source of the infection is the cat. However, careful examination of the cat does not confirm dermatomycosis. At the owner's request, the cat is bathed and treated with a prophylactic course of ketoconizole.

PROGNOSIS. Favorable. The chameleon had an uneventful recovery.

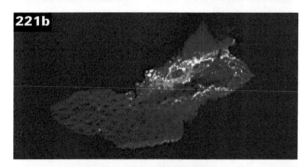

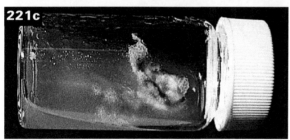

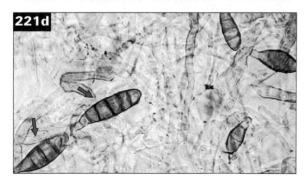

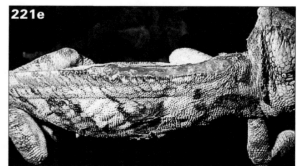

Case 222: **Mite infestation in a collared lizard**

CLINICAL PRESENTATION. A mature collared lizard has developed bright red-orange lesions adjacent to its axillae and just caudal to its hindlimbs (**222a** – photo courtesy Dr DR Mader).

INVESTIGATION. Inspection of the red-orange lesions with a small hand lens reveals a mass of mites (**222b**). These are removed with a moistened cotton-tipped applicator and transferred to a vial containing AFA solution (Frye, 1994). After the mites have been immersed in the AFA solution for a few hours, a few are mounted in Hoyer's mounting medium, cover slipped, and examined. Low-power microscopy confirms the parasites to be the lizard mite *Hirstiella trombidiiformes* (**222c**). This mite should be compared with the snake mite *Ophionyssus natracis* (**222d**).

DIAGNOSIS. Infestation with the chigger mite *H. trombidiiformes*.

PREVALENCE. Common.

MANAGEMENT. The lizard should be thoroughly cleansed to remove any mites that may have escaped the first collection. The lizard's integument is then washed with a solution of ivermectin (1 ml) mixed with propylene glycol (2 ml) and diluted with 500–1,000 ml of distilled water, applied as a fine spray. The lizard's cage is cleaned and sprayed with the same ivermectin solution.

Frequent surveillance for the presence of ectoparasites is important for detecting and preventing mite infestations. All new arrivals must be inspected; if they are harboring parasites, they must be treated before adding them to a colony.

PROGNOSIS. Favorable.

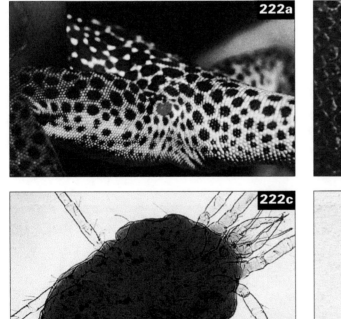

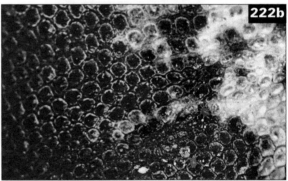

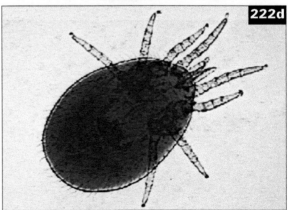

Case 223: **Intracoelomic mass, gradual weight loss, and marked bilateral buphthalmos in a Mexican beaded lizard**

CLINICAL PRESENTATION. An adult female Mexican beaded lizard with a history of gradual weight loss over a period of two years is presented. The lizard has continued to eat regularly during this time. The most striking feature is the extraordinary bilateral buphthalmos (**223a**) that the owner first noticed approximately two months prior to evaluation.

DIFFERENTIAL DIAGNOSES. Renal cell tumor; adrenal medullary tumor (e.g. pheochromocytoma); pyogranulomatosis (bacterial, mycotic, foreign body); parasitic cyst; intracoelomic fat-body steatitis.

INVESTIGATION. A firm swelling is palpated in the caudal coelomic cavity (**223b**). Whole body radiography reveals a rounded, soft tissue density mass in the caudal coelom (**223c**). Hematology and biochemistry determinations are unremarkable except for a PCV of 0.46 l/l (46%).

DIAGNOSIS. Renal tubular adenocarcinoma.

ETIOLOGY. Unilateral intracoelomic neoplasm.

PREVALENCE. Sporadic; more likely in older animals.

MANAGEMENT. The lizard is anesthetized by induction with 4% isoflurane–oxygen mixture delivered into a closed clear plastic chamber. When the lizard becomes unresponsive, it is removed from the chamber and a noncuffed endotracheal tube is inserted that is connected to the closed-circuit anesthesia machine. Isoflurane anesthesia is maintained at 3%. The lizard's knobby integument is scrubbed thoroughly and prepared for aseptic surgery.

At coeliotomy, the left kidney is about 6–8 times the size of the right kidney, and is firm, irregular, and lumpy. The left kidney and adrenal gland are excised after transfixing triple ligatures are placed around the left renal artery, vein, and ureter. At the owner's request, the beaded lizard is also spayed. The surgical specimens are photographed after they are incised (**223d**). Thorough exploration of the coelomic cavity for other pathology is

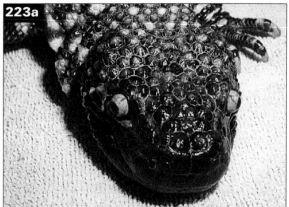

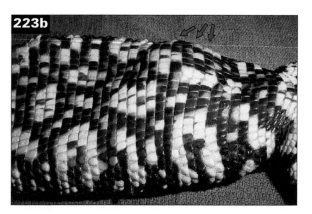

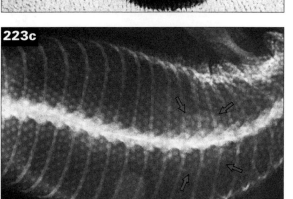

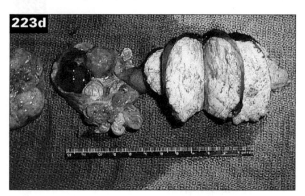

negative. Histopathology reveals an aggressive renal tubular cell adenocarcinoma, which has replaced most of the normal renal architecture (**223e**).

PROGNOSIS. Favorable. The lizard made an uneventful recovery and was eating raw egg yolks the morning after the surgery. The buphthalmos began to resolve almost immediately.

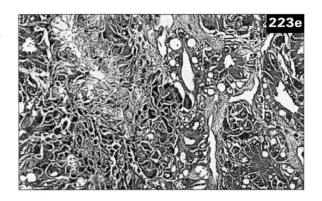

Case 224: **Unilateral curvilinear, pale gray deposit in the left eye of a Solomon Island prehensile-tail skink**

CLINICAL PRESENTATION. The left eye of an adult female prehensile-tail skink develops a semilunar-shaped collection of pale gray material. The skink is active and feeding well.

DIFFERENTIAL DIAGNOSES. Uveitis; lymphoreticular neoplasia.

INVESTIGATION. Direct ophthalmoscopy permits examination of the interiors of both eyes. The accumulation of leukocytes in the lower hemisphere of the left eye (**224**) does not impede inspection of the iris, crystalline lens, or retina. The affected eye's interior does not appear to be seriously inflamed. A whole blood sample is withdrawn from the ventral caudal vein for hematology and biochemistry determinations (below).

DIAGNOSIS. Hypopyon.

ETIOLOGY. Inflammation of the uveal tract.

PREVALENCE. Sporadic.

MANAGEMENT. A triple antibiotic ophthalmic ointment containing neomycin sulfate, bacitracin sulfate, and polymyxin B is instilled three times daily into the eye together with another ophthalmic ointment containing hydrocortisone. Within 48 hours the hypopyon is already diminished markedly; by the end of 96 hours the anterior chamber is clear. At this point, the topical hydrocortisone ointment is stopped, but the topical antibiotic therapy is continued for another 10 days.

PROGNOSIS. Favorable. The skink makes an uneventful recovery and its sight is preserved.

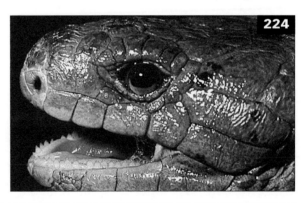

Hematology			Biochemistry		
PCV	0.34 l/l		Glucose	4.33 mmol/l	(77.9 mg/dl)
RBCs	1.66×10^{12}/l	$(1.66 \times 10^6/\mu l)$	Calcium	2.95 mmol/l	(11.8 mg/dl)
WBCs	12.8×10^9/l	$(12.8 \times 10^3/\mu l)$	Phosphorous	1.87 mmol/l	(5.79 mg/dl)
Heterophils	60%		TP	66 g/l	(6.6 g/dl)
Lymphocytes	24%		Albumin	23 g/l	(2.3 g/dl)
Plasmacytes	5%		Globulin	43 g/l	(4.3 g/dl)
Monocytes	5%		Uric acid	0.17 mmol/l	(2.87 mg/dl)
Azurophils	4%		AST	16 u/l	
Basophils	2%		ALT	130 u/l	
Eosinophils	0%		LDH	210 u/l	
Thrombocytes	Adequate				

Case 225: **Anorexia and lethargy in a green iguana**

CLINICAL PRESENTATION. A moderately thin, adult female green iguana has stopped eating and is lethargic. Its diet consists of moistened primate biscuits, mixed leafy green vegetables, and small amounts of soft fruit. After the primate biscuits were added to its diet, the iguana ate progressively less vegetables and fruit. Water is always available.

INVESTIGATION. Employing gentle palpation of the coelomic contents, multiple, hard, nontender swellings on either side of the caudal coelom are felt. Mild atrophy of the muscles over the pelvis is identified. Hematology and biochemistry studies disclose the above abnormalities.

Whole body radiography reveals multiple curved bone-density objects in the caudal coelomic cavity immediately in front of the pelvis (**225a, b**). These are located in the sites where the firm palpable swellings are detected. Because the radiological and physiologic chemical studies suggest chronic renal disease, the owner elects to have the iguana euthanatized and grants permission for a necropsy.

The most significant gross necropsy findings are confined to the kidneys. These consist of raised, firm, yellowish objects that are found within the dense connective tissues comprising the renal capsules (**225c, d**). Histopathology reveals multiple plaques of compact bone that are embedded within both renal capsules (**225e**).

DIAGNOSIS. Soft tissue mineralization.

ETIOLOGY. A diet composed mostly of primate biscuits contains excessive amounts of animal protein and preformed fat-soluble vitamins (especially vitamins A and D). The chronic ingestion of preformed vitamin D_3 promotes hypercalcemia and the deposition of calcium salts in nonskeletal sites, particularly some soft tissue organs (e.g. the renal capsules).

PREVALENCE. Sporadic.

PCV	0.18 l/l (18%) (with no nucleated RBCs identified)	
CPK	1,840 u/l	
Calcium	6.5 mmol/l	(26 mg/dl)
Phosphorus	3.5 mmol/l	(10.85 mg/dl)
Glucose	1.33 mmol/l	(23.9 mg/dl)
Potassium	7.8 mmol/l	(7.8 mEq/l)
Uric acid	0.43 mmol/l	(7.27 mg/dl)

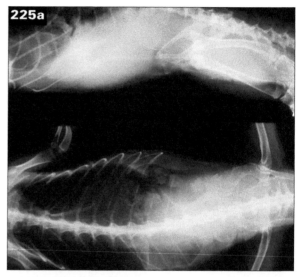

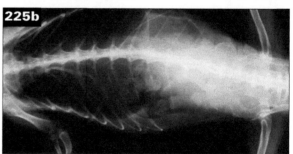

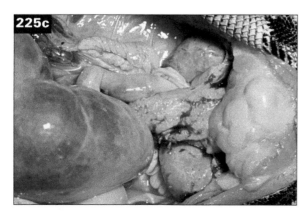

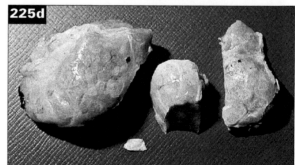

PROGNOSIS. Guarded to poor.

MANAGEMENT. Green iguanas are facultative folivores that utilize hindgut fermentation of complex carbohydrates (mostly cellulose) to simple sugars and fatty acids. This processing of plant material is analogous to the foregut fermentation of ruminants. Accordingly, folivorous lizards should be fed a diet consisting mostly of green, leafy plant material. When fed an appropriate diet and exposed to natural, unfiltered sunlight or its artificial ultraviolet equivalent, they are able to synthesize vitamin D_3.

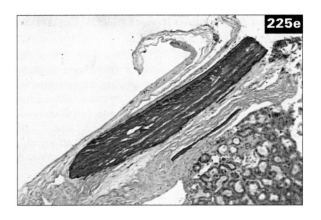

Case 226: **Chronic mandibular mass in a green iguana**

CLINICAL PRESENTATION. An adult male green iguana is presented for evaluation and treatment of a large, firm mass arising from the labial surface of its right mandibular dental arcade. The large, yellow-red-brown mass has been present for several months, but is not interfering with the iguana's eating. It has a broad base attached to the gingiva of the left mandible (**226a**) and it is movable. Surgical excision is recommended.

DIFFERENTIAL DIAGNOSES. Pyogranuloma (bacterial, mycotic, verminous); partially necrotic neoplasm.

DIAGNOSIS. Chronic oral pyogranulomatosis.

ETIOLOGY. Gram-negative pathogenic bacteria. *Citrobacter freundii*, *Serratia marcesens*, and *Pseudomonas fluorescens* were cultured from the mass after it was excised.

PREVALENCE. Common.

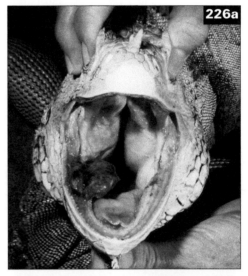

MANAGEMENT. The iguana is anesthetized and prepared for aseptic surgery. It is intubated with a Cole-type, uncuffed endotracheal tube to prevent aspiration of exudates. While the mouth is being held open, the mass is debulked by sharply excising down to its base, which is in the connective tissue of the mandibular gingiva. Three freeze-thaw cycles of cryotherapy are administered to the base from which the mass is removed, making certain that the surrounding healthy gingiva and integument are protected by masking-off the area from cryogenic spray. The cryosurgical treatment also controls hemorrhage from the vascular bed of gingiva from which the mass arises. The tissue is divided into two portions. The larger portion is used for microbiological culture and sensitivity; the smaller portion is formalin fixed and used for routine histopathologic processing and microscopic examintion.

PROGNOSIS. Favorable; an uneventful recovery is anticipated (**226b**).

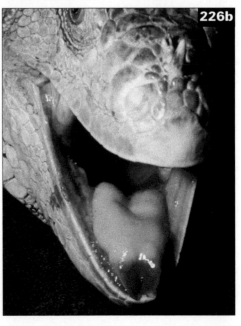

Case 227: **Quadrilateral limb-joint swelling and lameness in a green iguana**

CLINICAL PRESENTATION. An adult female green iguana presents with a history of progressive, painful, quadrilateral limb swelling and lameness. On gentle palpation, all four limbs are confirmed to be painful and, when flexed, they permit only very limited motion. The radiohumeral joints are particularly swollen and painful. The upper segments of each forelimb display significant muscle wasting.

DIFFERENTIAL DIAGNOSES. Rheumatoid arthritis; osteoarthritis; osteomyelitis; neoplastic osteopathology.

INVESTIGATION. A whole body radiograph and individual limb radiographs are made. The thoracic portion of the coelomic cavity has a ground-glass density and poorly aerated lung fields (**227a**). All of the radiographs demonstrate marked osteolysis, ranging from sclerotic remodeling of the distal humerus and proximal radius to massive outward cupping and expansion of the articular surfaces (**227b, c**). Blood is drawn for hematology and biochemistry determinations.

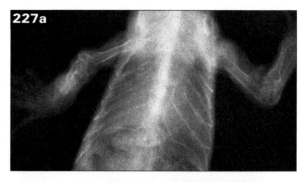

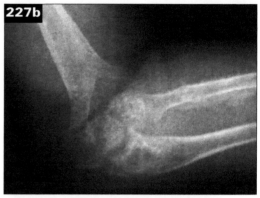

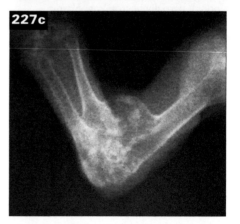

Hematology		
PCV	0.38 l/l	(38%)
RBCs	1.2×10^{12}/l	(1.2×10^6/µl)
Hemoglobin	126 g/l	(12.6 g/dl)
WBCs	19.2×10^9/l	(19.2×10^3/µl)
Lymphocytes	69%	
Plasmacytes	11%	
Heterophils	8%	
Monocytes	6%	
Azurophils	4%	
Basophils	2%	
Several lupus-erythematosus (L-E) cells identified		

Biochemistry		
Glucose	6 mmol/l	(108 mg/dl)
Calcium	3 mmol/l	(12 mg/dl)
Phosphorus	3.3 mmol/l	(10.23 mg/dl)
Potassium	5.6 mmol/l	(5.6 mEq/l)
TP	92 g/l	(9.2 g/dl)
Albumin	28 g/l	(2.8 g/dl)
Globulin	64 g/l	(6.4 g/dl)
Uric acid	0.4 mmol/l	(6.76 mg/dl)
AP	1 u/l	
AST	22 u/l	
ALT	18 u/l	
LDH	224 u/l	

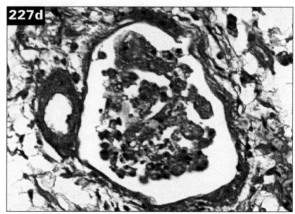

Histopathology of the kidneys reveals membranous thickening of Bowman's capsules in many of the glomeruli (**227d**). Interestingly, several lupus erythematosus (LE) cells were identified in stained peripheral blood films (**227e**). While awaiting the laboratory analyses, the iguana's condition deteriorates and its owner requests euthanasia. A necropsy is carried out.

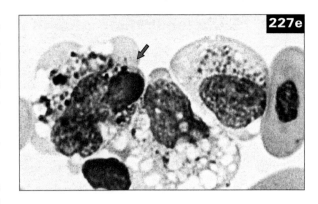

DIAGNOSIS. Autoimmune rheumatoid arthritis accompanied by chronic membranous glomerulonephritis.

PREVALENCE. Sporadic. As the population of captive reptiles grows older, an increase in the incidence of this disease is anticipated.

PROGNOSIS. Generally, the prognosis for rheumatoid arthritis in any species is guarded. Early in the course of the disease, before severe remodeling of the affected bones has occurred, steroidal and nonsteroidal antiinflammatory medications may reduce the acute or subacute inflammatory flare-ups that accompany this condition. However, once there is severe osteopathology, the bony alterations usually remain. Furthermore, the nonosseous changes in the kidneys tend to be cumulative, with the result being progressive renal insufficiency. Once a sufficient number of nephrons have been lost, renal function diminishes and end-stage kidney disease soon follows.

Case 228: **Worm in terrarium of two Madagascar panther chameleons**

CLINICAL PRESENTATION. A client brings a jar filled with water in which a 25 cm+ long nematode is swimming. This worm was found in the water pond portion of a terrarium that contains two chameleons. The owner is concerned about parasitism.

INVESTIGATION. Inspection of the nematode reveals that it is a 'horsehair' worm (**228**). These nematodes are members of the genus *Gordia*, which is classified within the Class Nematomorpha. They are parasitic only in insects, particularly crickets, grasshoppers, locusts, and cockroaches. They are not parasitic to reptiles or amphibians. Once they leave the body of their insect host, they become free-living, and they often are found in the water troughs of livestock.

DIAGNOSIS. Gordian 'horsehair' worms. Sometimes, these very long, thin worms are mistaken for parasitic ascarids or filarids.

PREVALENCE. Common, especially in environments were there is frequent exposure to wild crickets or grasshoppers.

PROGNOSIS. Excellent. These worms are not parasitic to reptiles or amphibians.

MANAGEMENT. If owners are concerned, they can be counseled to raise their own crickets in clean cultures, thus avoiding contamination with organisms parasitic to wild insects.

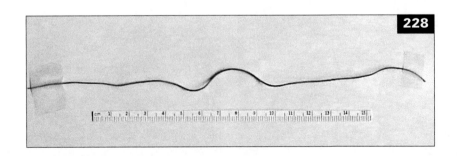

Case 229: **Coelomic distention in a green iguana**

CLINICAL PRESENTATION. A well-fleshed adult female green iguana has a gradual onset of coelomic distension over a period of two weeks. During this period the iguana remains alert, active, and has a normal appetite until two days prior to being evaluated.

DIFFERENTIAL DIAGNOSES. Egg yolk serocoelomitis (inflammation of the coelomic serosal surfaces); mycotic, bacterial, or viral serocoelomitis; nutrition-induced hypoproteinemia; hypoproteinemia secondary to cardiovascular, hepatic, renal, or enteric disease; protozoan or metazoan parasitism; lymphangiectasis; traumatic injury to one or more intracoelomic parenchymatous organs, especially an oviduct or segment of intestine; neoplasia.

INVESTIGATION. The coelom is grossly distended (**229a**). On percussion, a fluid wave on the opposite side of the body is readily created when one side is gently tapped with a finger. The iguana is reluctant to move because of its distended belly. Respiration is rapid and shallow. The oral and conjunctival mucosae are icteric. Ultrasonic Doppler blood flow investigation reveals muffled heart sounds and loud systolic ejection murmurs.

A whole body radiograph shows massive fluid accumulation that distends the abdominal portion of the coelom and compresses the lungs bilaterally (**229b**).

An aseptic percutaneous aspiration of the intracoelomic fluid yields abundant straw-yellow fluid with a SG of 1.1010. A total of 390 ml of this fluid is withdrawn, after which the iguana's respiration improves dramatically. Within 48 hours, the abdominal distension returns and the iguana is again breathing with difficulty. The owner requests euthanasia and a necropsy.

Necropsy confirms recurrence of excessive coelomic fluid. Numerous plaques of pale yellow fibrin cover the liver. Multilocular, thin, fluid-filled vesicles are attached to the mesentery (**229c**). The incised myocardium is riddled with discrete to coalescing firm, pale, nodular foci.

Histopathology confirms that the myocardial foci are chronic pyogranulomata, characterized by numerous multinucleated giant cells (**229d**). The liver is covered by

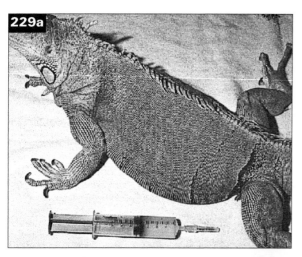

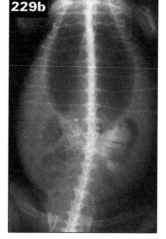

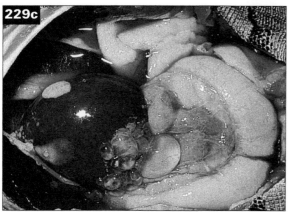

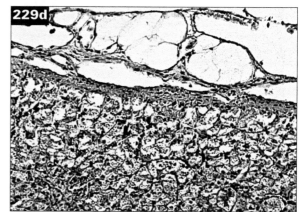

variably thick, multilocular, fluid-filled pseudo-membranes (**229e**). The aortic wall contains numerous, often coalescing, plaques of purple-staining mineralization (**229f**).

DIAGNOSIS. Fibrinous serocoelomitis, which is inflammation of the serosal surfaces of the coelom and its contents. It can be induced by any of several noninflammatory conditions (myocardial insufficiency, renal insufficiency, hepatic insufficiency, protein-wasting enteropathy); infections (viral, mycotic, bacterial); parasitic protozoan or metazoan parasitism; or traumatic injury to one or more internal organs, especially an oviduct or segment of intestine.

ETIOLOGY. Chronic myocardial pyogranulomatosis and severe aortic mural mineralization.

PREVALENCE. Sporadic; relatively common.

PROGNOSIS. Unfavorable.

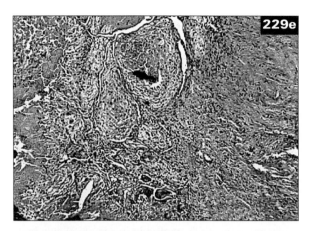

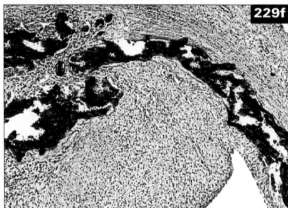

Case 230: **Large mandibular mass in an Australasian skink**

CLINICAL PRESENTATION. Six weeks prior to presentation, the owner of an adult male skink notices that it has developed a mass that protrudes from its lower right mandible (**230**). Over the six-week period, the mass has continued to slowly enlarge. The skink is active and eating regularly.

DIFFERENTIAL DIAGNOSES. Pyogranuloma: bacterial, mycotic, or verminous foreign body; neoplasm (osteoma, chondroma, etc).

INVESTIGATION. The mandibular mass is broad based, but still mobile when palpated. A radiograph of the skink's head ascertains the degree of any bone involvement. Hematology reveals a mild leukocytosis, heterophilia, and monocytosis. Other than these mild hematologic alterations, the balance of the hemogram and biochemistry values are unremarkable. A fine needle aspirate consists of inspissated pus and numerous heterophils and histiocytic macrophages.

DIAGNOSIS. Bacterial infection with pyogranulomatous inflammation.

PREVALENCE. Common in many captive reptiles.

MANAGEMENT. The lizard is anesthetized and prepared for aseptic surgical excision of the mandibular mass. The surgical specimen is submitted for microbiological culture and histopathology.

PROGNOSIS. Favorable.

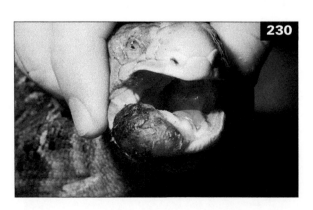

Case 231: **Severe vertebral distortion in a green iguana**

CLINICAL PRESENTATION. The owner of an immature green iguana notices that it is developing several marked curvatures in its vertebral column (**231a**). Periodic examinations reveal that the spinal deformity is growing increasingly severe. At the end of its second year, the iguana has assumed the shape of a horseshoe, with its head and pelvis being in close proximity. The iguana's respiration is rapid and shallow, reflecting the compression of the left hemithorax by the curved thoracic vertebrae.

INVESTIGATION. On auscultation, moist râles are heard over both lung fields. An ultrasonic Doppler blood flow study reveals markedly muffled heart sounds. Whole body radiographs reveal extreme curvature of the vertebral spine, with marked displacement of the coelomic contents (**231b**). The skeleton is well mineralized.

Although the iguana continues to eat well, it eventually experiences so much difficulty ambulating that its owners request euthanasia.

DIAGNOSIS. Kyphoscoliosis, the backward and lateral curvature of the vertebral spine.

ETIOLOGY. There is evidence that sometimes kyphoscoliosis in iguanas has a genetic component, or at least iguanas have a predisposition toward developing this severe musculoskeletal condition.

PREVALENCE. Common in green iguanas, especially those that are captive bred and farm raised.

MANAGEMENT. Constipation and urinary retention are common in severe cases of kyphoscoliosis in iguanas. These must be recognized and resolved by compassionate care employing stool softeners, enemas (when absolutely necessary), and meticulous attention to strict hygiene so that filth-borne dermatitis is prevented.

PROGNOSIS. Unless it is severe, kyphoscoliosis is not a fatal condition. However, if the cardiorespiratory, gastrointestinal, or genitourinary systems become severely compressed, their functions can be compromised, leading to illness and death.

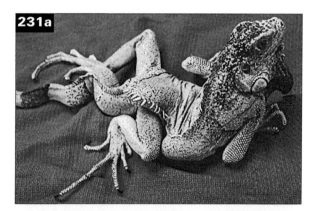

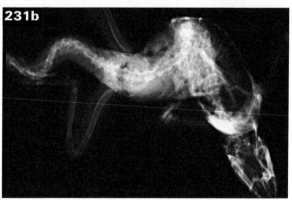

Case 232: **Nonsurgical retrieval of a large gastric foreign body in a small monitor lizard**

CLINICAL PRESENTATION. The owners of a juvenile monitor lizard see it swallow a large egg-shaped ornamental stone from its cage.

INVESTIGATION. Radiography is performed to assess the size and location of the ingested stone (**232a**).

DIAGNOSIS. Gastric foreign body.

MANAGEMENT. The lizard is sedated with a relatively short-acting anesthetic. Its mouth is opened and a suitable oral speculum or mouth gag inserted. A

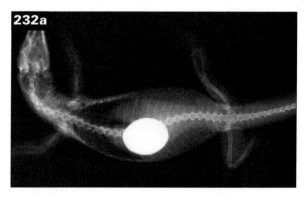

vulsellum or Doyen forceps, or a flexible mechanic's pick-up tool (**232b**), with the grasping jaws closed, is passed into the stomach. When able to feel the metal coming into contact with the stone, the jaws are opened and the stone grasped and extracted.

PROGNOSIS. Favorable.

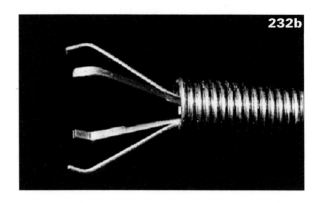

Case 233: **Severe lethargy in a female panther chameleon.**

CLINICAL PRESENTATION. Four days after the owners of an adult female chameleon notice that it is becoming progressively lethargic, refusing to accept living insect prey and, finally, unable to climb on the branches in its cage, they present it for evaluation. By the time the lizard is presented, it is already moribund and dies almost immediately after it is removed from the small transport carrier and placed onto the examination table.

INVESTIGATION. Inspection of the cadaver reveals a very thin chameleon with markedly atrophic paravertebral epaxial and coccygeal musculature. The chameleon's belly is bulging with firm rounded objects (**233a**). Necropsy reveals both oviducts are packed with numerous, foul-smelling, opaque, gray ova (**233b**). Rather than containing developing embryos, clear albumin, and yellow yolk, the eggs are uniformly turbid, gelatinous, and homogeneous. Microbiological culture yields *Salmonella urbana* in pure culture.

DIAGNOSIS. *Salmonella*-induced death and necrosis of the intraoviductal eggs, and intoxication of the lizard from absorption of amine-rich products of egg decomposition.

ETIOLOGY. Necrosis of intraoviductal shelled eggs.

PREVALENCE. Sporadic.

MANAGEMENT. Because reptile-associated salmonellosis in humans has been recorded many times, the owners of reptiles must be informed of the public health aspects, the importance of cage hygiene, and the necessity to seek medical assistance in case any family members become ill.

PROGNOSIS. Very guarded, even when diagnosed early. It is unlikely that the outcome would have been more favorable if the owners had presented their chameleon for examination earlier. The intraoviductal eggs were probably already dead days before the chameleon began to display illness. The decomposition of the dead and necrotic eggs would have already begun. Whether the infection with *S. urbana* contributed directly to the chameleon's illness, in addition to killing her eggs, is not known, but it is certainly possible.

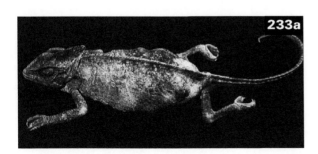

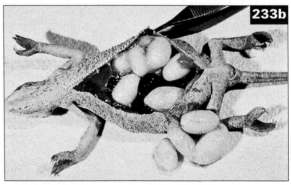

Case 234: **Identification of a ciliated protozoan organism in the feces of a green iguana**

CLINICAL PRESENTATION. While examining the feces of a green iguana, large numbers of ciliated protozoans that are very similar to *Paramecium* (**234**) are observed.

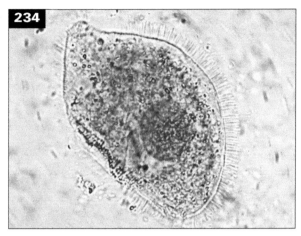

INVESTIGATION. A wet-mount specimen of fresh feces is prepared, stained with a drop of either merthiolate or Mayer's hematoxylin stain, cover slipped, and examined microscopically. *Nyctotherus iguanae* is identified.

PREVALENCE. *N. iguanae* is universal in healthy green iguanas, and this ciliated protozoan is essential for the digestion and fermentation of cellulose and other complex carbohydrates to simple sugars and fatty acids. Similar ciliated protozoans are involved in the conversion of carbohydrates in other folivorous reptiles and ruminants.

MANAGEMENT. The iguana should not be treated if only *N. iguanae* is identified in the feces. If an iguana is treated in error with an antiprotozoal agent such as metronidazole, the normal gut flora will have to be re-established by feeding the iguana feces from a normal healthy iguana. Therefore, routine dosing with metronidazole is contraindicated.

Case 235: **Chronic swelling and draining sinus tracts in the foot of a South American tegu**

CLINICAL PESENTATION. A second opinion is requested because an adult male tegu lizard has a chronic swelling of its left hind foot (**235a**). Periodically during the previous two years, tracts on the plantar and posterior heel area opened spontaneously and drained pus. Numerous different antibiotics were administered, with little improvement.

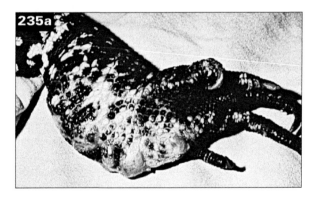

INVESTIGATION. A physical examination is carried out. Radiographs of the affected limb are obtained, a specimen of the exudate is collected for microbiological culture and sensitivity, and a blood sample is taken for hematology and biochemistry determinations. *Dermatophilus congolensis* in pure culture sensitive to a wide variety of bacteriocidal antibiotics is identified.

DIAGNOSIS. Dermatophiliasis.

ETIOLOGY. The invasion and infection of the skin and subcutaneous structures by the pathogenic microbe, *D. congolensis*.

PREVALENCE. Sporadic; infectious. Dermatophiliasis is a zoonotic disease transmissible to humans.

MANAGEMENT. A course of clindamycin (2.5mg/kg p/o q12h for 3 weeks) was ineffective, as was enrofloxacin (5 mg/kg p/o q12h for 2 weeks). Adding metronidazole (15 mg/kg p/o) was equally ineffective. An autogenous bacterin prepared from killed cultured organisms also failed to resolve the infection.

Finally, the tegu was anesthetized and the infected left hindlimb amputated at the coxofemoral articulation, creating a stump-free site. The surgical specimen was opened and it revealed multiple caseated lesions, each surrounded by very dense connective tissue capsules (**235b**). It is very likely that this encapsulation prevented an adequate microbiocidal inhibitory concentration of the various antibiotic agents that were administered to this tegu for over two years.

PROGNOSIS. Favorable, once the infected limb is amputated. The tegu made an uneventful recovery.

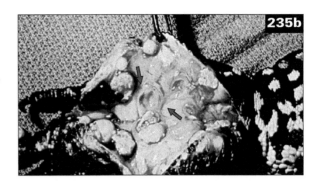

Case 236: **Fecal parasitic ovum identification in a monitor lizard**

INVESTIGATION. After appropriate dilution, mixing, and centrifugation, the wet preparation of a fecal sample from a monitor lizard is ready for microscopic examination and interpretation. Elongated, particularly thick, triple-walled embryonated ova are identified. The embryos are characterized by having tiny refractile hooklets at one end (**236**).

DIAGNOSIS. Acanthocephalan '(thorny-headed' worm) ovum. These parasites are most often identified in the feces of carnivorous reptiles.

MANAGEMENT. The lizard is treated with ivermectin (200 µg/kg i/m, repeated in 2 weeks).

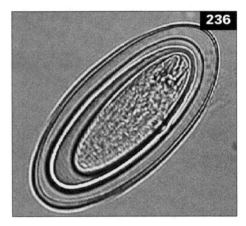

Case 237: **An adult male veiled chameleon with an object passed from its cloacal vent**

CLINICAL PRESENTATION. Dragging behind a male chameleon is a thin, elongated object that it passes from the cloacal vent. The object is pale grayish-pink to black and has a bulbous swelling at its free end (**237** photo courtesy Dr. F Faiolo). On close visual inspection, the object is identified as the chameleon's tongue. In this instance, the tongue passes entirely through the digestive tract undigested.

DIAGNOSIS. Glossophagy, the accidental swallowing of the tongue.

PREVALENCE. Sporadic.

MANAGEMENT. The chameleon is anesthetized and mild traction is applied to remove as much of the tongue as possible. A single ligature is applied and the exposed tissue is amputated.

A period of training is necessary to teach a tongue-less chameleon how to recognize and catch its insect prey.

PROGNOSIS. Favorable. The chameleon soon learns to apprehend insect prey by biting, rather than by catching with a tongue which is no longer there.

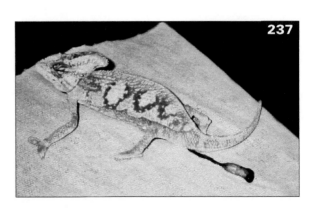

Case 238: **Partial unilateral hemipenial prolapse in a young green iguana**

CLINICAL PRESENTATION. The left hemipene of a subadult male green iguana has prolapsed (**238**). The prolapsed organ is still moist. In this instance it appears that the sand that is used as cage litter has adhered to the moist surface of the hemipene and has impeded its withdrawal into the hemipenial sheath and sulcus.

DIAGNOSIS. Foreign bodies (sand) adhering to the hempene.

PREVALENCE. Common.

MANAGEMENT. The exposed hemipenial tissue is cleansed gently to remove the grains of sand. A lubricating anti-inflammatory ointment is applied to the exposed hemipene. Using a glass rod or lubricant-moistened cotton-tipped applicator, gentle pressure is applied to the prolapsed hemipene and it is induced it to invert back into

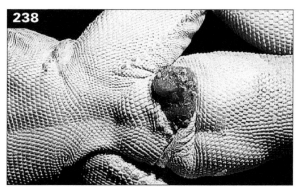

its sheath and sulcus. The coarse sand litter is replaced with dry leaves or other appropriate material.

PROGNOSIS. Favorable.

Case 239: **Multifocal round masses involving the costrochondral junctions of the ribcage in a green iguana**

CLINICAL PRESENTATION. An immature green iguana develops bilaterally symmetrical, swollen hindlimbs and mandible, and bulges along its ribcage (**239a**). The iguana is kept in an indoor terrarium with ambient room incandescent illumination. Its diet is mostly romaine lettuce and sliced bananas.

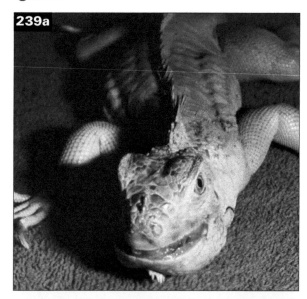

INVESTIGATION. A whole body radiograph and whole blood sample for hematology and physiologic chemistry determinations are obtained. The radiograph reveals soft tissue dense masses at each costrochondral junction (**239b**). Additionally, the long bones exhibit thinning of their cortices. Overall, the skeleton is poorly mineralized. A different green iguana's ribcage showing rachitic rosettes is illustrated in **239c**. The hematology is unremarkable except for hypocalcemia (1.28 mmol/l [5.12 mg/dl]) and hyperphosphatemia (2.68 mmol/l [8.3 mg/dl]).

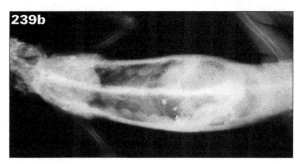

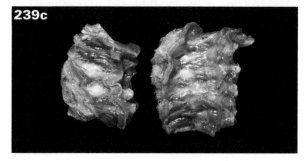

DIAGNOSIS. Rickets induced by hypovitaminosis D$_3$.

ETIOLOGY. Rickets is a condition characterized by a failure of the cartilaginous bony scaffold in young growing animals to properly mineralize.

PREVALENCE. Common.

MANAGEMENT. The diet is supplemented with exogenous, preformed vitamin D$_3$ and improved diet so that calcium-rich vegetables predominate. The iguana is allowed to sunbathe in natural, unfiltered sunlight outdoors whenever the weather allows. When the iguana cannot sunbathe, a source of ultraviolet illumination of a proper wave length (UVB 290–320 nm; UVA 320–400 nm) is added to its cage.

PROGNOSIS. Favorable once the diet and husbandry are improved.

Case 240: **Fecal parasitic ovum identification in a Gila monster lizard**

INVESTIGATION. After appropriate dilution, mixing, and centrifugation, the wet preparation of a fecal sample from a Gila monster lizard is ready for microscopic examination and interpretation. Round, thick, multiwalled embryonated ova with multiple refractile recurved hooklets are identified (**240**).

DIAGNOSIS. Cestode ovum.

MANAGEMENT. The lizard is treated with praziquantel (5–8 mg/kg i/m or p/o, repeated in 2 weeks).

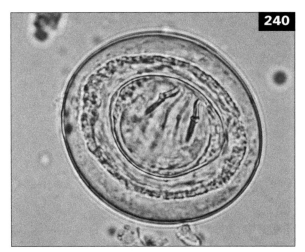

Case 241: **Fecal parasitic protozoan identification in an Australasian bearded dragon lizard**

INVESTIGATION. After appropriate dilution, mixing, and centrifugation, the wet preparation of a fecal sample from a bearded dragon lizard is ready for microscopic examination and interpretation. Small, round organisms with a single endocyst are identified (**241**).

DIAGNOSIS. Coccidiosis with *Isospora* species.

MANAGEMENT. The lizard is treated with sulfadimethoxine (90 mg/kg p/o the first day, and then 45 mg/kg p/o for the following 5 days). Hydration is maintained, if necessary, with parenteral fluid therapy. Fecal examination is repeated in two weeks, and the lizard retreated if necessary.

HUSBANDRY. Meticulous cage hygiene in order to prevent reinfection is essential.

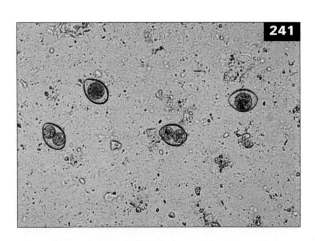

Case 242: **Change in right eye's appearance in a green iguana**

CLINICAL PRESENTATION. The appearance of an iguana's right eye suddenly changes. There is no prior history of trauma or illness.

INVESTIGATION. Direct ophthalmoscopy reveals that the lower hemisphere of the anterior chamber is filled with bright red blood (**242**) (photo courtesy Dr. A Abayon). The crystalline lens and fundus are normal. Physical examination of the iguana is negative except for the markedly altered right eye.

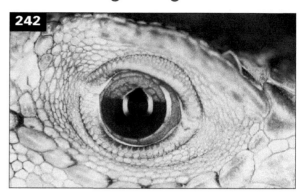

DIAGNOSIS. Acute hyphema (hemorrhage into the anterior chamber of the eye).

PREVALENCE. Sporadic.

MANAGEMENT. Treatment is not necessary. Acute hyphema usually resolves spontaneously as the blood is resorbed.

PROGNOSIS. Favorable

Case 243: **Sudden death in an adult female tegu lizard**

CLINICAL PRESENTATION. An adult female tegu is found moribund in its cage early one morning. The tegu had been in excellent health, eating well, and displaying no signs of illness. A review of the captive husbandry discloses nothing of concern.

INVESTIGATION. The tegu is in profound morbidity. The oral and conjunctival mucosae are very pale. When the tegu's toes are gently pinched, there is no reaction or attempt to pull them back. Ausculation does not detect any heart or breath sounds. An ECG detects only sinus rhythm of low amplitude. The tegu is clinically dead.

A whole body radiograph shows a large fluid density mass on the right side of the caudal coelomic cavity. The owners request a necropsy.

Necropsy reveals the right ovary protruding up through the fat-laden omentum (**243**). The connective tissue surrounding the right ovary is intact and encloses a large mass of clotted blood. On opening the periovarian tissue, approximately 20 ml of blood is found. Exploration of the right ovarian artery reveals a small full-thickness tear in its wall. The left ovary is unremarkable. The rest of the intracoelomic organs are normal.

DIAGNOSIS. Spontaneous rupture of the right ovarian artery and exsanguination into the right periovarian connective tissues.

ETIOLOGY. Idiopathic.

PREVALENCE. Sporadic.

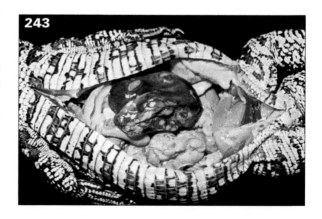

Case 244: **Fertile eggs deposited by a 'virgin' adult female green iguana**

CLINICAL PRESENTATION. Two freshly deposited shelled eggs from an adult female green iguana are presented for evaluation. The last time this iguana was in the company of a male was when it was seven months old, very small, and immature; the owner photographed it at that time (**244a**). In the intervening three years, this iguana was kept by itself.

INVESTIGATION. On opening the eggs, a developing embryo is found in each egg. Each embryo has pigmented eyes and tiny limb buds (**244b**). These embryos are processed histologically and the stained sections are examined microscopically. Astonishingly, brain, hepatic, intestine, renal, myocardial, and hematopoietic tissues are identified in each of these tiny early embryos (**244c–e**).

Located at the caudal portion of the oviduct are numerous glandular structures whose secretions nourish spermatozoa and facilitate their storage for lengthy periods.

DIAGNOSIS. Amphigonia retardata.

ETIOLOGY. Although it was believed that embryogenesis commences only after eggs are deposited and, thus, exposed to atmospheric oxygen, it is evident that substantial embryonic development of green iguanas occurs while the eggs are still in the oviduct. Obviously, this iguana was impregnated at an early age and stored living sperm for at least three years before reaching sexual maturity and producing fertile eggs. This is not an instance of parthenogenesis ('immaculate conception'); rather, immaculate deception accounts for this interesting embryonic development in the eggs of an erstwhile 'virgin' iguana.

PREVALENCE. Common.

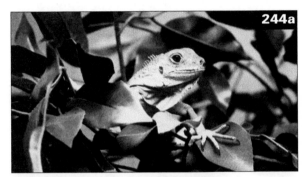

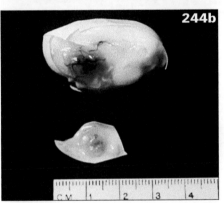

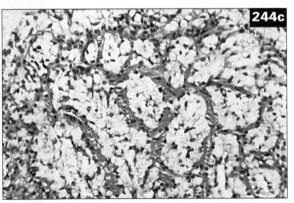

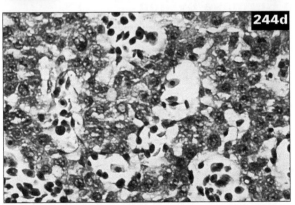

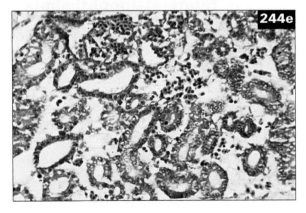

Case 245: **Sudden inability to use right hindlimb in a Meller's chameleon**

CLINICAL PRESENTATION. An adult male chameleon suddenly loses the use of its right hindlimb. There is no previous medical history. The chameleon is kept by itself in a spacious cage. Inspection of the cage does not support a contention that an item in the cage caused trauma.

The right hindlimb is flaccid, and the normally grasping apposed syndactylous toes of the right foot cannot be induced to close around a cotton-tipped applicator stick. The skin covering almost the entire length of the hindlimb is very dark; only a short segment shows the normal bright coloration (**245a**).

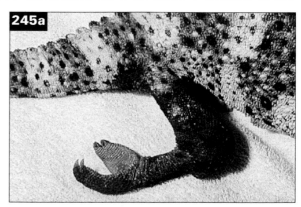

INVESTIGATION. Ultrasonic Doppler blood flow studies fail to reveal blood flow in the femoral artery. A radiograph of the affected limb is negative for fractures, osteolysis, or osteogenic production. A whole blood specimen is obtained, stained, and examined microscopically. The WBC count and differential are unremarkable. However, several microfilariae are identified (**245b**).

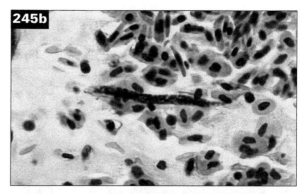

DIAGNOSIS. Verminous thromboembolism-induced ischemia and gangrene.

PREVALENCE. Sporadic.

MANAGEMENT. The chameleon is anesthetized and, after it is prepared for aseptic surgery, the right hindlimb is amputated at the coxofemoral joint by disarticulation, leaving no stump. Following surgery, the chameleon is injected with ivermectin (200 µg/kg i/m, repeated in 2 weeks).

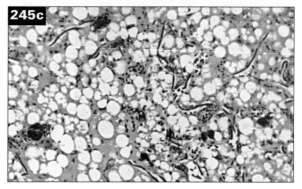

PROGNOSIS. Favorable. Chameleons and many other quadripedal lizards soon learn to ambulate well after losing one of their limbs. Once the circulating microfilariae and the adult filarids are eliminated, there should be no further verminous thromboembolic incidents. The liver from another chameleon illustrates microfilariae crowding the hepatic sinusoids (**245c**).

Case 246: **Bilateral anophthalmia in a Burmese python**

CLINICAL PRESENTATION. A juvenile Burmese python is evaluated because its owner discovers that the snake lacks eyes (**246**). A thorough inspection reveals a total absence of eyes

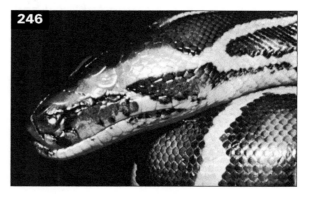

DIAGNOSIS. Bilateral anophthalmia.

ETIOLOGY. Anophthalmia is a developmental defect that probably has a genetic component.

PREVALENCE. Common in both the Burmese python and Royal python, both of which are popular pet snake species that are being bred in captivity. Inbreeding has reduced the genetic diversity of these taxa and, accordingly, has increased the prevalence of the defect. In some instances, only one eye is missing

MANAGEMENT. Sightless snakes, particularly pythons, do very well in captivity because they can rely on nonvisual

sense organs for the detection of prey. These include the sensitive tongue, which is used to perceive scent cues, and the labial pit organs, which are sensitive to thermal cues coming from the warmth of their prey.

PROGNOSIS. Favorable.

Case 247: **Iatrogenic traumatic avulsion of the tertiary spectacle and destruction of the underlying cornea in a rat snake**

CLINICAL PRESENTATION. A rat snake presents after its owner has tried to assist the snake in shedding the retained tertiary spectacle that covered its left eye. The owner had grasped the remnant of the retained spectacle with a forceps without previously moisturizing it. Traction on the remnant, which must have been tightly adhered to the subjacent cornea, caused the spectacle and cornea to be avulsed, leaving the iris and other contents of the eye totally exposed (**247a**).

INVESTIGATION. Direct examination of the affected eye confirmed that the cornea was avulsed, leaving the interior of the eye exposed and already dessicated.

DIAGNOSIS. Iatrogenic destruction of the left eye and its contents.

ETIOLOGY. Usually, when a snake is about to shed its old epidermis, a water-soluble shedding fluid, which moisturizes and lubricates the two surfaces comprising the new and old epidermal tissues, is secreted. If the snake (or lizard) is kept in an overly dry environment and/or if the cage lacks items on which it can rub its jaws and thereby loosen the old epidermis in order to begin the process of ecdysis, the moist epidermal surfaces soon dessicate and may be difficult to part from each other. The tertiary spectacles are derivatives of the epidermis and are normally molted during ecdysis.

PREVALENCE. Common.

MANAGEMENT. There are two methods for removing retained tertiary spectacles. One is to moisten a pledget of cotton or a small cotton sponge with a few drops of hard contact lens wetting and soaking solution, place the moistened cotton over the retained spectacle, and hold the cotton in place for a few minutes. The other method is to place the snake in a shallow container of tepid water for 30 minutes before attempting to remove any senescent epidermal remnants, then use a hand cloth or towel to remove remnants. If one or both tertiary spectacles fail to come away with the surrounding periocular epidermis, they can be loosened by gently inserting and sweeping a cerumen loop into and around the fornix that surrounds the eye (**247b**).

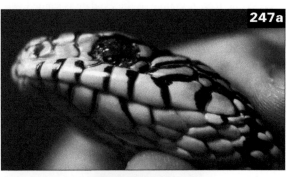

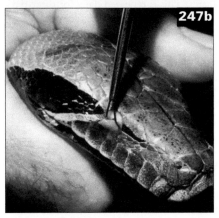

If the protection of the eye's interior is breached by having its cornea avulsed, thus exposing the uveal tract, lens, and retina, the eye is lost. If the cornea is avulsed, the eye should be enucleated and, if possible, the orbital defect covered with a sliding, full-thickness skin graft fashioned from the surrounding integument. If a skin graft is not practicable, the eye can be enucleated and the orbital defect covered with an antiseptic liquid dressing such as New Skin® (Medtech, Jackson, WY) or its equivalent.

PROGNOSIS. Effective treatment following enucleation will permit fibrous connective tissue to fill in the orbit. The orbit will be covered by the in-growth of integument from the periphery of the orbital defect and it will heal *per primum*. Therefore, although the eye is no longer functional, its cosmetic appearance can be enhanced.

Case 248: Oral lesions in a Central American boa constrictor

CLINICAL PRESENTATION. While in Nicaragua consulting on projects whose goal is sustainable captive breeding of selected reptiles, a wild-caught adult boa constrictor with oral lesions (248) is examined. The boa exhibits fractious behavior, which is typical for this subspecies. The boa's entire mouth is involved in an ulcerative process. Old ulcers containing caseated exudate that fills shallow ulcers, and freshly traumatized bleeding lacerations are identified.

INVESTIGATION. A sample of the exudate is stained with Gram's stain. The smear is teeming with gram-negative microorganisms.

DIAGNOSIS. Ulcerative stomatitis ('mouth rot').

ETIOLOGY. Trauma to the jaws and oral mucosae, with secondary bacterial infection and multiple ulcerations.

MANAGEMENT. The snake's oral cavity is gently but thoroughly cleansed with 0.75% povidone–iodine solution or 0.75% chlorhexidine diacetate solution until it is free of exudates. This is repeated daily for three days until the oral mucosa is no longer producing exudate. Enrofloxacin (10 mg/kg i/m) is given once daily for two weeks. Sterile saline is instilled intracoelomically (15 ml/kg q24h) for the entire length of time that the antibiotic therapy is administered.

Analysis of the snake's caging is highly instructive, because the snake is kept in a cage with walls, bottom, and top constructed with chicken-wire netting, and there is no closed area in which it can hide. As people walk past its cage, the snake repeatedly strikes out at them, thus further damaging its delicate oral tissues. When the snake is moved into a more appropriate enclosure, which is constructed of solid wood and is furnished with a large water container, natural dry-leaf litter, and a section of hollow log in which to hide, it no longer strikes out.

PROGNOSIS. Favorable.

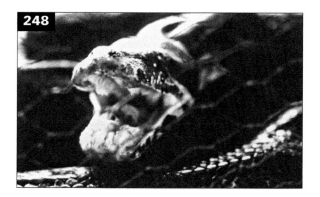

Case 249: Intraerythrocytic objects in the blood of a South American boa constrictor

CLINICAL PRESENTATION. A boa constrictor that was purchased immediately prior to being presented is evaluated. This boa constrictor was represented by the animal dealer as being a captive-bred snake. Physical examination is negative for gross abnormalities.

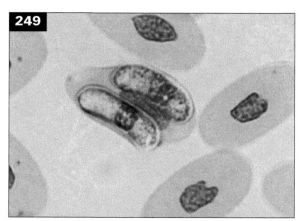

INVESTIGATION. A blood sample is taken and total WBC count, PCV, and differential count values determined. Although the WBC and PCV are within normal limits, many of the erythrocytes contain one or more sausage-shaped objects that often distort the cells and displace the erythrocyte nuclei (249).

DIAGNOSIS. Intraerythrocytic hemogregarine parasitiasis.

PREVALENCE. Very common.

MANAGEMENT. Hemogregarines are not usually pathogenic; therefore, it is not necessary to treat these harmless hemoprotozoans. However, the owner should be informed that it is highly unlikely that this snake was captive-bred because, in order to be infected, the snake would have to be exposed to the insect, mite or tick vectors that carry the infective stages of the hemogregarines.

Case 250: **Unilateral hemipenial prolapse in a false water cobra**

CLINICAL PRESENTATION. A mature male false water cobra is presented for evaluation of a total prolapse of its right hemipenis one day after its owner, believing that he could reduce the size of the prolapsed phallus and, perhaps, replace it within its sheath, inserted a hypodermic needle and withdrew what he estimates to have been at least 100 ml of whole blood from the snake's blood-engorged organ. When these 'therapeutic actions' proved to be ineffective, the owner sought professional assistance to preserve the reproductive potential of his prized breeder.

INVESTIGATION. The right hemipenis is erythemic and partially dessicated (**250**). Because of its size and dessication, it is immediately obvious that this phallic organ cannot be replaced within its postcloacal sheath, even if a relieving incision is created. In addition, it is doubtful whether the organ is still vital after being prolapsed and everted for at least 24 hours. A small volume of blood drawn for hematology determines that the PCV is 0.12 l/l (12%).

DIAGNOSIS. Unilateral hemipenial prolapse.

ETIOLOGY. Whereas male chelonians and male crocodilians have single penises, male snakes and lizards possess paired phallic organs, called hemipenes, each connected to its ipsilateral testis. These intromittant organs are employed one at a time during copulation. Only one hemipene is essential for successful reproduction.

MANAGEMENT. Aseptic surgical amputation is the preferred treatment for a dessicated prolapsed hemipene. General anesthesia is induced with ketamine and diazepam. An uncuffed endotracheal catheter is inserted and attached to a closed-circuit gas anesthesia machine adjusted to deliver a 3% isoflurane/oxygen mixture. The prolapsed hemipene is prepared for aseptic surgery. Mild digital traction is applied to the phallus so that its arterial, venous, and ejaculatory duct can be double ligated and transfixed with a through and through suture. The organ is amputated between the two transfixed ligatures. The very short transfixed and ligated stump is replaced into the right postcloacal hemipenial sulcus.

Because male snakes and lizards possess paired hemipenes, losing one does not, by itself, render a male who has lost one hemipenis sterile.

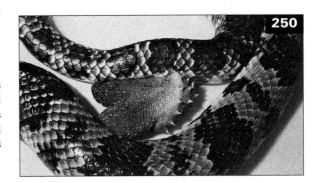

Case 251: **Spasmodic twitching in an adult female Burmese python**

CLINICAL PRESENTATION. An adult female Burmese python is evaluated because its owner notices that it is twitching spasmodically several times a minute and it is not eating. The twitching commenced on the day that the python deposited a clutch of 21 large eggs.

ETIOLOGY. It is entirely normal for brooding female pythons to twitch as they are curled about their clutches of eggs; by doing so, they contract their expaxial muscles and create additional warmth for incubating their eggs (**251**). The periodicity of their twitching is directly correlated to the ambient temperature of their immediate environment and that of the clutch of eggs.

PREVALENCE. Only brooding female pythons display this behavior.

MANAGEMENT. Brooding female pythons usually do not eat while incubating their eggs. They should, however, be provided with a source of clean drinking water. Also,

providing straw litter on which they can deposit their eggs and wrap about them will ensure a comfortable incubation site and lessen the likelihood that they will abandon their egg clutch.

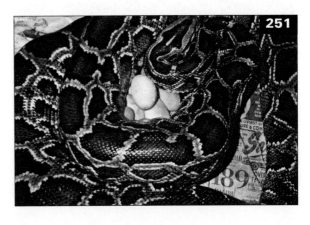

Case 252: **Postprandial regurgitation in a kingsnake**

CLINICAL PRESENTATION. A mature male Mexican kingsnake that previously was healthy and eating regularly is presented for examination because of regurgitation. The history reveals that the snake was sent to another collection on breeding loan. After a period of quarantine and repeated fecal examinations, it was placed with two females that were

healthy. On its return to the lending collection, the snake ate normally and seemed to be in good health. However, approximately three weeks after its return to the original collection, the snake began to regurgitate its meals about 24 hours after they were ingested. The regurgitated mouse meals were undigested. The snake appeared to be hungry and was eager to eat, but it was not able to digest its mouse prey. This behavior continued until the time that the snake was presented for examination.

DIFFERENTIAL DIAGNOSES. Gastric cryptosporidiosis; gastrointestinal obstruction from a foreign body (e.g. an ingested rock, litter material, a trichobezoar); gastrointestinal obstruction from an inflammatory lesion (e.g. granuloma); gastrointestinal obstruction from a mass of metazoan parasites (nematodes, cestodes); gastrointestinal obstruction from a neoplasm.

INVESTIGATION. Physical examination reveals a well-fleshed male snake with a firm, palpable swelling in the region of the stomach (**252a, b**). A radiograph confirms the presence of a soft tissue density in the region of the mid-body of the stomach (**252c**).

Collecting a gastric lavage specimen for cytologic examination can aid the diagnosis. A polyproplylene urethral catheter is lubricated with a water-soluble lubricant, attached to a 6 ml disposable syringe filled with Ringer's solution, and passsed into the stomach. Approximately 4 ml of the Ringers solution is instilled into the stomach. The gastric area is then 'fluttered' with the fingers of one hand for a few seconds to distribute the Ringer's solution and dislodge some cells, and as much of the fluid as possible is aspirated into the syringe. The recovered gastric lavage specimen is centrifuged and decanted. A few drops of the 'button' that remains in the centrifuge tube are placed onto a freshly polished glass slide. A drop of merthiolate (Mayer's hematoxylin can be substituted) is added before cover-slipping and examining the stained wet mount specimen microscopically. Numerous round organisms measuring 3–6 microns are seen (**252d**). These are consistent with *Cryptosporidium serpentis*.

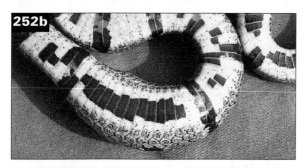

252a

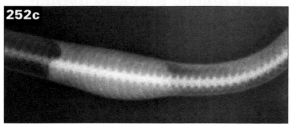

252b

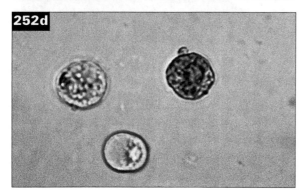

252c

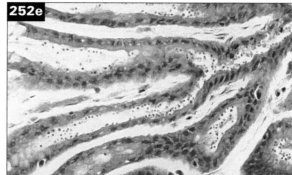

252d

252e

A few drops of what was left of the pellet in the centrifuge tube are tested with a *Cryptosporidium*-specific antigen immunoassay (ProSpectT®, Alexon-Trend). Although this testing system was developed for use in mammals, it is highly specific and useful in reptiles (Frye *et al.*, 1999).

Histologic sections characteristic of gastric cryptosporidiosis are illustrated (**252e, f**). In snakes the gastric mucosae are most often infected. In lizards, cryptosporidiosis involves other sites such as the stomach, intestine, kidney, and salivary glands (Frye *et al.*, 1999).

DIAGNOSIS. Gastric cryptosporidiosis due to *C. serpentis* infection.

ETIOLOGY. Although gastric cryptosporidiosis has been described as hypertrophic gastritis (Brownstein *et al*, 1977), in fact hypertrophy of the muscular tunics and atrophy of the gastric mucosae occur simultaneously.

PREVALENCE. Increasingly common because snakes are moved from one collection to another without adequate quarantine.

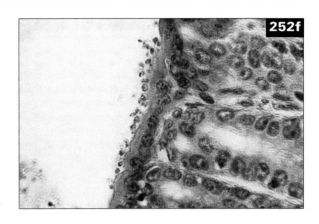

MANAGEMENT. Because there has yet to be a safe and effective treatment for cryptosporidiosis in reptiles, the kingsnake was euthanatized and subjected to a complete necropsy, which confirmed the diagnosis of gastric cryptosporidiosis.

Case 253: **Peracute cephalic edema in a Central American boa constrictor**

CLINICAL PRESENTATION. While doing field research in Nicaragua, a wild boa constrictor with a massively swollen head is observed. The intermandibular soft tissues, extending down to the neck, are greatly indurated and edematous (**253a**). Several wasps are observed stinging the boa, and two large ticks are attached to the integument covering the snake's left cervical region, immediately caudal to the swollen jaw.

INVESTIGATION. The boa is caught and physically restrained so that the stinging wasps could be killed and the two ticks removed. The very acute reaction to the wasp stings is immediately apparent.

DIAGNOSIS. Acute hyperimmune reaction to wasp venom.

PREVALENCE. Sporadic.

MANAGEMENT. Ready access to medications is limited due to being in the field, away from a laboratory or pharmacy; therefore, the immediate goal is to reduce the swelling and maintain an open airway. The only injectable drug that is available is diphenylhydramine. The boa's estimated body weight is approximately 10 kg. A dose of 0.5 ml is injected intravenously into the ventral caudal vein, and 1.0 ml is injected into the epaxial muscles along the snake's vertebral column.

A whole blood sample is collected and a blood film is made and stained. Microscopic examination reveals many of the eosinophils to be degranulated (**253b**).

PROGNOSIS. Favorable. The boa's cephalic swelling subsides over a period of two hours and, after making certain that it is out of immediate danger, it is released back into the rain forest.

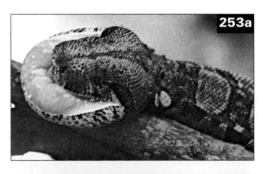

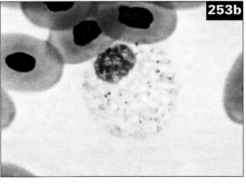

Case 254: **Serocoelomitis in essentially any oviparous or ovoviviparous reptile**

CLINICAL PRESENTATION. One or more yolked eggs of any sexually mature female chelonian, crocodilian, oviparous (or ovoviviparous) lizard, or snake can rupture. Concomitant rupture of an oviduct results in the spillage of yolk lipid (as well as albumin and products of conception) into the coelomic cavity. The clinical signs vary with the amount of spillage, the length of time that the egg contents have been free within the coelom, and whether there is concurrent infection, as well as inflammation, associated with the spillage.

The clinical manifestations observed in reptiles that are affected by egg yolk serocoelomitis reflect the organs whose blood supply is obstructed by emboli that contain yolk lipid. For example, if the myocardium is affected, myocardial ischemia and infarction are observed (**254a**); similarly, if the cerebral vessels are obstructed, central nervous system disorders are seen (**254b, c**).

ETIOLOGY. Egg yolk is highly reactive and, if it spills into the coelomic cavity, it induces a severe cell-mediated inflammatory reaction. Mesothelial cells and histiocytic macrophages are mobilized and stimulated to engulf this antigenic material. These macrophages phagocytize the lipid-rich yolk in an attempt to remove it. During this process, yolk lipid can enter the splanchnic venous circulation and become widely disseminated throughout the body, which leads to the formation of yolk lipid emboli that obstruct small- to medium-diameter blood vessels in the myocardium, brain, lung, etc.

MANAGEMENT. Treatment consists of coeliotomy; thorough, repeated coelomic lavage with sterile saline or Ringer's solution, with the goal of removing as much yolk lipid as possible; and antibiotic and anti-inflammatory therapy.

PROGNOSIS. The prognosis for female reptiles affected with egg yolk serocoelomitis varies with its severity. Generally, because the inflammatory reaction to yolk is so severe, the prognosis is guarded.

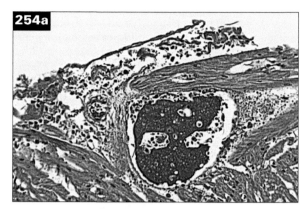

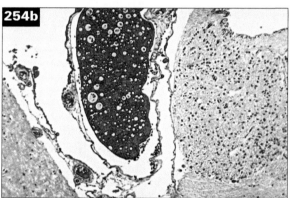

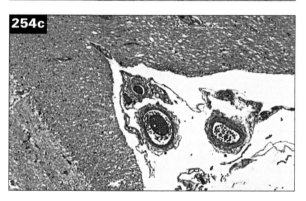

Case 255: **Red lesions in the coelom of a royal (ball) python**

CLINICAL PRESENTATION. The cadaver of a royal (ball) python that refused to eat for over one year is presented for necropsy. The skeletal muscles appear wasted. The coelomic adipose bodies that are normally present in healthy royal pythons are lacking. Numerous raised, glistening, dark pink-to-red lesions are scattered throughout the coelomic cavity where the adipose bodies would usually be found (**255a**). Otherwise, the necropsy is unremarkable.

DIFFERENTIAL DIAGNOSES. Serous atrophy of adipose bodies; protozoan or metazoan parasitic cysts; pyogranulomata; metastatic neoplastic implantations.

INVESTIGATION. Tissue samples are collected for routine histopathology. Microscopically, the normally plump, fat-laden adipose tissue is seen as aggregates of markedly shrunken adipocytes that are characterized by scanty cytoplasmic lipid bound by thin connective tissue membranes. Numerous small blood vessels penetrate between these depleted adipocytes (**255b**).

DIAGNOSIS. Serous atrophy of adipose (fat) tissue.

ETIOLOGY. Depending on the amount of stored adipose tissue that is available as a source of energy, many reptiles can withstand a prolonged period of anorexia or food deprivation. However, eventually that source becomes depleted. As their cytoplasmic lipid is exhausted, the adipocytes shrink and the adipose tissue is replaced gradually by fibrovascular connective tissue elements. This replaced tissue has an entirely different appearance than normal fatty tissue; rather than being pale yellow and voluminous, the atrophied adipose tissue is seen as multiple glistening, raised, dark pink or red foci (**255a**). Starvation causes the fat stores to be used for energy.

PREVALENCE. Common when reptiles and amphibians are poorly nourished.

PROGNOSIS. Favorable if the affected reptile or amphibian begins to eat normally. This condition is reversible once an adequate food intake is restored, so that excess energy can be stored as lipid within the adipocytes comprising the fat bodies.

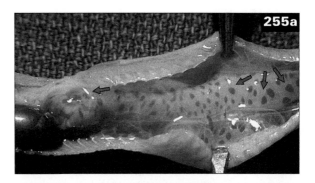

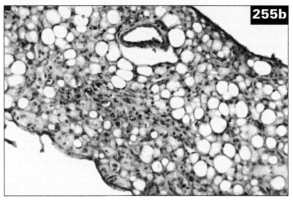

Case 256: **Cloacal swelling and inflammation in an Australasian blood python**

CLINICAL PRESENTATION. A mature female python has a severely swollen and inflamed cloaca (**256**). The cloaca and the soft tissues surrounding the anal vent were inflamed for approximately one week.

INVESTIGATION. A specimen of exudate is collected for cytology, Gram staining, and microbiological culture and antibiotic sensitivity testing.

DIAGNOSIS. Bacterial cloacitis due to an infection with *Pseudomonas aeruginosa*.

ETIOLOGY. Inflammation of the cloaca and anal vent area can be due to any of the following causes: bacterial infection; mycotic infection; metazoan parasitism (mite infestations; gastrointestinal nematodes); trauma; chemical injury.

MANAGEMENT. The inflamed tissues must be cleaned thoroughly with a mild but effective disinfectant such as chlorhexidine diacetate at a concentration of 0.75%. The tissues are dried and a combination antibiotic/anti-inflammatory ointment applied. If the inflammation is severe, parenteral broad-spectrum bacteriocidal and physiologic fluid therapy is indicated. Particulate litter material is removed and replaced with clean cotton

toweling so that the treated tissues will not attract and accumulate litter particles.

Proper cage hygiene is essential in preventing infections. The cage litter should be clean and dry. Fecal and urinary wastes, shed skin remnants, etc. must be removed promptly. Because mite and parasitic intestinal helminth infestations can also contribute to cloacal and perianal irritation and inflammation, examinations for ecto- and endoparasites should be routine.

PROGNOSIS. Favorable. The python made an uneventful recovery.

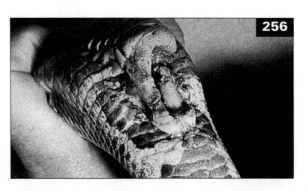

Case 257: **Multiple pale, raised lesions in the oropharnyx of a red-tailed boa constrictor**

CLINICAL PRESENTATION. An immature red-tailed boa constrictor with a myriad number of grayish-white, slightly raised lesions within its oropharyngeal mucosae (**257a**) is presented by its owner, a practicing physician, who has treated his snake for ulcerative stomatitis with a variety of aminoglycoside antibiotics.

Without obtaining a microbiological culture and sensitivity testing, the owner began his treatment with ten days of penicillin-streptomycin sulfate. When this therapy was not effective, he switched to gentamicin sulfate injections for another ten days, followed by a course of amikacin sulfate injections. These treatments consisted solely of antibiotic injections; no fluid therapy or additional warmth were provided to the snake. Within about three days after receiving the amikacin injections, the snake became severely depressed and refused to eat or drink. At this point the physician decided to seek veterinary assistance.

INVESTIGATION. A whole blood specimen is drawn from the ventral coccygeal vein for hematology and biochemistry analyses.

Several hundred individual to coalescing small, pale gray, raised lesions are identified within the oral and pharyngeal mucosae. Histopathology confirms severe renal gout (**257b**).

DIAGNOSIS. Aminoglycoside intoxication-induced nephropathy, hyperuricemia, and visceral gout.

ETIOLOGY. The hyperuricemia was induced by the inappropriate use of nephrotoxic aminoglycoside antibiotics without providing fluid therapy to maintain renal perfusion.

PREVALENCE. High, especially when fluid-therapy does not accompany aminoglycoside (and other potentially nephrotoxic) antibiotic therapy.

MANAGEMENT. Before commencing antibiotic therapy, a culture and sensitivity is obtained in order to ascertain which antibiotic, if any, would be most likely to be effective. When treating an ill reptile, appropriate fluid therapy must be given to maintain hydration and renal perfusion. This is particularly important when employing any drug that is nephrotoxic. Additional cage warmth is provided in order to maintain synthesis of immunoglobulins. This synthesis is temperature-dependent; therefore, additional cage warmth facilitates immunoglobulin synthesis.

PROGNOSIS. Unfavorable because uric acid is relatively insoluble once it has been deposited in soft tissues.

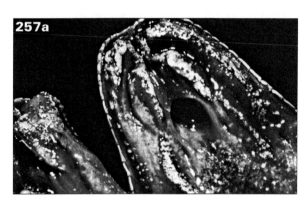

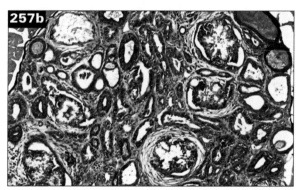

Test	Result		Normal values	
PCV	0.44 l/l	(44%)	0.185 l/l	(18.5%)
WBCs	19.4×10^9/l	$(19.4 \times 10^3/\mu l)$	6.7×10^9/l	$(6.7 \times 10^3/\mu l)$
Heterophils	71%		9%	
Lymphocytes	11%		51%	
Monocytes	12%		2%	
Azurophils	6%		–	
Calcium	1.63 mmol/l	(6.52 mg/dl)	2.5–5.5 mmol/l	(10–22 mg/dl)
Phosphorous	2.6 mmol/l	(8.06 mg/dl)	0.8 mmol/l	(2.48 mg/dl)
Potassium	14.8 mmol/l	(14.8 mEq/l)	3.0–3.7 mmol/l	(3.0–3.7 mEq/l)
Glucose	4.9 mmol/l	(88.2 mg/dl)	0.6–3.9 mmol/l	(10.8–70.2 mg/dl)
TP	90 g/l	(9.0 g/dl)	46–80 g/l	(4.6–8.0 g/dl)
Uric acid	0.65 mmol/l	(10.98 mg/dl)	0.07–0.34 mmol/l	(1.18–5.75 mg/dl)

Case 258: **Enterohepatitis in a red-tailed boa constrictor**

CLINICAL PRESENTATION. A mature South American red-tailed boa constrictor displays icterus, profound depression, weakness, dehydration, and bloody, mucus-laden diarrhea. Palpable firm masses are detected within the caudal coelomic cavity.

DIFFERENTIAL DIAGNOSES. Protozoan enteritis (entamoebiasis, giardiasis, trichomoniasis, etc); severe bacterial enteritis with enterotoxemia (salmonellosis, etc); severe mycotic enteritis; severe ulcerative colitis; chemical intoxication (corrosive or otherwise toxic substance); gastroenteric neoplasm, (leukemia, adeno-carcinoma); ischemic, gangrenous enteritis.

INVESTIGATION. Radiography reveals greatly thickened small and large intestines and a swollen liver. A specimen of the bloody stools is collected, stained with merthiolate or Mayer's hematoxylin as a wet mount and examined microscopically. A small volume of whole blood is drawn for hematology and biochemistry analyses.

While waiting for the stool specimen to be properly stained and examined, fluid-replacement therapy with lactated Ringer's solution is infused intravenously via the ventral coccygeal vein. The snake died a few hours after its initial admission and permission for a necropsy was granted.

Microscopy of the stained fecal wet mounts and the lumenal contents of the affected segments of intestine reveals the presence of large numbers of protozoan trophyzoites, as well as bi-, tri-, and quadrinucleated cyst forms of amoebic protozoans admixed with the bloody and fibrinous enteric exudates. The quadrinucleated cysts are morphologically indistinguishable from *Entamoeba histolytica*, the amoeba of humans.

Gross pathology reveals markedly thickened and hemorrhagic intestines and multiple pale, wedge-shaped foci within the liver (**258a, b**). Histopathology confirm fibrinonecrotic enteritis in which myriad numbers of amoebic organisms of both trophyzoite and cyst forms are identified (**258c**). The liver has multiple areas of infarction, and amoebae are found between hemorrhagic and necrotic hepatocellular cords and sinusoids.

DIAGNOSIS. Entamoebic enterohepatitis.

ETIOLOGY. *Entamoeba invadens* infection.

PREVALENCE. Common in reptile collections where their drinking water is contaminated with the feces of turtles and/or crocodilians.

MANAGEMENT. Snakes and lizards affected with *E. invadens* must be isolated from the general captive reptile population and treated with metronidazole. For boid snakes (boas, pythons, anacondas) the dosage of metronidazole is 250 mg/kg p/o, repeated in 14 days, and for colubrid, viperine, crotalid, and elapid snakes it is 25–40 mg/kg p/o repeated in 14 days, in both groups accompanied by aggressive supportive nursing, bacteriocidal antibiotics, fluid therapy, and additional ambient warmth.

Entamoebiasis in reptiles can be prevented if good water hygiene is maintained. Generally, *E. invadens* is a commensal organism that lives in the gut of aquatic and semiaquatic chelonians and crocodilians, and although it can be pathogenic for these hosts, it usually is not. However, when the water supply for snakes and lizards is contaminated with the cysts forms of *E. invadens*, it becomes virulently pathogenic.

PROGNOSIS. The prognosis for recovery from entamoebic enterohepatitis is guarded because of the severe tissue damage that occurs early in the progress of this disease. If diagnosed sufficiently early, this condition can be treated effectively.

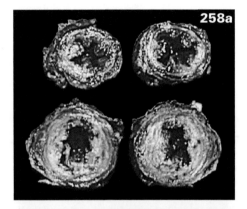

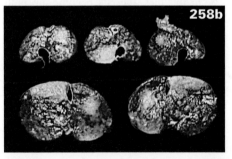

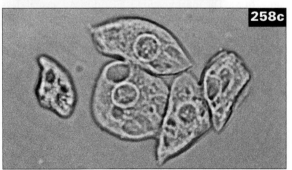

Case 259: **Bilateral palpable, firm swellings in the tail of a South American boa constrictor**

CLINICAL PRESENTATION. A young adult boa constrictor has developed bilateral firm swellings on either side of its tail, extending cranially along either side of the posterior vertebral column. Its diet consists of laboratory rats. About a month prior to evaluation it began refusing to eat, and now it is showing signs of reluctance to move.

INVESTIGATION. Gentle palpation of the boa constrictor reveals lumpy masses throughout the body, both intra- and extracoelomically. The most pronounced firm and swollen areas are found on either side of the posterior body, both cranial to and caudal to the cloacal vent. After preparing the skin of the tail as for aseptic surgery, a fine needle biopsy specimen is aspirated, formalin fixed, and processed for histology. Microscopic examination reveals the presence of markedly abnormal and inflamed body fat.

The owners request euthanasia and a necropsy. Masses of dry, yellow, waxy body fat are identified beneath the skin and between the dorsolateral epaxial and coccygeal muscles (**259**). The intracoelomic fat bodies are also severely altered.

DIAGNOSIS. Steatitis (panniculitis; inflammation of body fat) secondary to dietary overload of polyunsaturated lipid(s) contained in the bodies of obese rats eaten by this snake.

ETIOLOGY. Hypovitaminosis E. Vitamin E, an essential anti-oxidant in lipid metabolism, is depleted when overwhelming amounts of polyunsaturated or rancid fats are eaten. This snake is the mascot of the Department of Nutrition in a major university. One of the research projects being conducted by the department involves feeding laboratory rats a diet limited to sunflower seeds and tap water. On this diet, the rats become morbidly obese. During the course of the study, some of the test rats are killed and small pieces of their tissue are obtained for various tests. The cadavers of these massively obese rats are then fed to the mascot boa.

PREVALENCE. Sporadic; related to the captive diet fed.

MANAGEMENT. Captive carnivorous reptiles should be fed natural diets comprising healthy prey.

PROGNOSIS. Unfavorable. Once body fats are inflamed and are altered by the formation of the water-insoluble pigment, ceroid, the granulomatous inflammation becomes permanent.

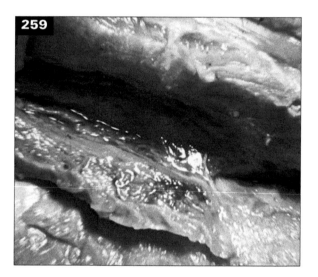

Case 260: **Solution to a problem of bandaging the tail of a South American red-tailed boa constrictor**

CLINICAL PRESENTATION. The skin on the tail of a South American red-tailed boa constrictor is moist and severely inflamed from immediately caudal to the anal vent to the tip (**260a**). The inflammation is first noticed several days prior to presentation. The boa is active and is eating well.

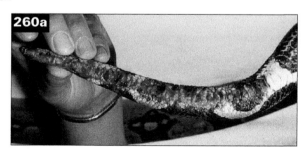

INVESTIGATION. Specimens for microbiological culture and sensitivity testing and a blood sample for hematology are obtained. The culture yields a mixed gram-negative and gram-positive flora. The hemogram reveals only a modest leukocytosis, with mild heterophilia.

DIAGNOSIS. Bacterial pyodermatitis.

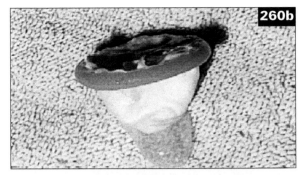

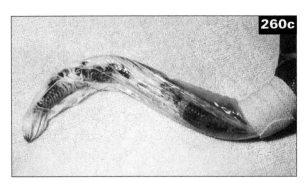

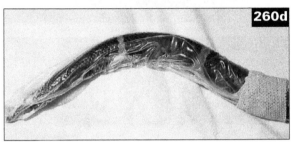

ETIOLOGY. Bacterial infection.

PREVALENCE. Common.

MANAGEMENT. A moist dressing containing an antimicrobial ointment must be placed on the snake's tail, but the snake has crawled out of all of the dressings applied so far. The following technique facilitates applying bandages to a snake: obtain a package of non-lubricated condoms; fill the reservoir tip of one of the condoms with water-soluble silver-sulfadiazine ointment (**260b**); roll the ointment-filled condom over the tail (**260c**); massage the ointment onto the inflamed skin until it is thoroughly distributed; tape the open end of the condom to the healthy normal tissue using elastic tape, securing it only sufficiently tight to prevent it from slipping off; cut the ends of the tape with a slight radius so that the tape will not unravel as the snake crawls about its enclosure (**260d**); leave the taped, ointment-filled condom in place for a week before changing; repeat bandaging with condom, as necessary;

Parenteral bacteriocidal antibiotic and fluid therapy is also required.

PROGNOSIS. Favorable. The snake tolerates its condom bandage very well and makes an uneventful recovery (Frye, 1992).

Case 261: **Pale yellow objects passed by a female garter snake**

CLINICAL PRESENTATION. The owner of an ovoviviparous (live-bearing) garter snake brings in a jar containing eight elongated, firm, yellow objects that the snake passed during the evening before. He requests an identification of the objects. The snake appears healthy and is eager to eat live goldfish that are offered to it.

INVESTIGATION. The eight objects are firm and gelatinous (**261**). They are homogenous on cut section and are identified as 'slugs', which are the failed products of conception.

DIAGNOSIS. Spontaneous abortion of eight early products of conception.

ETIOLOGY. Ovoviviparous snakes retain their unshelled fertilized eggs within their oviducts during their gestation period. When gestation fails, these products of conception are passed through the proctodeum and out the cloacal vent.

PREVALENCE. Sporadic.

MANAGEMENT. No treatment is necessary.

PROGNOSIS. Favorable.

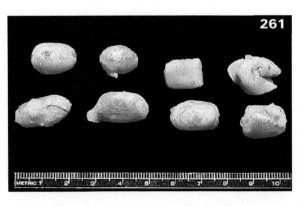

Case 262: **Raised subepidermal lesions in a California mountain kingsnake**

CLINICAL PRESENTATION. Small white swellings first develop beneath the scales surrounding the eyes of an adult California mountain kingsnake (**262a**). Within a week, similar swellings are seen in the skin covering its flanks and tail (**262b**).

INVESTIGATION. Using a fine hypodermic needle, specimens of material beneath the scales of the eyes, flank, and tail are aspirated aseptically. One sample is used for microbiological culture and sensitivity and the other for cytology. Microbiology yields *Citrobacter freundii* in pure culture. Cytology reveals an exudate composed of mixed heterophil granulocytes and mononuclear lymphoplasmacytes, and foamy histiocytic macrophages with engulfed cellular detritus.

DIAGNOSIS. Disseminated bacterial pyodermatitis.

PREVALENCE. Sporadic, depending upon husbandry practices.

MANAGEMENT. Aggressive bacteriocidal therapy is employed using one or more antibiotics, together with supportive nursing including fluid therapy and provision of additional cage warmth.

PROGNOSIS. Guarded, because it is likely that the wide distribution of the inflammation and infection has already 'showered' the vascular system with infective microemboli. The snake subsequently died and, on necropsy, massive inflammation is identified in the liver, lungs, and kidneys (**262c**).

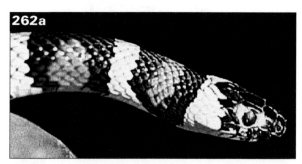

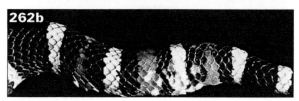

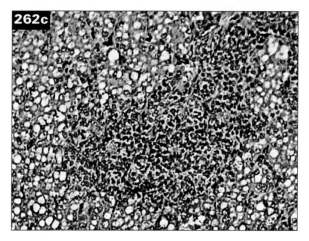

Case 263: **Black organisms in the mouth of an indigo snake**

CLINICAL PRESENTATION. Small, shiny black organisms are present within the oral cavity of a wild-caught indigo snake (**263a**). The snake is open mouth breathing; otherwise, physical examination is unremarkable. The snake's diet consists of wild-caught amphibians.

INVESTIGATION. The organisms are readily removed with a dry cotton tipped applicator. They are immersed immediately in AFA solution prior to being submitted for parasitological identification (Frye, 1994). AFA not only fixes and preserves small invertebrate specimens, it also relaxes them and, thus, facilitates their clearing, staining, and mounting for microscopy.

DIAGNOSIS. The oral objects are identified as flukes classified within the genus *Ochetosoma* (**263b**).

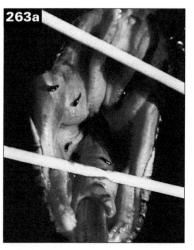

ETIOLOGY. Like others within the order Trematoda, ocheosomids utilize an indirect life cycle that requires several intermediate hosts before they mature. Once the fluke ova are passed in the feces of the final or definitive host, they are ingested and hatch into miracidia within a suitable intermediate aquatic snail host. Soon, xiphidiocercariae develop further into daughter sporocysts. After developing and finally leaving the snail, cercaria penetrate and encyst in the soft tissues of amphibian larvae. The infected frog, toad, or tailed amphibian larvae are then eaten by either another amphibian or by a reptile. Here they develop into sexually mature, final-stage flukes after about 35 days (Schell, 1970).

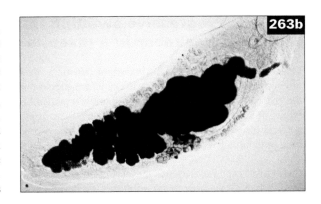

MANAGEMENT. The oropharyngeal flukes are removed from the snake and it is returned to its owner with advice to feed the snake small rodents and fowl chicks, rather than wild-caught amphibians.

With the advent of highly effective trematocidal drugs such as albendazole and praziquantel, it is now possible and practicable to treat parasitized reptiles specifically for their helminths. However, because ochetosomid flukes are minimally pathogenic and are readily seen without magnification, they can be removed easily without having to resort to medication even when they are located within the oropharynx of snakes. Thus, the goal is to prevent their infestation by avoiding their intermediate amphibian hosts.

Case 264: **Swelling in the cranial coelomic cavity in a Children's python**

CLINICAL PRESENTATION. A juvenile Children's python has developed a marked swelling in the cranial portion of its coelomic cavity and is becoming progressively weaker, refusing to climb or move about its cage.

DIFFERENTIAL DIAGNOSES. Aortic stenosis; cardiomyopathy; myocardial abscess or pyogranulomatosis; cardiac or mediastinal neoplasm; parasitic cyst.

INVESTIGATION. Physical examination reveals a swelling in the region of the heart (264a). This swelling is pulsatile and synchronous with the heartbeat. Ultrasonic Doppler blood flow investigation reveals very loud (VI/VI) aortic ejection murmurs. An ECG discloses a first-degree heart block and atrial fibrillation (264b). The owner requests euthanasia and grants permission for a necropsy. The heart is markedly enlarged. The aortic valve cusps are greatly thickened, leaving only a very narrow passage for blood to pass into the aorta from the single ventricle (264c).

DIAGNOSIS. Aortic stenosis.

PREVALENCE. Sporadic; this is a developmental anomaly.

PROGNOSIS. Unfavorable.

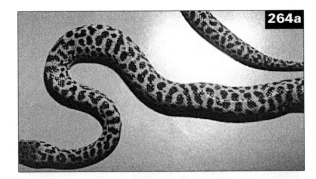

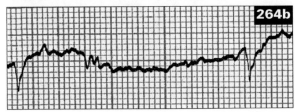

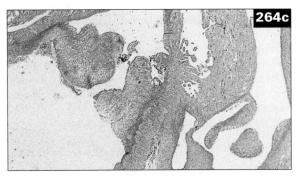

Case 265: **Progressive swelling in the region of the heart, and profound weakness in a juvenile Burmese python**

CLINICAL PRESENTATION. An immature python with a progressively and rapidly enlarging swelling in the region of the heart is evaluated. The snake is profoundly weak, and is reluctant to move about in its cage. There is no prior medical history. The snake was eating killed laboratory mice until just a few days before presentation.

DIFFERENTIAL DIAGNOSES. Developmental anomaly; cardiomyopathy induced by sublethal viral infection during early embryonic development.

INVESTIGATION. The swelling in the region of the heart (**265a**) is pulsatile and synchronous with the heartbeat. Ultrasonic Doppler blood flow investigation reveals severely muffled heart sounds. An ECG discloses a first-degree heart block (**265b**). The snake dies a few hours after being hospitalized for additional studies. Permission for a necropsy is granted. On opening the pericardial sac, a markedly enlarged, very flabby heart is revealed. Histologic examination discloses myocardial hypoplasia affecting both the atria and solitary

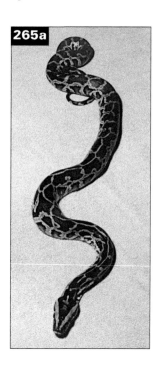

ventricle. Myocardial fibers are wispy and widely separated by edema fluid (**265c**).

DIAGNOSIS. Severe congenital myocardial hypoplasia and edema.

ETIOLOGY. Idiopathic.

PREVALENCE. Sporadic.

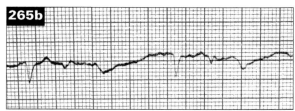

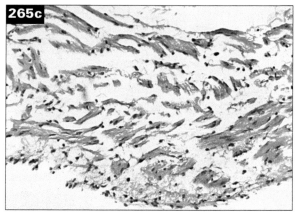

Case 266: **Firm caudal swellings in a water snake**

CLINICAL PRESENTATION. Firm bilateral swellings develop in the caudal coelomic cavity of an adult female water snake (**266a**). Until two weeks prior to presentation, the snake was in apparently good health and was eating her diet of live goldfish and fish-scented dead mice.

INVESTIGATION. Routine presurgical hematology and biochemistry determinations are unremarkable except for mild hemoconcentration (PCV = 0.4 l/l [41%]), an elevated uric acid (0.37 mmol/l [6.25 mg/dl]), and elevated potassium (5.8 mmol/l [5.8 mEq/l]). Radiography reveals soft tissue swellings cranial to the tail and cloaca.

DIAGNOSIS. Bilateral renal *Aspergillus*-related renal mycetomata.

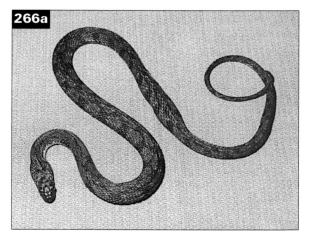

PREVALENCE. Sporadic.

MANAGEMENT. The snake is anesthetized and an exploratory coeliotomy performed. Both kidneys are grossly swollen, pale, and have a granular appearance (266b). A small wedge biopsy is taken from one of the kidneys and touch impressions made from the freshly excised tissue. These are stained with a rapid metachromatic blood stain. The rest of the biopsy sample is formalin fixed and submitted for histopathology. The impression smears and the stained histologic slides contain branching septate hyphae admixed in mixed inflammatory leukocytes (266c). Given the results of the biopsy and the evidence of renal insufficiency, the owners request euthanasia. Necropsy reveals that the normal parenchyma of both kidneys is replaced by mycotic granulomatous inflammatory tissue. The fungus is identified as *Aspergillus* species.

PROGNOSIS. Unfavorable – guarded.

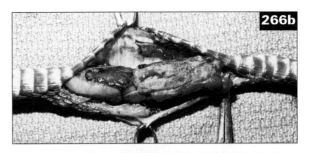

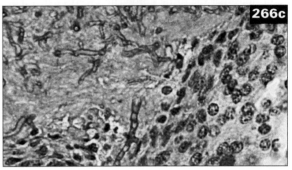

Case 267: **White plaque on the corneas of a desert tortoise and an emydid turtle**

CLINICAL PRESENTATION. An adult desert tortoise and a turtle are evaluated because their owners found unilateral, amorphous, opaque white plaque covering the entire cornea of their left eyes (267a, b). The tortoise and turtle very recently emerged from hibernation and, other than their eye lesions, they seem to be normal.

DIFFERENTIAL DIAGNOSES. Posthibernation coagulative keratopathy; post-traumatic or postinflammatory exuberant fibroplasia or pannus; superficial/interstitial/stromal cholesterol/calcium keratopathy.

INVESTIGATION. Only one eye is affected in each chelonian. Direct ophthalmoscopy cannot effectively reveal the interior of the globe because of the opacity of the corneal plaque. The corneae and sclerae are not inflamed, but the plaques are adhered tightly to the subjacent corneal surface.

DIAGNOSIS. Idiopathic coagulative keratopathy.

PREVALENCE. Sporadic.

MANAGEMENT. Treatment with an ophthalmic ointment containing a proteolytic can be used atraumatically to lyse these tenacious proteinaceous plaques. However, because these enzymes are most effective at mammalian body temperatures, they tend to be significantly less effective in ectothermic animals such as reptiles and amphibians.

An alternative approach is to apply the juice of a fresh papaya to the affected eye two or more times daily. Fresh papaya contains papain, which is a proteolytic enzyme.

Papain is effective at room temperatures, and its use will not adversely affect healthy, normal tissues.

PROGNOSIS. By treating coagulative keratopathy with fresh papaya, it is possible to dissolve proteinaceous deposits without having to resort to surgical excison.

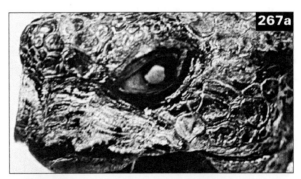

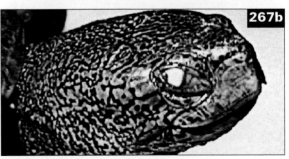

Case 268: Severely misshaped carapace and inability to use its limbs in a soft-shelled turtle

CLINICAL PRESENTATION. An immature male soft-shelled turtle is examined because it refuses to walk and has developed a grossly misshapen carapace. The turtle is kept in a shallow aquarium, and is fed raw boneless fish fillets, raw boneless beef, and raw boneless poultry. It has eaten this diet for at least six months. On examination it is obvious that the turtle's problem involves much more than a failure in locomotion. The edges of the normally soft and pliable carapace are curved upward, and all four of the turtle's limbs remain immobile when touched gently (268a). The shell is overly pliable. When the turtle is gently picked up, its limbs droop and they cannot be retracted by the turtle.

DIFFERENTIAL DIAGNOSES. Hypovitaminosis D_3 (rickets); diet-associated osteomalacia due to a diet deficient in calcium or too rich in phosphorus (secondary nutritional hyperparathyrodism); renal-associated osteomalacia ('renal rickets'); primary hyperparathyroidism due to a functional parathyroid adenomatous tumor that is secreting abnormal amounts of parathormone.

INVESTIGATION. Whole body radiographs reveal a severely osteopenic skeleton. All four of the limb bones have multiple folding-type fractures.

DIAGNOSIS. Secondary nutritional hyperparathyroidism due to a relative insufficiency of available calcium and a relative over-sufficiency of phosphorus. It is also possible that a deficiency of vitamin D_3 exacerbated the severe $Ca:PO_4$ imbalance.

ETIOLOGY. As the turtle tried to walk or move, it sustained multiple fractures because the softened bones in its limbs were not able to oppose the forces placed upon them. In a turtle with a well-mineralized skeleton, the soft, leathery carapace is supported by the widely flattened ribs. This turtle's ribs are extremely soft and, therefore, the carapace curves upward.

Under normal, wild conditions, soft-shell turtles consume small fish and invertebrates consisting of snails, insects, and worms. In doing so, they also consume the gut contents and skeletal elements of the fish, the gut contents of the invertebrates, and the calcareous shells of snails. The boneless flesh of beef and poultry is rich in phosphorus but very deficient in calcium. Under most circumstances, the ratio of calcium to phosphorus should be at least 2:1. However, a diet composed solely of boneless meat could have a calcium to phosphorus ratio of 1:40. When this kind of diet is consumed, the calcium that is stored in the skeleton is slowly leached in an attempt to maintain normal $Ca:PO_4$ homeostasis. The parathyroid gland is stimulated to secrete parathormone. Calcium is excreted by the kidneys while phosphorus is retained. This only exacerbates hyperparathyroid activity and skeletal demineralization.

PREVALENCE. High.

MANAGEMENT. Treatment must address the dietary mineral imbalance by initially supplementing calcium, correcting the diet to reflect a more normal $Ca:PO_4$ ratio, and providing vitamin D_3 either by exposure to the proper wavelength of ultraviolet illumination or by ingestion of preformed activated dihydrocholesterol.

Soft-shell turtles are aquatic; therefore, they do not fare well when they are kept dry because the delicate integument covering their leathery carapace and plastron becomes dessicated and, subsequently, cracks. They can, however, be kept in shallow containers of water. Prey that contains bone, such as whole small fish, are nutritious and avidly consumed. Alternatively, artificial diets formulated from farm raised trout or ornamental koi carp contain vitamin D_3 and an adequate $Ca:PO_4$ ratio and are also recommended. These products are made in both floating and sinking varieties; the sinking form is the easiest for a recuperating soft-shelled turtle to prehend and ingest (268b) (photo courtesy Dr SL Barten).

PROGNOSIS. Once the diet has been corrected and supplementation has been initiated, recovery can be remarkably rapid. Improvement usually occurs within 4–6 weeks; the turtle will be able to walk, and its carapace will regain its more normal flattened contours.

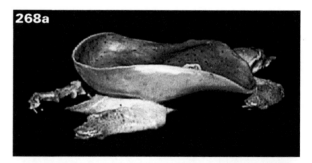

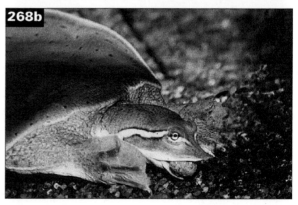

Case 269: **Multifocal cutaneous ulcerations in soft-shelled turtles**

CLINICAL PRESENTATION. Several immature soft-shelled turtles presented for evaluation because they had developed multiple red lesions on their leathery integument. Although most of these lesions were located on the plastron, a few were located on the carapace as well. Some turtles from this collection had died after their red lesions progressed into abscesses and ulcers.

DIFFERENTIAL DIAGNOSES. Bacterial dermatitis (any of several bacterial pathogens); mycotic dermatitis (any of several fungal pathogens); viral dermatitis (poxvirus etc); parasitic dermatitis (infestation with leeches, protozoans, etc); chemical dermatitis (chemical burns, necrosis).

INVESTIGATION. Samples of the lesions were taken as aseptically as possible and touch impressions for Gram staining were prepared. Some samples were subcultured in thioglycolate broth slants for enrichment for 24 hours before streaking them onto blood agar plates. One sample was air fixed for cytology. A whole blood specimen was withdrawn from each turtle and submitted for routine hematology.

A gram-negative organism was identified in a smear made from a representative cutaneous lesion. Microbiology yielded *Citrobacter freundii* in pure culture, sensitive to several bacteriocidal antibiotics. Mycotic stains and culture were negative. Cytology was negative for parasites, viral inclusions, and other evidence of viral infection.

DIAGNOSIS. Septicemic cutaneous ulcerative disease (SCUD).

ETIOLOGY. SCUD was first described (Kaplan, 1957) as an infectious disease in soft-shelled chelonians. It can also occur in aquatic and semi-aquatic turtles. Early in its progress, SCUD is seen as multifocal, punctate petechial hemorrhages, which soon coalesce into larger ecchymoses that eventually become shallow abscesses. Within a few days to a week, the fibrinonecrotic pseudomembranes that form over the abscesses loosen and fall away, leaving an ulcer (**269a–c**). Hidden from external view are insidious inflammatory foci that spread hematogenously to the liver, lungs, spleen, kidneys, etc.

PREVALENCE. Common in soft-shelled turtles.

MANAGEMENT. Antibiotic therapy with at least one broad-spectrum bacteriocidal (not bacteriostatic) antibiotic was given straight away while awaiting the results of the microbiological and other laboratory tests. Fluid therapy was given to the affected turtles. The turtles were housed individually in shallow pans or trays filled with clean water that was changed at least twice daily. All affected turtles were isolated from apparently healthy turtles. Even healthy turtles that have been exposed to infected turtles were treated as if they were actually infected.

PROGNOSIS. Guarded, because SCUD becomes aggressively septicemic early in its course. **NB:** Because *Citrobacter freundii* is a zoonotic pathogen, care MUST be taken when handling infected and/or suspected cases of SCUD. The tank water from infected turtles must be discarded in a sanitary manner so that cross-contamination is avoided.

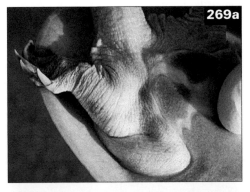

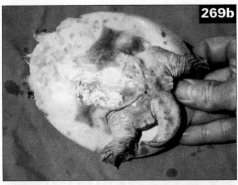

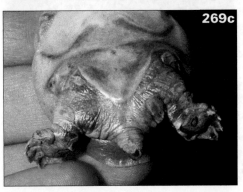

Case 270: **Profound morbidity in a Pacific pond turtle**

CLINICAL PRESENTATION. A moribund adult Pacific pond turtle is presented for evaluation on the 11th day of progressive lethargy after being in excellent health. On the day of presentation, the turtle becomes comatose and fails to respond to external stimuli.

INVESTIGATION. A small whole blood sample is obtained and the laboratory results are shown below.

The hematology and few minimal biochemistry results that could be determined with the small volume of blood that was available reveal several strikingly abnormal values. The TP is elevated. Abnormalities in plasma protein are often associated with either significant dehydration or the pathologic production of mono- or polyclonal globulin fractions due to plasmacytic immunoinflammatory disorders or neoplasia. The globulin fraction is markedly elevated and the glucose is extremely elevated.

The turtle died almost immediately following examination. A complete necropsy showed no gross lesions. Representative thin pieces of tissues are collected from all major parenchymatous organs. Histopathology reveals an almost total lack of normal pancreatic islets of Langerhans. A careful review of multiple stained serial sections of pancreas identifies only a single islet that is not completely surrounded and infiltrated by plasmacytes. Photomicrographs of stained pancreatic sections are shown (**270a–c**).

DIFFERENTIAL DIAGNOSES. Hyperproteinaemia is often induced by dehydration or a marked increase in the globulin fraction of the plasma protein. In a normally hydrated animal, it usually suggests a significant humeral immune response to an antigenic challenge; often infection. Hyperproteinaemia can also be induced by the malignant proliferation of plasmacytes (multiple myeloma), in which case a monoclonal spike is usually revealed when the serum is subjected to electrophoresis.

Hematology		
RBCs	2.9×10^{12}/l	$(2.9 \times 10^6/\mu l)$
WBCs	8.7×10^9/l	$(8.7 \times 10^3/\mu l)$
Lymphocytes	29%	
Heterophils	42%	
Azurophils	19%	
Monocytes	7%	
Basophils	3%	
Biochemistry		
TP	85 g/l	(8.5 g/dl)
Albumin	28 g/l	(2.8 g/dl)
Globulin	57 g/l	(5.7 g/dl)
Albumin:globulin ratio	2.13:1.00	
Glucose	46.8 mmol/l	(842.4 mg/dl)

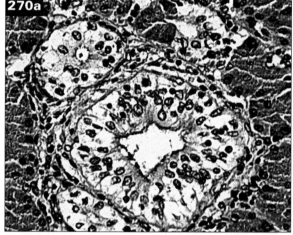

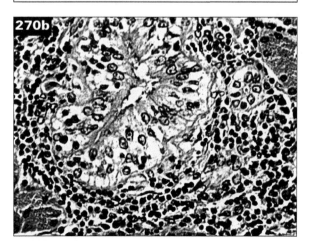

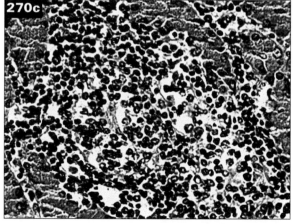

In this instance the history of a relatively brief illness that led to severe progressive lethargy ending in coma and death could have been traced to any of the above differentials. However, severe hyperglycemia is not usually associated with tumor cachexia. Clearly, the definitive diagnosis has to rest on histopathologic examination of the tissues; however, while awaiting the pathology results, some features of this case suggest a tentative diagnosis. The turtle was severely hyperglycemic and it was probably diabetic at the time of its presentation. A plasma glucose level of 46.8 mmol/l (842.4 mg/dl) is several times greater than normal (usually <5.6 mmol/l [100.8 mg/dl]). The TP and globulin fraction were also significantly elevated. This pattern suggests, but does not confirm, an immune-mediated disorder of the pancreatic islet tissue.

DIAGNOSIS. Diabetes mellitus secondary to subacute immune-mediated autoimmune insulitis.

ETIOLOGY. Spontaneous diabetes mellitus in reptiles has been recorded several times. As in mammals, the etiology of this severe metabolic disorder in reptiles can probably be linked to any of the following: genetic predisposition; toxic insult; inflammation resulting in the loss of islets of Langerhans; trauma; verminous or calcareous obstruction of the biliary system; neoplasia leading to the destruction of insulin-secreting cells within the pancreas.

PREVALENCE. Sporadic, spontaneous.

PROGNOSIS. Because of its extreme morbidity, only a very guarded prognosis can be advanced to the owner.

Case 271: **Cottony white substance within an old, partially healed carapacial fracture in a box turtle**

CLINICAL PRESENTATION. An owner requests a physical examination of a recently acquired turtle with no pertinent medical history. The only abnormality in this well-fed box turtle is an old, partially healed, full-thickness caudal carapacial fracture, the fissure of which contains a fluffy material. Careful inspection of the fissure discloses a cottony white growth arising from the detritus (**271a**).

DIFFERENTIAL DIAGNOSES. An opportunistic pathogenic fungal infection; an opportunistic saprophytic fungal infection.

INVESTIGATION. A small piece of the cottony white material is lifted and placed onto a slide with a drop of 10% potassium hydroxide or lactophenol cotton blue and examined microscopically. Another small piece of the cottony substance is inoculated into a dermatophyte test medium (DTM) vial, incubated at room temperature, and observed for fungal growth. A small piece of the growth is selected, mounted with lactophenol cotton blue, and examined microscopically.

DIAGNOSIS. Fungal macroconidia consistent with *Microsporum* species are identified arising from the fungus growing in the exudate curetted from the base of the lesion (**271b**).

PREVALENCE. Sporadic, opportunistic.

MANAGEMENT. The fissure is thoroughly cleansed with dilute povidone–iodine solution, air dried, and painted with a stock solution of povidone–iodine solution.

PROGNOSIS. Favorable.

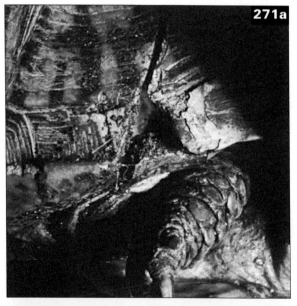

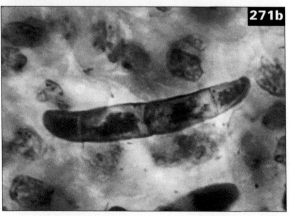

Case 272: **Tenesmus in a California desert tortoise**

CLINICAL PRESENTATION. A robust looking adult male California desert tortoise is examined because of frequent tenesmus, as if attempting to pass urine or stools. The tortoise has been in captivity for many years and is kept in a large yard where it eats lawn grass. In addition, the tortoise is fed canned dog food, which it prefers to vegetables. There is no significant prior medical history and there are no external abnormalities. However, direct digital palpation and ballottement of the coelomic contents with fingers inserted into the inguinal 'pockets' immediately cranial to the hindlimbs reveal the presence of multiple, large, firm intracoelomic objects.

INVESTIGATION. Radiography of the tortoise in dorsal recumbency reveals the presence of three round to irregular, oval, dense objects within the coelom (**272**). The radiodensity and appearance of these objects are consistent with urinary calculi.

Routine presurgical hematology (WBC count and differential and PCV), and biochemistry (AST, ALT, LDH, TP, globulin, albumin, glucose, uric acid, calcium, phosphorus, and potassium), are all within normal values for this species.

DIAGNOSIS. Multiple urinary calculosis. Because the tortoise is a male, the objects could not be anomalous shelled ova.

ETIOLOGY. Cystic urolithiasis can occur in captive terrestrial herbivorous chelonians due to any of the following: a diet rich in animal protein, especially with respect to purines and pyrimidines; water deprivation; pre-existing and/or intercurrent inflammation of the urinary bladder; a foreign body that serves as a nidus around which urates accumulate to form one or more urinary calculi.

Although many terrestrial chelonians will feed opportunistically upon invertebrates, small mammals, and ground-nesting birds and their eggs, and even carrion, their natural diet consists mainly of plants, including grasses and legumes, which contain modest to moderate amounts of phytoprotein. Also, terrestrial chelonians possess the ability to recycle a significant portion of their urine by resorbing water via their urinary bladder mucosae. When fed a diet rich in protein, particularly animal protein, and/or when they are deprived of adequate drinking water, the formation of urate calculi is promoted.

MANAGEMENT. The tortoise is prepared for aseptic surgery and a generous square plastrotomy is created (Frye, 1972). The three urinary calculi are removed via a cystotomy incision. Following exploration of the coelomic cavity, the plastrotomy incision is closed.

Dog food should be eliminated from the tortoise's diet and fresh green vegetables added to the mostly lawn grass menu. The tortoise must have access to a shallow container of fresh water at all times.

PROGNOSIS. Favorable once the calculi are removed and the diet is corrected. The tortoise made an uneventful recovery.

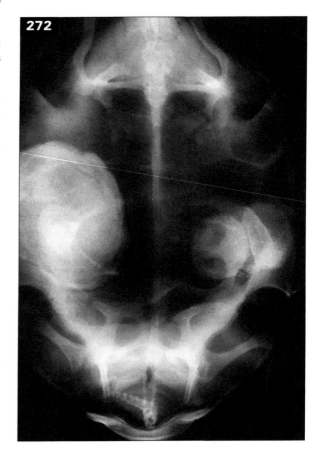
272

Case 273: **Severe bilateral swollen eyelids and conjunctivae in a snake-necked turtle**

CLINICAL PRESENTATION. An adult African snake-necked turtle is examined because both pair of its eyelids and conjunctivae are severely inflamed and swollen and held tightly shut in blepharospasm (**273a**).

DIFFERENTIAL DIAGNOSES. Foreign bodies within the conjunctival sac(s); bacterial blepharitis; mycotic blepharitis; viral blepharitis; chemical injury to the eyelid tissues; traumatic injury to the eyes and eyelids.

INVESTIGATION. The eyelids are opened gently and a small amount of conjunctival secretions collected and applied to microscope slides. These impressions are stained with a rapid Romanowsky-type stain and examined microscopically. A blood sample is withdrawn for a CBC.

Microscopy reveals large numbers of heterophil leukocytes and large macrophages with engulfed cellular debris within their cytoplasms (**273b**). Clear, nonstaining glassy diatoms are present free within the exudate (**273c**).

DIAGNOSIS. Diatom-associated blepharoconjuctivitis.

ETIOLOGY. Conjunctival foreign bodies.

PREVALENCE. Depends on husbandry practices and the quality of the water in which the turtles swim.

MANAGEMENT. Under mild sedation appropriate for restraining the turtle, each eyelid is opened and it and the underlying conjunctival sac is flushed with repeated lavages of sterile saline solution. Once the conjunctival sacs are flushed thoroughly, an antibiotic and inflammatory ophthalmic ointment is instilled. Within 24 hours, the turtle is able to open its eyelids.

The aquarium or tank that houses the turtle is thoroughly cleaned. The water should be changed frequently to reduce the population of diatoms in the water column. Diatoms, which are algal organisms with glass-like silica skeletons, are ubiquitous in aqueous environments; they rarely induce medical conditions unless a large number are present in the water. Their silica conformation is scabrous and, therefore, induces inflammation of delicate tissues.

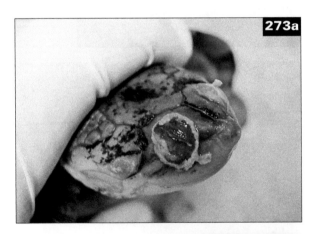

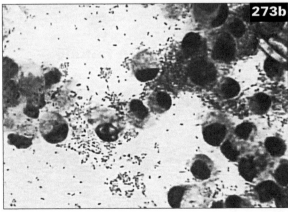

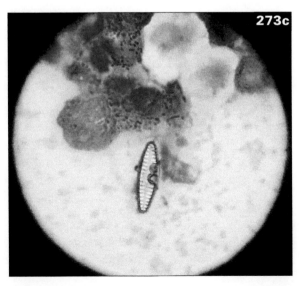

Case 274: **Foul odor emanating from a box turtle**

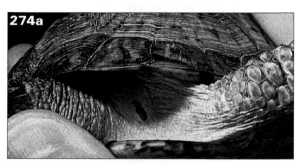

CLINICAL PRESENTATION. The owner of a mature box turtle suddenly notices a foul odor coming from her pet.

INVESTIGATION. The particularly foul odor appears to be emerging from a small elliptical orifice located between the neck and forelimb (**274a**). An alligator forceps inserted to probe the depths of this hole extracts a living fly maggot. After lavaging and probing the interior of this opening, 32 fly larvae are extracted (**274b**).

DIAGNOSIS. Myiasis (fly strike).

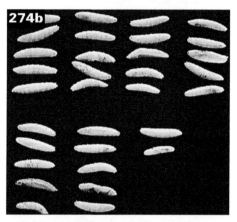

PREVALENCE. Myiasis most commonly occurs during warm weather, and it even affects chelonians that do not have pre-existing cutaneous wounds (**274c**).

MANAGEMENT. All the maggots must be removed because their excreta contain toxic amines that are injurious when absorbed. If necessary, the aperture of the fly-strike wound is opened in order to facilitate removal of the maggots. Once it is certain that no more larvae remain, the wound is rinsed thoroughly. A water-soluble antibiotic ointment is deposited into the cavity and, if necessary, a short Penrose drain inserted and secured to the edges of the wound. Physiologic fluid and broad-spectrum antibiotic therapy complete the treatment.

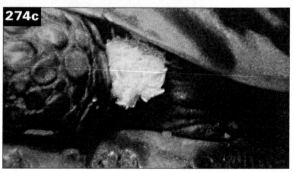

If practicable, terrestrial chelonians should be housed in screened enclosures in order to prevent attack by flies and their larvae. If this is not possible, an insect-repellent can be sprayed onto the chelonians' skin to lessen fly strike. Daily inspection of outdoor tortoises is advised.

PROGNOSIS. Favorable if all the maggots are removed promptly and if the wound pocket is flushed, treated with antibiotics, and drained (as necessary).

Case 275: **Dried object projecting from anus of a mature female ornate box turtle**

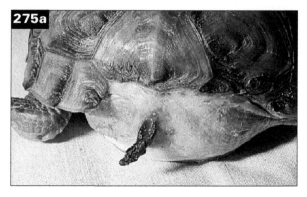

CLINICAL PRESENTATION. An adult female box turtle with an object projecting from its anus (**275a**) is presented for examination. This object was first seen two days prior to the turtle being evaluated.

INVESTIGATION. The object is a dried segment of rectum that appears to have prolapsed and become traumatized and dessicated. The anal sphincter tone is intact. Presurgical screening hematology and a biochemistry panel are all within normal limits for this species.

DIAGNOSIS. Rectal prolapse.

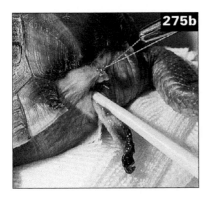
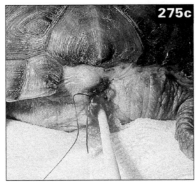
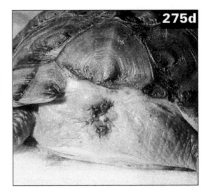

ETIOLOGY. Spontaneous.

PREVALENCE. Sporadic.

MANAGEMENT. The box turtle is anesthetized and the surgical site prepared for aseptic surgery. Mild traction is applied to the prolapsed rectum and a surgical probe inserted that will serve as a stent (275b). Individual tacking stay sutures are placed into the rectum cranial to the prolapse to prevent it from retracting back into the pelvic canal. A healthy segment is selected. The necrotic portion is amputated, leaving a cuff of vital rectum. Leaving the probe in place, this healthy rectal tissue is anastomosed to the distal-most segment that is still attached to the anal ring with four equally placed, full-thickness, nonabsorbable sutures (275c, d). The sutures are removed in approximately four weeks.

PROGNOSIS. Favorable. The turtle made an uneventful recovery, and the sutures were removed in four weeks.

Case 276: **Inability to pass feces in a California desert tortoise**

CLINICAL PRESENTATION. The owner of a male California desert tortoise notices that it is straining to pass feces, but none is produced.

INVESTIGATION. A large bolus of feces is palpated and balloted within the caudal coelomic cavity. Whole body radiography reveals three metal wood screws embedded within the mass of feces contained within the colon (276). Hematology and biochemistry tests are unremarkable.

DIAGNOSIS. Ingested metallic objects in the large intestine.

PREVALENCE. Common when foreign objects are present within the captive environment.

MANAGEMENT. Because the tortoise has not passed its stools for several weeks and is straining, the wood screws must be removed via plastrotomy and enterotomy. The tortoise is anesthetized and intubated with a noncuffed endotracheal catheter. The catheter is secured so that it will not become dislodged. The catheter is connected to a closed-circuit gas anesthesia machine delivering isoflurane or sevoflurane and anesthesia is maintained with a 3–4% gas/oxygen concentration. The tortoise is prepared for aseptic surgery. A plastrotomy incision is created and an enterotomy performed to remove the fecal bolus with the embedded wood screws. The stool bolus is radiographed to confirm that all three screws are removed. The enterotomy and plastrotomy incisions are closed.

Any foreign material that can be ingested from the tortoise's enclosure should be removed. Using a magnet secured to a pole is an effective method for collecting ferrous metal objects.

PROGNOSIS. Favorable.

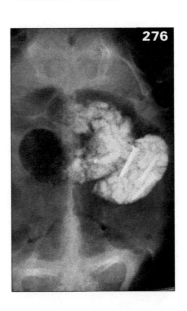

Case 277: **Spherical intraurocystic object in a California desert tortoise**

CLINICAL PRESENTATION. A well-nourished adult female desert tortoise with no prior medical history is presented because of tenesmus. The owner first noticed this behavior several days prior to requesting an examination.

INVESTIGATION. Palpation and ballottement of the coelomic contents with fingers inserted into the inguinal pockets immediately cranial to the hindlimbs disclose the presence of multiple firm, round objects. One object in particular is freely mobile within the urinary bladder. Whole body radiography reveals a large, elongated cystic calculus, a spherical object with a thin mineralized rim, and a colon filled with stools in which mineral fragments are embedded (**277a**). Hematology and biochemistry studies are unremarkable

DIAGNOSIS. Retained shelled egg and urinary calculus within the coelomic cavity, and a bulky bolus of inspissated feces mixed with calcareous material.

ETIOLOGY. Migration of a shelled egg through the proctodeum followed by retrograde passage into and through the urodeum and, finally, into the urinary bladder. This migration is usually induced by trauma, which forces the egg(s) from the proctodeum into the urodeum and, thence, into the urinary bladder.

PREVALENCE. Sporadic; usually induced by trauma.

MANAGEMENT. The tortoise is prepared for aseptic surgery. A generous plastrotomy is created and a cystotomy performed. A very large urinary calculus and a discolored shelled egg are removed from the urinary bladder (**277b**). After the cystotomy incision is closed, an enterotomy is performed to remove a bolus of inspissated feces that is admixed with gravel and sand. The plastrotomy incision is closed.

PROGNOSIS. Favorable. The tortoise made an uneventful recovery and produced a clutch of fertile eggs the following year.

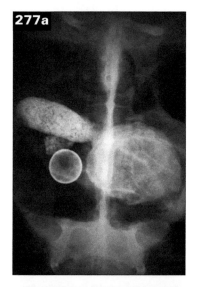

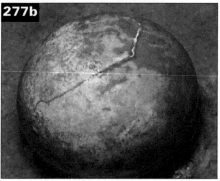

Case 278: **Autoamputation in a Pacific pond turtle**

CLINICAL PRESENTATION. An adult Pacific pond turtle is evaluated because its left forelimb dropped off distal to the humerus, leaving a raw stump with bone exposed (**278a**).

INVESTIGATION. Impression smears of the stump are obtained, air dried; and stained with Gram's stain and Fite's modification of acid-fast stain. These reveal myriad numbers of acid-fast microorganisms (**278b**). Once these organisms are identified, the owner elects to have the turtle euthanatized because of concerns for zoonotic disease. The only significant gross and microscopic abnormalities involve the left forelimb. The edges and deeper tissues near the site of the autoamputation contain multiple granulomata in which acid-fast

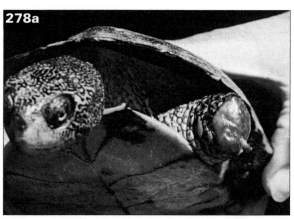

microorganisms are found engulfed within large histiocytic macrophages.

DIAGNOSIS. Mycobacteriosis; lepromatous leprosy.

ETIOLOGY. *Mycobacterium* species.

PREVALENCE. Sporadic.

MANAGEMENT. Because there is a dangerous public health potential with mycobacteriosis, treatment is not attempted. Antimycobacterial therapy is possible but, due to the potential risk of acquiring a serious zoonotic disease, the difficulty of oral dosing relatively small chelonians for the prolonged length of time that these treatments require, and the expense of the medications, euthanasia is an understandable and justifiable option in this instance.

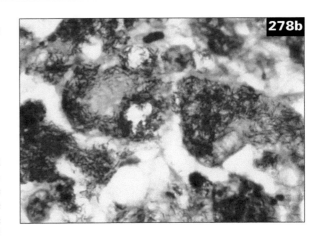

Case 279: **Chronically excoriated carapacial lesions in an African spurred tortoise**

CLINICAL PRESENTATION. An immature spurred tortoise has excoriated lesions that undermine several of the dorsal carapacial scutes (dorsal and dorsolateral keratinous shell plates). The lesions are dry and dusty (**279a**) (photo courtesy Dr N Brotons).

DIFFERENTIAL DIAGNOSES. Mycotic dermatitis; bacterial dermatitis; thermal injury; acariasis.

INVESTIGATION. The undermined and loosened scutes are gently lifted away and the dusty keratinous debris that accompanies these loosened scutes is collected in dry vials and saved for laboratory analysis. Portions of the material are preserved in AFA solution for an hour, then transferred by pipette onto glass slides that are flooded with a few drops of Hoyer's mounting medium (Frye, 1994), cover slipped, warmed until all the bubbles are eliminated, and examined microscopically. Some of the thicker scutes are preserved in 10% neutral buffered formalin solution, decalcified with formic acid, processed histologically, and examined microscopically (**279b, c**).

DIAGNOSIS. Subepidermal acariasis.

ETIOLOGY. Parasitic mites.

PREVALENCE. Sporadic.

MANAGEMENT. Once the loosened carapacial scutes are removed, the underlying epithelial tissue is gently scrubbed with 0.75% chlorhexidine diacetate solution. This is repeated daily for several weeks. Soon, the keratin at the periphery of each lesion regenerates and gradually covers the denuded scutes.

All the animals in a collection should be inspected regularly for any mite infestation. Treatable medical conditions must receive effective treatment without delay.

PROGNOSIS. Favorable. The tortoise had an uneventful recovery.

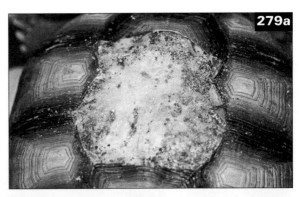

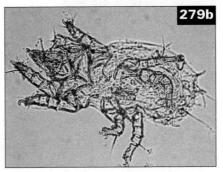
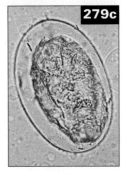

Case 280: **Ventral cervical swellings in a group of four Galapagos tortoises**

CLINICAL PRESENTATION. Four adult Galapagos giant tortoises that are on display at a major municipal zoo are examined because each has developed large, firm swellings in the region of the ventral neck (**280a**).

DIFFERENTIAL DIAGNOSES. Fibrous goiter; granulomatous inflammation; neoplasia.

INVESTIGATION. A careful review of the diet being fed to these four tortoises reveals that, because of budgetary concerns, instead of their usual diet of large alfalfa (lucerne) hay pellets and mixed salad greens, they have been fed white head cabbage almost exclusively for several months.

The tortoises' ventral cervical swellings are identical in that each is firm on palpation, not tender, and partially mobile. Two of the tortoises are prepared for aseptic surgery, and the skin and subcutaneous tissues overlying the cervical swellings are infiltrated with 2% lidocaine. Fine-needle biopsy cores are obtained for histopathologic processing and microscopic examination.

Histopathology identifies hypothyroidism characterized by a change in the thyroid follicular pattern from the normal, in which follicles lined by cuboidal epithelial cells are filled with abundant, pink-staining colloid (**280b**), to one in which the follicles are lined by tall columnar epithelial cells containing very scanty colloid (**280c**).

DIAGNOSIS. Fibrous goiter; hypothyroidism.

ETIOLOGY. Diet-induced hypothyroidism. Budgetary considerations aside, these tortoises should have been provided a nutritious diet. Substituting white head cabbage for their usual diet of hay pellets and salad greens induced a state of hypothyroidism because cabbage contains, as part of its chemical components, isothiocynate and sodium and potassium salts of isothiocyanic acid, which are constituents of many cruciferous plants (cabbages, mustards, etc). Some members of this family of edible plants contain more isothiocyanate; others contain less. These goitrogens compete for iodine in the synthesis of the thyroid hormone, thyroxin, and, therefore, provoke a deficiency of thyroid hormone.

PREVALENCE. Sporadic, depending on the captive-diet fed.

MANAGEMENT. Once recognized, diet-induced hypothyroidism is treated with iodine supplementation with sodium iodide or potassium iodide, or by adding kelp to the diet as a natural source of iodine (as well as other halogens).

PROGNOSIS. Favorable once iodine replacement therapy is initiated and the diet that induces the condition is corrected. However, although the thyroid function can be restored, the fibrous component of the goiters may not resolve completely.

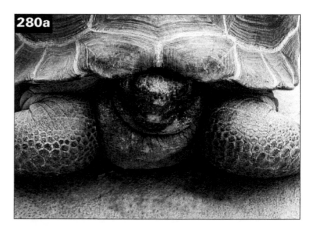

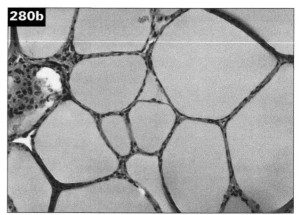

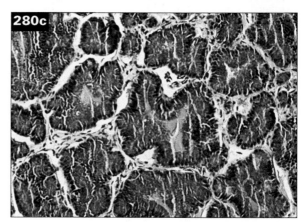

Case 281: **Continual straining in a South American red-legged tortoise**

CLINICAL PRESENTATION. An adult female red-legged tortoise is presented for examination because of almost continual tenesmus (straining) for approximately one week. This tortoise is housed with a male of the same species, and they were seen copulating several times during the past few months.

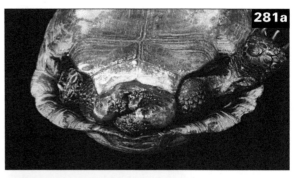

INVESTIGATION. The caudal-most portion of the plastron is abraded, and the cloacal membranes partially prolapsed from the cloacal vent (**281a**). Whole body radiography reveals the presence of four mineralized shelled eggs. The egg that is closest to the pelvis is fractured at one end, with the sharp shell fragments pointing caudally (**281b**). These eggs are readily palpated when balloted with finger tips inserted into the inguinal 'pockets' in front of each hindlimb.

A whole blood sample is drawn for routine presurgical evaluation. The hematology and biochemistry results of these tests are unremarkable.

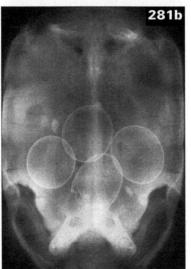

DIAGNOSIS. One of four mineralized shell eggs within the oviduct is fractured.

ETIOLOGY. Intraoviductal shelled egg fractured by the forceful mating activities of a conspecific male tortoise.

PREVALENCE. Common.

MANAGEMENT. It is obvious that the sharp shell edges of the hind-most fractured eggshell will (or already have) impinge on the delicate inner surfaces of the oviduct (**281c**); therefore, surgery is mandatory. The tortoise is anesthetized, intubated, and prepared for aseptic surgery. A generous plastrotomy is created. A salpingotomy is performed to remove the four eggs through a single incision. The salpingotomy is closed with two layers of absorbable sutures. The coelomic cavity is explored thoroughly and the plastrotomy incision closed (Frye and Schuchman, 1974). The tortoise with its three intact eggs is sent home with the owner one day after surgery. These three eggs are incubated, and one of them hatches about three months later.

Due to their sexually aggressive nature, adult male tortoises should not be housed with gravid female tortoises. When copulating with a gravid female, the male's penis can damage any shelled eggs with which it comes into contact, either directly or by imparting kinetic energy to those in front of the egg being struck (in a cue ball fashion).

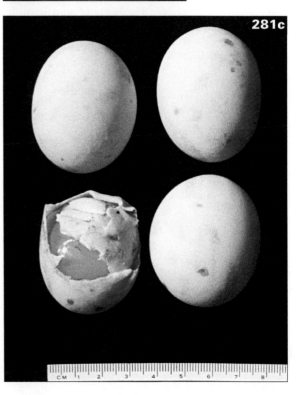

PROGNOSIS. Favorable. The tortoise had an uneventful recovery and produced several clutches of fertile eggs during the years following her surgery.

Case 282: **Asymmetrical swimming posture in a painted turtle**

CLINICAL PRESENTATION. An adult female painted turtle is evaluated because it is swimming in the water tank with its left side deeper in the water than its right side (**282a**).

DIFFERENTIAL DIAGNOSES. Unilateral pneumonia (or at least pneumonia that is more severe on one side); pyogranulomatosis due to bacterial or mycotic infection; unilateral lung collapse; unilateral hydrothorax; verminous pneumonia; pulmonary or mediastinal neoplasm.

INVESTIGATION. Dorsoventral and anterior–posterior whole body radiographs are made (**282b, c**). A transtracheal or intratracheal wash is obtained, and specimens for cytology and microbiological culture and sensitivity testing are collected.

DIAGNOSIS. Bacterial pneumonia and consolidation of the left lung.

PREVALENCE. Common.

MANAGEMENT. A course of bacteriocidal antibiotic therapy is commenced. Supplemental oxygen enhances oxygenation of tissues, facilitates the turtle's breathing, and reduces the heart rate. This turtle died several weeks after it was presented for evaluation. Necropsy revealed that the left lung was completely consolidated and fibrotic.

PROGNOSIS. Unfavorable. The lungs of aquatic turtles serve not only as organs of respiratory gas exchange, they also serve as hydrostatic organs by which buoyancy is maintained and diving is facilitated.

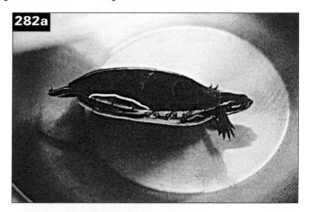

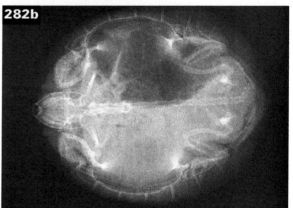

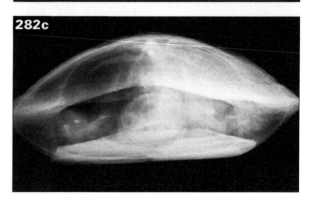

Case 283: **Tenesmus in an adult female Texas tortoise**

CLINICAL PRESENTATION. Several days after tenesmus began, an adult female Texas tortoise is presented for evaluation. The tortoise refuses to eat and she was seen excavating shallow holes in the turf of her enclosure, then backing into these depressions and straining as if to pass stools or eggs.

INVESTIGATION. Using both hands, one or two fingers of each hand are inserted into the inguinal 'pockets' immediately cranial to each hindlimb, and the caudal coelom is balloted by gently rolling the tortoise semi-clockwise and semi-counterclockwise. Digital ballottement reveals several firm objects within the coelom. A ventrodorsal radiograph shows four very large shelled ova and one partially disintegrated, fractured shelled ovum within the coelom (**283a, b**). The large intestine contains feces within which are embedded calcareous or rocky objects. The shelled eggs measure 35 mm, 32 mm, and 31 mm. However, the pelvic inlet measures only 18 mm in cross-sectional diameter, as does the distance between the overhanging caudal-most carapace and plastron.

A whole blood sample for hematology and biochemistry determinations is taken (right).

DIAGNOSIS. Egg binding due to cross-sectional mismatch between shelled eggs and distal urogenital passages. In addition, there is radiographic evidence of yolk-lipid serocoelomitis.

Egg binding occurs when a female is unable to pass her shelled ova. In some instances, oviductal egg rupture causes the contents of the egg to spill into the coelomic cavity, which induces yolk-lipid serocoelomitis.

ETIOLOGY. The etiology can be any of the following: anomalously large or misshapen shelled eggs; anatomic mismatch of shelled ova size with the cross-sectional pelvic diameter; extramural obstruction of the oviduct by an enteric fecal bolus or foreign material within the pelvic canal (e.g. sand, gravel, cage litter materials); oviductal inertia due to hypocalcemia or hypoestrogenism.

PREVALENCE. Common.

MANAGEMENT. The tortoise is anesthetized and the plastron prepared for aseptic surgery. A plastrotomy, exploratory coeliotomy, salpingotomy, and intracoelomic lavage are performed to remove the widely disseminated egg yolk lipid.

PROGNOSIS. Unfavorable to very guarded because of the widely distributed egg yolk lipid and the massive inflammation within the coelomic cavity and its contents.

Hematology

PCV	0.37 l/l	(37%)
WBC	16.4 × 10⁹/l	(16.4 × 10³/µl)
Heterophils	61%	
Lymphocytes	28%	
Azurophils	3%	
Monocytes	8%	
Thrombocytes	Adequate	

Comment: several large macrophages with engulfed lipid are identified.

Biochemistry

Glucose	5.2 mmol/l	(93.6 mg/dl)
Calcium	2.8 mmol/l	(11.2 mg/dl)
Phosphorus	2.77 mmol/l	(8.59 mg/dl)
Sodium	133 mmol/l	(133 mEq/l)
Potassium	3.9 mmol/l	(3.9 mEq/l)
Uric acid	0.4 mmol/l	(6.76 mg/dl)
TP	68 g/l	(6.8 g.dl)
Albumin	21 g/l	(2.1 g/dl)
Globulin	47 g/l	(4.7 g/dl)
AST	122 u/l	
ALT	44 u/l	
LDH	102 u/l	
AP	86 u/l	

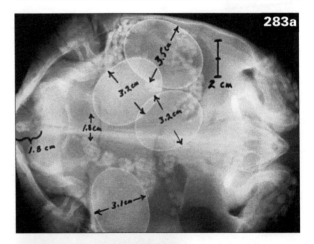

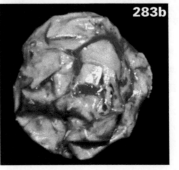

Case 284: Installation of pharyngostomy and esophagostomy tubes in chelonians

CLINICAL PRESENTATION. Mandibular and maxillary fractures prevent a tortoise from prehending its food. After the fractures are repaired surgically, a decision is made to install an esophagostomy tube so that the tortoise can return to a positive nitrogen balance without having to use its healing mouthparts.

MANAGEMENT. Placement of pharyngostomy and esophagostomy tubes is a relatively short-term method for providing a patient that is not eating or drinking a channel by which soft foods and fluids can be placed into the stomach without inducing stress, which occurs when the animal is forcefully restrained. The procedure is commonly used in progressive management.

The tortoise is anesthetized, intubated, and maintained on isoflurane or sevoflurane at 3–4%. The lateral cervical area is prepared for aseptic surgery. The external carotid and jugular arteries are located; this is facilitated by using an ultrasonic Doppler blood flow detector (284a). A curved Rochester, Kelly, or Doyen forceps is inserted into the pharynx and the jaws are opened slightly so that the curved jaws lie against the inner surface of the pharyngeal or esophageal lumen, respectively. Using a number 15 scalpel blade, a stab incision is made into the lumen of the passage. A fine-pattern Metzenbaum scissors is used to lengthen the stab incision, making certain that it is in the lumen of the pharynx or esophagus (284b). A rubber urethral catheter is inserted into the incision and advanced to a premeasured distance that places it into the stomach (284c). In order to secure the tube, a piece of adhesive tape is placed, creating a 'butterfly' to which the skin can be sutured (284d), thus securing the tube and keeping it from becoming dislodged. One or two sutures are inserted. The free end is directed up and over the carapace so that it can be taped in place (284e). The tube is flushed with a small volume of water to confirm that it is properly situated in the stomach. A plug is inserted into the expanded end of the catheter. These feeding tubes can be left in place for four to six weeks, if necessary.

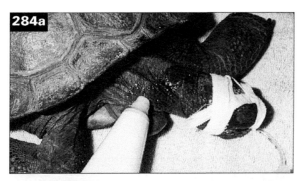

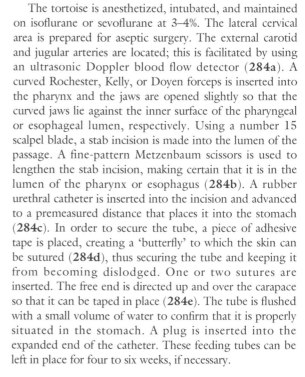

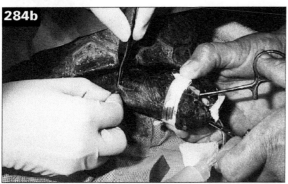

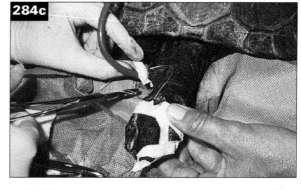

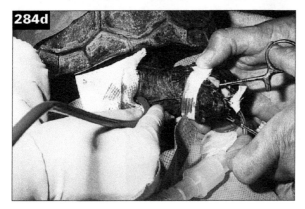

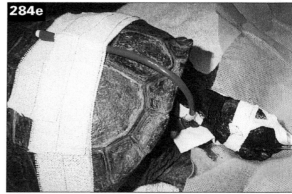

Case 285: **Gastrointestinal foreign bodies in an adult California desert tortoise**

CLINICAL PRESENTATION. An adult desert tortoise with a history of consuming foreign material present in its environment exhibits increasing lethargy and anorexia.

INVESTIGATION. Whole body radiography reveals multiple irregularly shaped dense metallic foreign bodies within the gastrointestinal tract (285). A whole blood sample is drawn and submitted for hematology and blood lead level determination. The hematology results are unremarkable except for mild anemia (PCV 0.26 l/l [26%], 3 nucleated RBCs/high-power field). The lead level in this tortoise's blood is 10.19 μmol/l (210.9 μg/l) (a control tortoise's blood has 1.24 μmol/l [25.67 μ/gl]).

DIAGNOSIS. Lead intoxication.

PREVALENCE. Sporadic to common, depending on husbandry practices.

MANAGEMENT. 10–40 mg/kg EDTA diluted in lactated Ringer's solution is injected i/v daily until the level of lead in the blood is reduced to 1.2 μmol/l or less. 20 ml/kg of the Ringer's solution is infused once every 24 hours. The ingested lead fragments are removed if possible by employing gastrointestinal lavage or by administering nonaqueous cathartics so that additional lead is not absorbed.

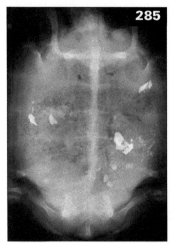

All sources of lead must be removed from the tortoise's enclosure. Old painted wood, storage batteries, fishing weights, etc. must be eliminated.

PROGNOSIS. Favorable.

Case 286: **Severe morbidity in an Asiatic box turtle**

CLINICAL PRESENTATION. One of two Asian box turtles recently imported from Southeast Asia suddenly displays very severe depression and appears to be dead. However, when a limb is pulled gently, the turtle slowly retracts it back into its shell. This turtle dies very shortly after physical examination and before any diagnostic testing can be performed. The other turtle appears healthy (286a).

INVESTIGATION. A whole blood specimen is obtained from the cadaver and stained with a rapid Romanowsky-type blood stain. Microscopic examination of the blood film reveals myriad numbers of corkscrew-shaped, spirochaete-like microorganisms in the plasma (286b). There is no microbiological culture.

DIAGNOSIS. Spirochetemia.

ETIOLOGY. Septicemia.

PREVALENCE. Sporadic; becoming more likely with increased international trade in nonindigenous reptiles.

MANAGEMENT. The living turtle is treated with piperacillin (50 mg/kg i/m q24h) plus fluid therapy (20 ml/kg q24h).

PROGNOSIS. Favorable if diagnosed and treated early in the course of infection.

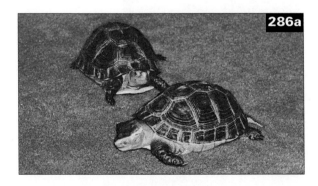

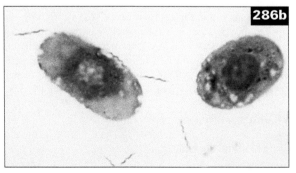

Case 287: **Tenesmus in a California desert tortoise**

CLINICAL PRESENTATION. An adult gravid female desert tortoise exhibits severe, nearly continuous, straining without producing stools, urine, or shelled eggs.

INVESTIGATION. Ballottement of the caudal coelomic cavity reveals the presence of several firm, freely movable objects. Whole body radiography discloses six well-mineralized shelled eggs. Three of these eggs share their calcareous shells (287a). Routine presurgical hematology and biochemistry determinations are unremarkable.

DIAGNOSIS. Tenesmus induced by three normal and three anomalous (conjoined) intraoviductal shelled eggs.

PREVALENCE. Egg binding is common; the incidence of conjoined shelled eggs is sporadic.

MANAGEMENT. The tortoise is anesthetized, prepared for aseptic surgery, and a generous plastrotomy and salpingotomy created. The three normal and three anomalous shelled eggs are removed (287b). The salpingotomy incision is closed in two layers. After exploring the coelomic cavity, the plastrotomy is closed.

PROGNOSIS. Favorable.

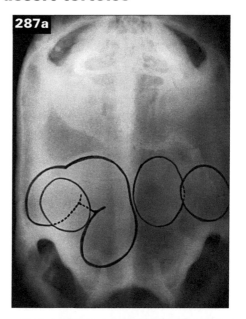

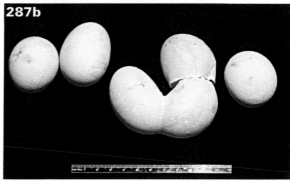

Case 288: **Phallus observed in a female Hermann's tortoise**

CLINICAL PRESENTATION. The owner of an adult female tortoise notices a black, spade-shaped organ intermittently protruding from the cloacal vent. The tortoise deposited at least one clutch of eggs in the previous years.

INVESTIGATION. A whole body radiograph reveals numerous shelled eggs within the coelomic cavity (288a). The tortoise appears healthy, and it is eating well. Routine hematology and biochemistry tests are unremarkable. The owners request identification of the organ that intermittently protrudes from the tortoise's cloacal vent, particularly when it is picked up (288b) (photo courtesy Dr O Grazioli).

DIAGNOSIS. Pseudohermaphroditism.

PREVALENCE. Sporadic.

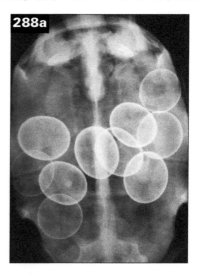

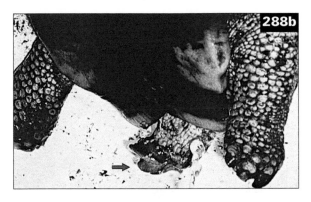

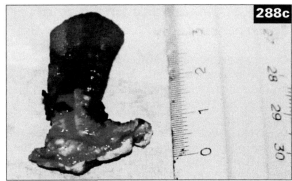

MANAGEMENT. The tortoise is anesthetized and the contents of the cloacal vault explored. The protruding organ is identified as a large, firm, heavily pigmented phallus. The owners grant permission for the excision of this organ. Double-transfixed ligatures are placed and the phallus is removed in its entirety (**288c**). The organ is submitted for histopathologic processing and it is confirmed to be a normal phallus.

PROGNOSIS. Favorable. The tortoise makes an uneventful recovery and eventually deposits over a dozen eggs.

Case 289: **Gasping and respiratory distress in an adult male California desert tortoise**

CLINICAL PRESENTATION. An adult male California desert tortoise is evaluated as an emergency because it suddenly begins to gasp with its mouth open. The oral mucosae are cyanotic, and the tortoise is reluctant to move. The tortoise was healthy until it was fed several fresh, ripe figs a few hours prior to presentation.

INVESTIGATION. Whole body radiography reveals massive gastrointestinal tympany. The stomach and intestine contain large volumes of gas, which cause compression of the right lung field (**289**).

DIAGNOSIS. Acute gastrointestinal dilation (tympany).

ETIOLOGY. Induced by the ingestion of fresh ripe figs that are fermented.

PREVALENCE. Sporadic.

MANAGEMENT. The tortoise is placed into a closed oxygen chamber for 30 minutes to provide it with supplementary oxygen. A urethral catheter is passed into the stomach. A large volume of gas escapes from the tortoise's stomach, and 0.5 ml of simethicone solution is then administered through the same catheter. Once the tortoise is breathing more normally, a second 0.5 ml dose of simethicone is administered. The catheter is replaced with a larger-diameter feeding tube. The tortoise is suspended upside down and its stomach flushed with tepid water. Once the stomach is rinsed free of its ingesta, another catheter is inserted into the copradeum portion of the cloaca. A tepid water enema is given until clean, feces-free water runs out. A third 0.5 ml dose of simethicone solution is then administered and the catheter removed . The simethicone is used to lyse the gas bubbles in the alimentary tract.

PROGNOSIS. Favorable, once the source of the gas fermentation is removed and oxygenation is restored.

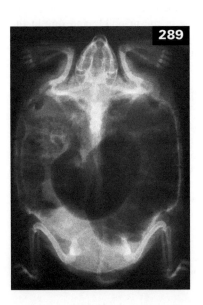

Case 290: **Necropsy findings after the sudden death of a juvenile spurred tortoise**

CLINICAL PRESENTATION. A juvenile spurred tortoise, which had been fed a diet rich in animal protein (dog food, cat food, mealworms, and scanty vegetables), dies suddenly and is presented for necropsy examination.

INVESTIGATION. Multiple pale foci in the liver and periarticular lesions are seen on necroscopy (**290a**). Representative samples of affected tissues are placed in 10% buffered formalin solution and in absolute methanol. Urate crystals dissolve in formalin but are preserved in absolute methanol. Sections are processed for routine histopathology. Microscopic examination reveals numerous 'star burst'-like gouty tophi containing urates in the liver and kidneys, and in and around joints (**290b**).

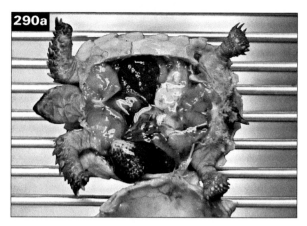

DIAGNOSIS. Visceral and periarticular gout.

PREVALENCE. Common.

MANAGEMENT. Adequate fresh water must be provided in a vessel that is readily accessible, and a diet appropriate for this species must be fed (mostly leafy green vegetables and only a modest amount of animal protein). If a patient is treated with an aminoglycoside antibiotic or other chemical that is known to be nephrotoxic, it important to give supplementary hydration and not rely on the animal drinking sufficient water to maintain normal renal perfusion.

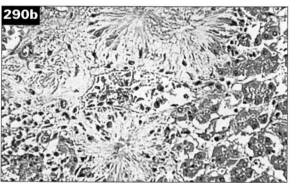

Case 291: **Ununited mandibular fracture in a California desert tortoise**

CLINICAL PRESENTATION. An adult male California desert tortoise with a history of having its fractured mandible and maxilla treated by the insertion of two stainless steel orthopedic wires (one in the mandible and one in the maxilla) eight months previously, is referred for a second opinion because of a failure of the mandibular fracture to heal (**291a**). During the intervening eight months, the owners were hand-feeding the tortoise a soft diet of moistened alfalfa (lucerne) hay pellets. Aside from the unhealed fractures, the tortoise appears in good health, is well fleshed, and is active.

INVESTIGATION. Dorsoventral and lateral radiographs of the head are obtained.

DIAGNOSIS. Trauma.

PREVALENCE. Common.

MANAGEMENT. The tortoise is anesthetized and its upper and lower jaws prepared for aseptic surgery. Two trocar-

tip Kirschner wires are inserted transversely into the mandible in parallel approximately 3–4 mm apart (**291b**). The two wires are cut, leaving approximately 2–3 mm protruding beyond the skin surface on each side of the mandible (**291c**), taking care to avoid piercing the tongue. A volume of cold-setting dental acrylic cement is added with a sufficient volume of the methylethyl ketone catalyst to a discarded syringe cap (**291d**). This is mixed thoroughly to a consistency of thick cream. Soft acrylic is applied to the skin, and the ends of the Kirschner wires are covered (**291e**). While still soft, the acrylic is smoothed with a tongue depressor (**291f**). The outer surface of the maxilla is cleansed and another layer of dental acrylic applied, leaving the original layer *in situ*. With an emery board, the cutting edge of the dental acrylic is sanded so that the tortoise can shear its vegetable diet. A postoperative radiograph is obtained (**291g**). The two Kirschner wires and dental acrylic splints are left in place until the mandible has healed.

PROGNOSIS. Favorable.

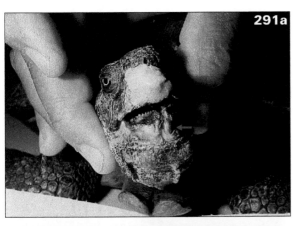

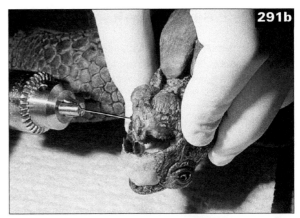

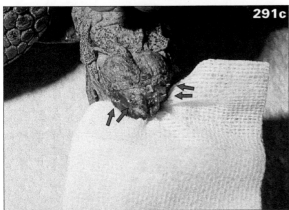

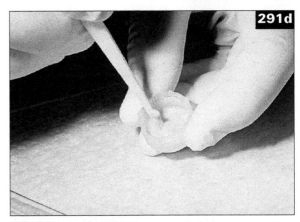

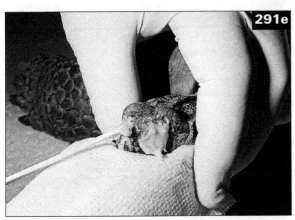

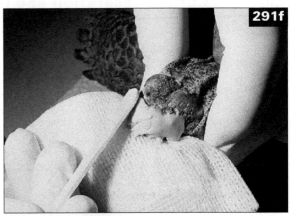

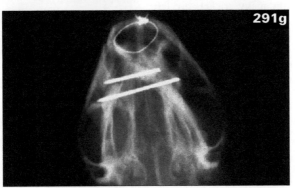

Case 292: **Sudden lethargy and morbidity in a Pacific pond turtle**

CLINICAL PRESENTATION. A Pacific pond turtle is examined after it had exhibited sudden lethargy that soon progressed to a moribund state. The turtle was unresponsive to gentle stimulation with fingers and prodding with a wooden applicator stick. The inguinal 'pockets' immediately in front of each hindlimb were distended.

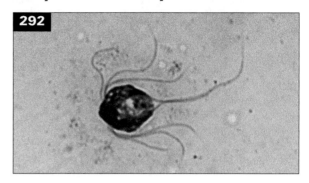

INVESTIGATION. Ultrasonic Doppler blood flow detection revealed a steady heart beat, but the turtle was not breathing. A whole body dorsoventral radiograph disclosed a uniformly homogeneous 'ground-glass' fluid density throughout the coelomic cavity. The fluid was aspirated via percutaneous needle aspiration, centrifuged, and the concentrated material made into a wet mount and stained with Mayer's hematoxylin. Microscopic examination of the wet mount revealed numerous protozoan organisms with six well-defined flagella (**292**). These were identified as *Hexamita* species.

DIAGNOSIS. *Hexamita*-induced serocoelomitis.

PREVALENCE. Sporadic.

MANAGEMENT. If identified early in the course of infection, *Hexamita* infection can be treated with metronidazole (50–100 mg/kg p/o) plus physiologic fluid therapy. Intracoelomic lavage will cleanse the inflamed serosal surfaces and will help reduce the population density of the organisms.

PROGNOSIS. Unfavorable unless the pathogens are discovered early and treated effectively.

Case 293: **Corneal laceration and iris prolapse in a red-eyed tree frog**

CLINICAL PRESENTATION. A pet red-eyed tree frog is presented as an emergency case for evaluation of a massive injury to its left eye (**293**).

INVESTIGATION. The iris of the left eye has prolapsed through a full-thickness corneal laceration. The exposed iris has already became dessicated by the time that the frog is presented for examination.

ETIOLOGY. This frog shares a terrarium with other frogs. The terrarium is furnished with plastic plants and a few dried wooden branches. The prey insects fed to these frogs consist almost entirely of domestic crickets (*Gryllus domesticus*). Depending on how many crickets are left from the last feeding, a few more are placed into the terrarium every few days. There is no fresh vegetable matter for the crickets to eat. Feeling the effects of hunger, one or more of the surviving crickets attacked this frog and severely damaged its eye by biting and penetrating the left cornea.

PREVALENCE. Depends on whether or not prey crickets are provided with an adequate food supply.

MANAGEMENT. Surgery is required. The frog is anesthetized by applying one drop of alfaxalone/alfadolone to its dorsal integument. Once the frog is unresponsive to external stimuli, its left eye is enucleated and the orbital defect covered with a liquid antiseptic plastic dressing (NewSkin® Medtech, Jackson, WY).

When living prey insects such as crickets are placed into a cage with their predator amphibians or reptiles, an appropriate food source must be provided for them so that any surviving insects will be able to eat and not have to resort to attacking their erstwhile predators.

PROGNOSIS. Favorable. The frog made an uneventful recovery and soon learned to accommodate to its monocular vision.

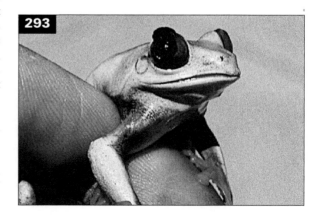

Case 294: **Mass arising from digit of an African bullfrog**

CLINICAL PRESENTATION. An adult African bullfrog is presented for examination and evaluation of a cauliflower-like, fungating, pink mass arising from the distal phalanx of the first digit of its left forelimb (**294a**). The frog was in captivity for several years and thrived on a diet of mixed small invertebrates and small laboratory mice. The frog appears to be healthy and active.

DIFFERENTIAL DIAGNOSES. Pyogranuloma due to infection with a bacterial pathogen (e.g. *Mycobacterium* species); mycotic granuloma; parasitic granuloma; foreign body granuloma; extra-articular gouty granuloma; neoplasm.

INVESTIGATION. On physical examination, which includes an ultrasonic Doppler blood low investigation, the only abnormality identified is the digital lesion. This mass is firm and freely moveable; when palpated, it appears to be mildly painful.

DIAGNOSIS. Articular and periarticular (including visceral) gout.

ETIOLOGY. Articular, periarticular, and extra-articular (including visceral) gout can be caused by any of the following: water deprivation/dehydration; spontaneous renal failure; dietary overload with purine and pyrimidine-rich foodstuffs; inappropriate use of aminoglycoside antibiotics without appropriate fluid therapy to maintain renal perfusion; some nephrotoxic chemical and plant substances; a genetic predisposition for developing gout.

MANAGEMENT. Aseptic surgical amputation of the distal phalanx of the first digit on the right manus is the preferred treatment. The frog is anesthetized with alfaxalone/alfadolone applied topically to its dorsal integument, starting with five drops and observing for relaxation. Once the frog is relaxed, a final three drops are applied. Once the frog becomes unresponsive to external stimuli, the affected digits and manus are prepared for aseptic surgery. The distal phalanx of the first digit on the right manus is amputated distal to a single transfixed ligature at the base where it joins the palm of the manus.

Immediately following surgery, multiple impressions are made from the freshly incised cut surfaces of the mass. These are fixed in absolute methanol, stained with a Romanowsky stain, and examined microscopically with both plain and cross-polarized illumination. Once microcrystals that are consistent with urates are identified, the surgical specimen is immersed in absolute methanol and processed histopathologically. Absolute methanol is used because urates will dissolve if the tissue specimens are preserved in formalin or other aqueous fixatives. Microscopic examination of stained serial sections confirms the presence of urate microcrystals (**294b**).

This frog is neither water deprived nor dehydrated. There is no evidence of intercurrent renal disease. A careful review of its medical history does not reveal prior treatment with aminoglycoside antibiotics. There is no indication of the frog having been exposed to nephrotoxic chemical or plant agents. It is possible, however, that its diet, which included numerous small mice that might have contained sufficient purine- and pyrimidine-rich organ tissues (liver, spleen, kidneys, etc.), induced hyperuricemia and, thus, precipitated the deposition of urate crystals in the frog's tissues.

PROGNOSIS. Favorable, with an uneventful recovery. The prognosis is positive because, except for the digital gouty mass, the bullfrog is healthy and vigorous. Once its diet is changed, further urate accumulations should be obviated.

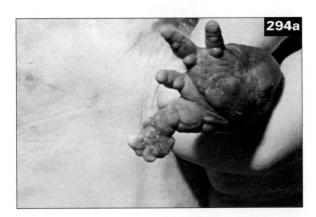

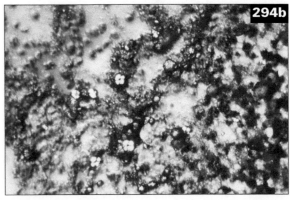

Case 295: **Argentine horned frog with a massively swollen body**

CLINICAL PRESENTATION. An immature Argentine horned frog that was purchased from a pet shop as a recently metamorphosed froglet is presented for evaluation because it has gradually become massively swollen and, finally, is unable or refuses to move or eat. The frog is kept in a terrarium furnished with damp sphagnum moss that is washed and wrung out to partially dry at least once weekly. Initially, the frog's diet was live small guppies. Then, as the frog grew, small ornamental goldfish that are kept in an aquarium and are fed commercial flaked fish food, were eaten. For the first few months the frog grew rapidly and appeared to be in excellent health. However, after several more months, the owner noticed that the frog was growing ever more bloated and more reluctant to move. Finally, the frog ceased to eat when provided with its usual goldfish prey.

INVESTIGATION. Physical examination reveals a well-fed frog with gross accumulation of fluid beneath the skin of its belly and what appears to be a similar accumulation of ascitic fluid within its coelomic cavity (**295a, b**). Ultrasonic Doppler blood flow investigation discloses markedly abnormal heart sounds with prominent grade IV/VI holosystolic atrioventricular and aortic murmurs. Samples of the fluids obtained from beneath the skin and within the coelomic cavity via percutaneous aspiration are clear and have a SG of 1.005. Cytology reveals that the fluid is essentially devoid of cells.

At this point the frog is euthanatized and a complete necropsy is carried out (**295c**). This reveals several significant abnormalities, which include marked mineralization of the myocardium (**295d**), kidneys (**295e**), liver, and alimentary tract.

Although the diet contained adequate protein, it is unlikely that it was properly digested or assimilated; also, it is likely that much of the protein that was present in the stools was lost before it could be absorbed. The myocardial function was impeded because the heart was so severely mineralized that it could not pump blood effectively. Because the frog refused to move, its lack of muscular activity would have reduced the amount of lymph that returned to the heart. The liver was similarly affected, with calcium-rich mineralized connective tissue largely replacing normal hepatocellular tissue. The renal parenchyma was severely mineralized, leaving the glomeruli, renal tubules, and collecting tubules crowded and displaced. The intestine was massively mineralized; this affected its ability to absorb essential protein.

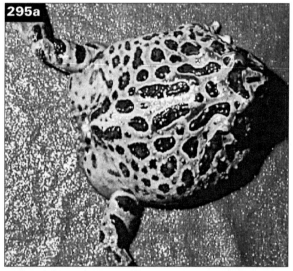

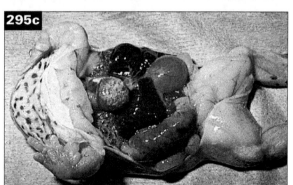

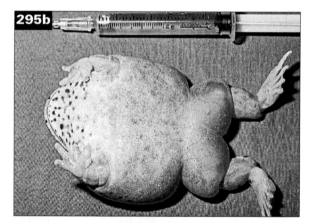

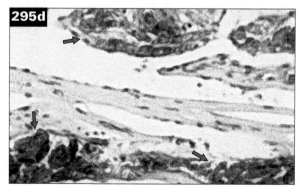

DIAGNOSIS. Hypercalcemia secondary to iatrogenic hypervitaminosis D_3.

ETIOLOGY. Dhe history reveals the etiology of this interesting case. Analysis of the flaked fish food that was fed to the prey goldfish offered to the frog disclosed an unusually rich content of vitamin D_3. Thus, as the frog ate its goldfish prey, it was slowly, but consistently, accumulating a toxic level of vitamin D_3.

Both the subcutaneous and intracoelomic fluid accumulations (anasarca and ascites, respectively) are consistent with transudates, based on their very low SG and relative lack of cells. The most likely etiology of the low SG of the fluid is diminished protein content. Hypoproteinemia can be induced by any of the following etiologies: lack of available dietary protein; inability to digest and assimilate ingested protein; hepatic failure leading to diminished plasma protein synthesis; renal dysfunction causing urinary loss of protein; myocardial dysfunction, particularly failure of the heart to return venous blood to the central pool; any obstruction that prevents normal return of lymph to the central circulation; protein-wasting enteropathy that results in protein being lost in the feces.

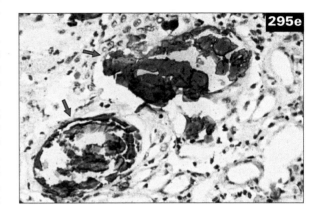

Case 296: **Urinary bladder prolapse in an Argentine horned frog**

CLINICAL PRESENTATION. An otherwise healthy, mature Argentine horned frog is examined because its urinary bladder has prolapsed (**296a**).

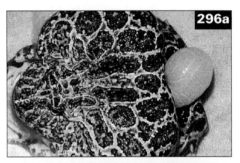

INVESTIGATION. A stool specimen containing enteric parasites that could cause the frog to strain excessively and, thereby, forcibly evert its bladder was not available for analysis.

MANAGEMENT. The frog is placed into a shallow container, and a few drops of alfaxalone/alfadolone are applied to its dorsal integument. Once the frog relaxes, a few more drops of alfaxalone/alfadolone are applied to its dorsal integument to achieve surgical anesthesia. The skin of the perineum and each flank is prepared for aseptic surgery. With the frog in ventral recumbency, the urinary bladder is emptied of any residual urine by aspiration. The urinary bladder is inverted by placing mild pressure on the now deflated organ with a sterile glass rod or cotton-tipped applicator moistened with saline until the urinary bladder is replaced into its normal position within the coelomic cavity (**296b**). If necessary, one or two small episiotomy-like relieving incisions can be created to facilitate replacement of the indurated bladder. Once the urinary bladder is in its normal location, several through and through, full-thickness interrupted horizontal or vertical mattress urocystopexy sutures are inserted on each side of the frog's belly to secure the urinary bladder to the muscular body wall and prevent its reprolapse (**296c**) (Frye, 1989, 1993).

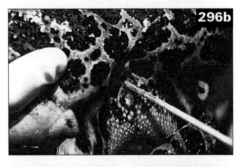

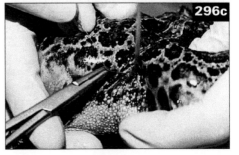

PROGNOSIS. Favorable. The frog made an uneventful recovery and did not reprolapse its urinary bladder.

Case 297: **Unilateral corneal discoloration and opacity in a tree frog**

CLINICAL PRESENTATION. A small pet tree frog has a multipunctate to diffuse pale gray to white discoloration and opacity involving most of its right eye (**297**). The frog has been fed a diet consisting of small to medium-sized crickets and mealworms for approximately two years. The corneal opacification was first noticed four months prior to presentation.

DIFFERENTIAL DIAGNOSES. Cataract; post-traumatic corneal fibrosis; postkeratitis corneal scarring; interstitial cholesterol and calcium keratopathy.

INVESTIGATION. Direct ophthalmoscopy demonstrates that the opacities are located within the substance of the cornea and not on its surface or within or on the crystalline lens.

DIAGNOSIS. Interstitial cholesterol and calcium keratopathy.

ETIOLOGY. Diet-associated hypercholesterolemia with deposition and secondary calcification of the cornea. These conditions are believed to be related to a diet containing lipid-rich insects, especially domestic crickets (*Gryllus domesticus*), waxworms (*Galleria* species), and meal-beetle larvae (*Tenebrio molitor*).

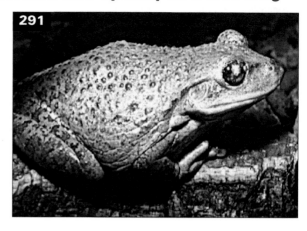

PREVALENCE. Common in long-term captive frogs and toads fed cultured crickets, waxworms, and mealworms.

MANAGEMENT. If the diet can exclude cholesterol-rich cultured insects, and is changed to earthworms and small flying insects, the keratopathy might be arrested before it grows worse and completely impedes light transmission.

PROGNOSIS. Unfavorable.

Case 298: **Severe ulcerative dermatitis in a colony of African clawed frogs**

CLINICAL PRESENTATION. A university research colony of approximately 5,000 African clawed frogs is maintained in a series of indoor tanks, each holding approximately 500 frogs. Suddenly, every morning, the caretaker finds numerous frogs dead or moribund.

INVESTIGATION. Representative living and freshly dead frogs are selected for microbiological culture and sensitivity, and necropsy. The most severely affected frogs have dermal ulcerations on their rostrums and feet. The skin and superficial muscles of many frogs are completely eroded, with the mandibular bone and digits exposed (**298**). Water samples and affected frog tissue samples are cultured microbiologically, and they yield pure cultures of the fish pathogen *Aeromonas salmonicida*. When this is announced, the animal caretaker staff are questioned. One of the caretakers admits to having gone fishing and, after catching more fish than he could use, he brings fresh salmon to the frog colony, grinds it in a food mill, and feeds it to all of the frogs. This breech of animal colony protocol occurs three days before the first sick and dead frogs are observed.

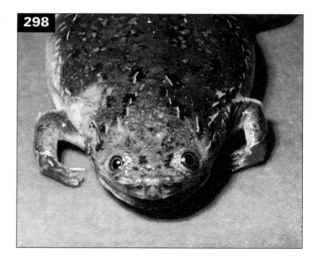

DIAGNOSIS. Aeromoniasis.

ETIOLOGY. *A. salmonicida* infection.

PREVALENCE. Common in water-borne bacterial infections affecting aquatic amphibians.

MANAGEMENT. Because so many frogs are being housed in the colony and because of their delicate mucoid skin, individual frogs are not treated. Rather, all frogs exhibiting illness or integumentary lesions are removed and isolated. The water flow into and out of the water tanks is increased substantially to increase the dilution of pathogens in the water column. Just these two simple measures resolve the epidemic of aeromoniasis in the colony. The incidence of affected frogs drops immediately and, within 10 days, the outbreak is finished. Water samples are collected again and they no longer yield *A. salmonicida* on culture.

Flawless hygiene, especially in order to maintain high-quality tank water, is imperative in colonies of aquatic amphibians. Once a feeding regimen is established, it should not be modified without appropriate authority and quality assurance to ensure that it is safe and nutritious.

PROGNOSIS. Devastatingly severe unless there is improved husbandry.

Case 299: **Massive trauma to the left hindlimb of a western toad**

CLINICAL PRESENTATION. A good Samaritan brings in an adult female western toad that has sustained a crushing injury when a heavy rock falls on it. The toad is active and alert. Except for the injury to the left hindlimb, which is completely crushed (**299a**), the toad appears healthy and vigorous. There is no hemorrhage.

ETIOLOGY. Trauma.

PREVALENCE. Sporadic.

MANAGEMENT. The toad is anesthetized by applying a few drops of alfaxalone/alfadolone to its dorsal integument, and prepared for aseptic surgery. The left hindlimb is amputated by disarticulating it at the coxofemoral joint. The surgical incision is closed with absorbable sutures. Two coats of NewSkin® (MedTech) liquid plastic antiseptic dressing are applied to seal the sutured incision. The toad is released when it has recovered from anesthesia and is fully able to ambulate.

PROGNOSIS. Favorable. The toad was released into the author's backyard and made an uneventful recovery (**299b**). Immediately after surgery, the toad tended to walk in circles; however, it was able to walk in a straight line and eat insects and earthworms in a short period of time following surgery.

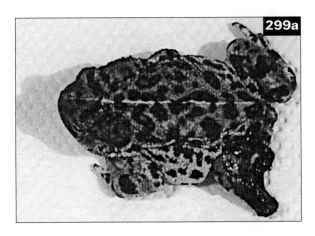

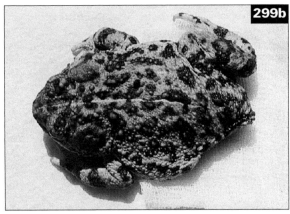

Case 300: **Chronic dermal ulceration in a Pacific tree frog**

CLINICAL PRESENTATION. Multiple, deep, dermal ulcerations develop in the ventral skin of the hindlimbs of a pet Pacific tree frog (**300**). The frog is kept in a terrarium furnished with damp sphagnum moss, which is rinsed weekly, and several small pots of living house plants.

INVESTIGATION. A sterile swab specimen is obtained from one of the ulcers, and an impresssion smear made for Gram-stained cytology, which reveals gram-negative microorganisms

A second swab specimen is obtained for microbiology. It is subcultured in thioglycolate broth to enhance growth of gram-negative microorganisms. After 24 hours, it is streaked out onto blood agar and incubated at room temperature under a reduced oxygen atmosphere. The culture yields *Aeromonas hydrophila*.

DIAGNOSIS. Subacute to chronic *A. hydrophila* infection.

PREVALENCE. Very common in captive amphibians.

MANAGEMENT. The integument of most amphibians is semipermeable; therefore, it is possible to administer many medications by applying them onto the dorsal skin. When applying bacteriocidal antibiotic to the frog's skin, the dosage is calculated based on its body weight. This often requires an accurate metric scale that is calibrated in grams.

PROGNOSIS. Favorable to guarded. The reason for adding the adjective 'guarded' is that many strains of *A. hydrophila* produce potent endotoxins that can induce rapid death even before gross lesions appear. In this instance, the *A. hydrophila* is not as virulent as many others are and, therefore, induces much less pathology without endotoxemia.

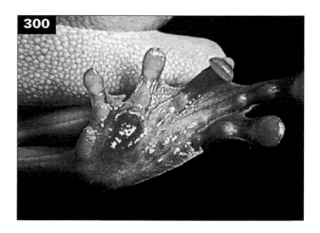

Case 301: **Unusual eye appearance in an American bullfrog**

CLINICAL PRESENTATION. A household cat attacks an adult American bullfrog, which causes superficial lacerations on the left side of the bullfrog's head extending from just in front and below the left eye to over the left tympanum and shoulder. A partially healed corneal scar is identified in the upper edge of the left cornea. The iris and crystalline lens are prolapsed into the lower portion of the left anterior chamber (**301**).

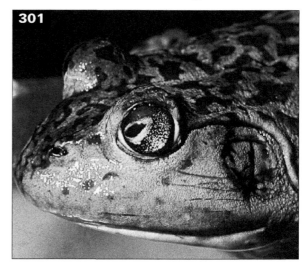

DIAGNOSIS. Unilateral prolapse of the crystalline lens.

ETIOLOGY. Trauma; cat scratches.

PREVALENCE. Sporadic.

MANAGEMENT. Because the lacerations are healing well, no medical treatment is required.

PROGNOSIS. Favorable. The frog still has monocular vision and, while hospitalized, demonstrates that it can detect, attack, and ingest prey crickets. Therefore, it is released to an outdoor pond.

Summary questions and answers

Q1. What are the major signs of intussusception in an iguana?

Q2. How can traumatic avulsion of a tertiary spectacle be avoided when treating a snake for a retained spectacle?

Q3. Are snakes that are cage mates of a snake infested with ochetosomes at risk of being infested? If so, why?

Q4. In a snake with gastric cryptosporidiosis, what are the principal clinical signs?

Q5. How could the normally pathogenic fungus *Microsporum* possibly grow on the detritus within an old shell fracture of a box turtle?

Q6. What are the primary functions of the parietal eye?

Q7. What is the relationship between morbid obesity and diabetes mellitus in many obese captive monitor lizards?

Q8. Why is it imperative to provide fresh vegetable matter in cages where live insects are fed as prey to reptiles and amphibians?

Q9. How do eyeless pythons find their prey?

Q10. Why should large amounts of white head cabbage not be fed to reptiles?

Q11. Injectable or orally administered ivermectin is recognized as an excellent acaricidal agent for killing mites and ticks. Why is it applied only topically to chelonians?

Q12. What features of an iguana suffering from rheumatoid arthritis are consistent with other autoimmune disorders?

Q13. Why should green iguanas affected by kyphoscoliosis not be used for breeding captive-bred iguanas?

Q14. When using a mechanic's pick-up tool to grasp gastric foreign bodies, why must the tool be inserted with the four grasping jaws closed?

Q15. Why are so many antibiotics ineffective in resolving abscesses or pyogranulomata in a tegu's swollen foot?

Q16. What distinguishing characteristic makes the ova of *Capillaria* so readily identifiable?

Q17. Why is the presence of raised subepidermal swellings around a kingsnake's eyes, as well as in other distant integumentary sites, such an unfavorable prognostic sign?

Q18. How does pseudohermaphroditism differ from true hermaphroditism?

Q19. How does the ingestion of fresh ripe figs relate to gastric tympany in a desert tortoise?

Q20. In a Central American boa constrictor displaying signs of a massive hyperimmune reaction to wasp stings, what other drug medication, besides an antihistamine such as diphenylhydramine HCl, would be useful if it was available?

A1. Vomiting, regurgitation of ingesta; a palpable sausage-shaped mass in the coelom; gas-filled loops of intestine.

A2. Moisturize first with contact-lens wetting solution.

A3. No. These trematodes (flukes) have an indirect life cycle and require one or more intermediate hosts in order to infect their definitive snake hosts.

A4. Postprandial regurgitation of meals after approximately 24–36 hours; swelling in the region of the stomach.

A5. The infection can be an example of opportunism. If the fungus is not especially pathogenic, it is possible to treat it effectively.

A6. It serves as a dosimeter by which the diurnal reptiles that possess it regulate their basking behavior; it influences hypothalmic hormone interactions with some endocrine glands.

A7. A lipid-rich diet, lack of exercise, and chronic obesity tend to promote chronic active pancreatitis. With recurrent bouts of pancreatitis, more and more islets of Langerhans are lost. Eventually, there is insufficient insulin to metabolize glucose and, therefore, diabetes ensues.

A8. So that the insects will have a source of food and, therefore, not have to attack their predators.

A9. They employ nonvisual cues: heat-sensing labial pits detect warmth and the tongue and vomeronasal organ detect the scent of prey.

A10. White head cabbage and some other members of the Brasssica family of vegetables contain significant amounts of sodium and potassium isothiocyanate, which is antagonistic to thyroxin synthesis by the thyroid; therefore, when excessive amounts are consumed, hypothyroidism can be induced.

A11. Ivermectin, when injected or ingested, is highly toxic to chelonians; therefore, it is applied topically as a dilute solution, which is safe and effective for treating chelonian ectoparasitism.

A12. Lupus erythematosus (L-E) cells in the peripheral blood; membranous glomerulonephritis; hyperglobinemia.

A13. Kyphoscoliosis appears to be a developmental characteristic that has a genetic component; therefore, affected iguanas should not be used as breeders.

A14. To avoid traumatizing the esophagus and stomach. The jaws are opened only after the tool is within the stomach; until then, the four jaws remain safely closed within the tubular sheath.

A15. Each of the individual abscesses or pyogranulomata are surrounded by very dense connective tissue capsules. These may help prevent further dissemination of the infection, but they also inhibit the absorption of antibiotics into these foci of infection.

A16. The plug-like opercula that closes each end of the ovum.

A17. Finding widely dispersed inflammatory lesions is highly suggestive of septicemia and widespread dissemination of infection to vital internal organs.

A18. True hermaphrodites possess gonadal tissue of both genders. Pseudohermaphrodites possess one or more secondary or accessory organs of the opposite sex, but possess gonadal tissue of only a single gender.

A19. Figs contain much readily fermentable simple and complex fruit sugars, which promote excessive gas formation by the microorganisms responsible for digestion.

A20. An injectable adrenal corticosteroid.

Bibliography

References

Brownstein DG, Strandberg JD, Montali RJ, Bush M, Fortner J (1977) Cryptosporidium in snakes with hypertrophic gastritis. *Veterinary Pathology* **14**, 606–617.

Campillo NJB, Frye FL (2002) Preliminary report of subepidermal carapacial mite infestation in an African spurred tortoise, *Geochelone sulcata*. *Proceedings of the Association of Reptilian and Amphibian Veterinarians Annual Meeting*, Reno, p. 17.

Frye FL (1989) Non-invasive urocystopexy for repair of urinary bladder prolapse in an Argentine horned frog, *Ceratophrys ornata*. *Proceedings of the Third International Colloquium on the Pathology of Amphibians and Reptiles*, Orlando, p. 113.

Frye FL (1992) Use of a condom as an occlusive bandage in snakes: a new wrinkle on an old resource. *Journal of Small Exotic Animal Medicine* **2(1)**, 13–14.

Frye FL (1993) Non-invasive urocystopexy and colopexy for repair of urinary bladder and colorectal prolapses in reptiles and amphibians. *Proceedings of the American College of Veterinary Surgeons Forum*, San Francisco, pp. 384–385.

Frye FL, Schuchman SM (1974) Salpingotomy and caesarian delivery of impacted ova in a tortoise. *Veterinary Medicine/Small Animal Clinician* **69(4)**, 454–457.

Frye FL, Kass L (1991) Characterization of cell type in subacute basoeosinophilic myelogenous leukemia in a snake. *Herpetopathologia* **2(1)**, 63–71.

Frye FL, Barten SL, Pepin DW, McNeely H, Vasser JR (1994a) Histological, histochemical, and immunohistochemical characteristics of disseminated malignant mesothelioma in a corn snake (*Elaphe g. guttata*). (Abstract) *Proceedings of the Second World Congress on Herpetology*, Adelaide, p. 91.

Frye FL, Pepin DW, McNeely H, Hadfy LB, Corcoran JH, Vasser JR (1994b). Functional pancreatic glucagonoma in a rhinoceros iguana (*Cyclura c. figgensi*) characterized by immunohistochemistry. (Abstract) *Proceedings of the Second World Congress on Herpetology*, Adelaide, p. 92.

Frye FL, Kaiser HE (1995) Spontaneous autoimmune pancreatitis and diabetes mellitus in a turtle, *Clemmys marmorata*. *Anti-Cancer Research* **15(5A)**, 1752.

Hildebrandt J-P (2001) Coping with excess salt: adaptive functions of extrarenal osmoregulatory organs in vertebrates. *Zoology* **104**, 209–220.

Kaplan HM (1957) Septicemic cutaneous ulcerative disease in turtles. *Proceedings Animal Care Panel* 7, 273–277.

Kass L, Frye FL (1995) Acute erythroblastaemia and characterisation of cell type in an iguana, *Iguana iguana*. *Herpetopathologia* **2(2)**, 161–169.

Korabiowska M, Brinck U, Frye FL, Harshbarger JC, Schauer A, Kaiser HE (1998) Comparative immunohistochemical and photometric analysis of snake melanomas. *In Vivo* **11**, 420–415.

Leonardi L, Grazioli O, Mechelli L, Frye FL (2002) Gastric mucinous adenocarcinoma in a diamond python (*Morelia spilotes spilotes*). *Proceedings of the Association of Reptilian and Amphibian Veterinarians Annual Meeting*, Reno, p. 63.

Textbooks

Cooper JEC, Jackson OF (1981) *Diseases of the Reptilia. Two Volumes*. Academic Press, New York and London.

Frye FL (1991) (ed) *Biomedical and Surgical Aspects of Captive Reptile Husbandry. Two Volumes*. (2nd edn). Krieger Publishing Company, Malabar.

Frye FL (1994) *Reptile Clinician's Handbook: A Compact Clinical and Surgical Reference*. Krieger Publishing Company, Malabar, pp. 97–100.

Frye FL, Williams DL (1995) *Self-Assessment Colour Review of Reptiles and Amphibians*. Manson Publishing, London.

Hoff GL, Frye FL, Jacobson ER (1984) (eds) *Diseases of Amphibians and Reptiles*. Plenum Press, New York.

Ippen R, Schroeder H-D, Elze K (1985) *Handbuch der Zootierekrank-heiten, Volume I, Reptilien*. Akademie Verlag, Berlin.

Mader DR (2006) (ed) *Reptile Medicine and Surgery* (2nd edn). WB Saunders, Philadelphia.

Marcus LC (1981) *Veterinary Biology and Medicine of Captive Amphibians and Reptiles*. Lea & Febiger, Philadelphia, p. 17.

Schmidt-Nielsen K (1997) *Animal Physiology: Adaptation and Environment*. Cambridge University Press, Cambridge.

Section 4
ORNAMENTAL FISH

Gregory A Lewbart

Classification of cases by species

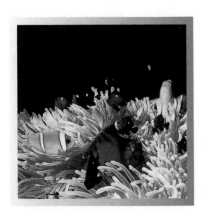
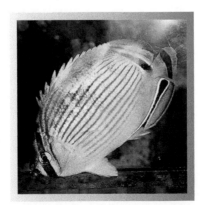
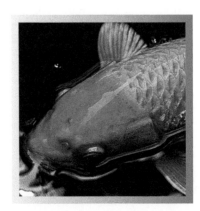

Introduction

The first English language texts on fish medicine written by veterinarians did not appear until the early 1990s. Since then, there has been remarkable growth in the field with regards to numbers of veterinarians treating fish, clinical technology and advances, and peer-reviewed clinical and basic research studies. In 1989 the first full-time public aquarium veterinarian was hired at the National Aquarium in Baltimore. Within ten years, nearly every major aquarium in the United States had at least one staff veterinarian and many employed two or more. While these aquariums also house mammals, birds, reptiles, and invertebrates, the bulk of the clinical load is fish. Within the last decade several internship programs have become established to train aquarium and aquaculture veterinarians. Two university residency programs now exist to prepare veterinarians for board certification in zoological medicine (American College of Zoological Medicine), with an emphasis in aquatic animal medicine.

As our knowledge of fish diseases, therapeutics, and water quality increases, more and more veterinarians will be qualified to work responsibly with these animals. Peer-reviewed articles on the clinical management issues of pet fish now appear in many veterinary, aquaculture, and fisheries biology journals. Nearly every major North American veterinary conference includes fish medicine in the program and several veterinary schools now offer continuing education courses on this subject. In addition, a growing number of textbooks and review articles contain valuable information on pet fish medicine (Hartman *et al.*, 2006). All veterinarians, even if they have never worked on a fish, have a broad understanding of disease processes, diagnostics, animal husbandry, and chemotherapeutics. The opportunity to apply this knowledge to a client's pet fish problem can be a rewarding experience. Currently, some exotic animal clinicians report that fish patients generate 10% or more of their income.

The keeping of fish as pets is a hobby with a long history. In recent years, particularly during the past decade, ornamental pond fish including koi and goldfish have become increasingly popular in various parts of the world. In fact, more pet fish are kept as pets in the United States than any other single group of animals including dogs, cats, small mammals, birds, and reptiles (Wise *et al.*, 2002).

While many hundreds of fish species are maintained in captivity, the bulk of pet fish fall into four basic categories: marine tropical species; koi and goldfish; freshwater tropical species; and freshwater temperate species. There are four major sources of pet fish in the ornamental fish industry. They include the following: wild caught and shipped immediately; wild caught and conditioned or 'grown out'; indoor aquaculture; and outdoor aquaculture. In some cases a combination of the above may be employed.

While it appears that freshwater tropical fish sales are flat or in a slight decline, outdoor pond numbers and the species that inhabit them are increasing dramatically. Marine reef systems, with an emphasis on coral reef invertebrates and fish, are an area of rapid growth in the pet fish/aquarium industry.

Until the 1980s, except in rare instances, most of the medical care and husbandry practices were performed by the hobbyists themselves or with the help of the local pet store clerk or aquarium maintenance person. Many of these people are very knowledgeable and conscientious, but there are no minimal training standards, as there are in the veterinary profession. Additionally, veterinarians understand the principles of medicine, surgery, and animal husbandry. The same fundamental disciplines such as critical care, microbiology, parasitology, nutrition, pathology, and surgery that are applied to terrestrial animals can be applied to pet fish. Preventive medicine is a valuable, though currently underutilized, service that we can offer to our clients.

Fish clinicians should identify a laboratory that is familiar and comfortable with handling fish samples, especially those related to clinical pathology and microbiology. In some cases this may require involvement with more than one laboratory.

With literally hundreds of species kept in captivity, from a variety of (sometimes) unrelated families, it is understandable that clinicians will not be familiar with every species of fish with which they are presented. However, fish clinicians who are likely to deal with fish should (1) be familiar with zoonoses and be able to speak intelligently to their clients on this topic; (2) cultivate a list of colleagues with which to share information and seek consultation; and (3) have a thorough understanding of the natural history, anatomy, and physiology of the major groups of pet fishes (e.g. goldfish, koi, cichlids, livebearers, anabantoids).

Medications

There are currently no drugs approved by the US Food and Drugs Administration (FDA) for use in pet fish in the United States, although a small number are approved for use in fish intended for human consumption. The FDA is currently examining the wide availability of prescription drugs, especially antibiotics. (For more information on the FDA and the use of drugs in aquaculture, consult the following web address: (www.fda.gov/cvm/.) With the relatively recent (2004) passing of the Minor Use and Minor Species (MUMS) Animal Health Act, it is possible that some dramatic changes will be seen in the availability of drugs for use in pet fish. (It is likely that these changes will mean more 'approved' or 'indexed' drugs.) Such measures will necessitate sound pharmacokinetics, efficacy, and safety studies to support clinical use of antimicrobials and other chemotherapeutants in fish. Relatively little research related to pharmacology has been reported in ornamental fish. What little information exists is based on clinical efficacy and *in vitro* trials using a number of different antimicrobials. A recently published on-line database contains valuable information on pharmacokinetics in fish (Reimschuessel *et al.*, 2005). Many commonly employed veterinary compounds, including antibiotics, parasiticides, and disinfectants, should be on hand and available for use with pet fish patients. The fish practitioner should also be aware of the wide use of over-the-counter (OTC) drugs by pet fish hobbyists. An effort should be made to learn about these OTC compounds and have a basic understanding of their ingredients and impact on the patient and its environment.

History taking

A complete history should be taken on each patient or each population of patients. Fish should first be given a gross 'in tank' or 'in pond' inspection if appropriate, followed by a thorough physical examination. There are several good references on what questions to ask a client with sick pet fish (see Bibliography section). The clinician will require such important information as: How long has the client owned the fish? How experienced is the client with aquarium or pond management? What and how often are the fish fed? Have any new fish been introduced into the aquarium or pond recently and, if so, were they quarantined? Have the fish been treated with any medications? Armed with answers to these and other background questions the veterinarian or technician is ready to analyze the water quality.

Water analysis

In the majority of cases the aquarium or pond water should be tested. An accurate and properly functioning test kit is probably the fish clinician's most valuable diagnostic tool. The basic pet fish diagnostic laboratory must be equipped to test for temperature, ammonia, nitrite, nitrate, pH, dissolved oxygen, and total alkalinity. Test kits that measure copper and chlorine are also desirable. Most professional diagnostic laboratories can perform heavy metal and miscellaneous toxin testing. Several companies manufacture test kits that accurately and inexpensively test the appropriate water quality parameters.

Biopsy and other sampling techniques

In many cases, and especially those dealing with a client's pet fish, the clinician may want to take some antemortem tissue samples for examination. Many procedures can be performed rapidly with little risk to the piscine patient. Naturally, larger fish fare better and generally provide more diagnostic samples than smaller fish, and the overall condition of the animal is a factor in how it will respond to biopsy techniques.

If a water quality problem has been ruled out but a parasitic or bacterial infection is suspected, the following simple procedures can be performed: a skin scraping; a fin clip; and, in most cases, a gill snip. An anesthetic agent such as tricaine methanesulfonate (MS-222) or eugenol (clove oil) can be used to restrain the fish and make these procedures easy and safe. MS-222 is purchased in a crystalline form and can be used to produce a working stock solution of 10 grams per liter of clean, dechlorinated water. By making dilutions from this stock solution, the clinician can accurately formulate safe and effective anesthetic solutions. Each liter of stock solution should be buffered with about 5–10 grams of sodium bicarbonate (baking soda). The stock solution should be stored in a glass or plastic bottle away from light at room temperature. When prepared and stored in this manner, the stock solution is good for about 30 days, perhaps longer. Final concentrations of between 100 and 150 mg/liter will anesthetize most fish within a matter of 3–5 minutes. Several studies have investigated clove oil (which may contain several isomers of eugenol) as a fish anesthetic (see Bibliography section). Clove oil is available on an OTC basis at most pharmacies in the United States. Eugenol is not completely soluble in water and should be diluted with ethanol at a ratio of 1:9 (clove oil:ethanol) to yield a working stock solution of approximately 100 mg/ml, since each ml of clove oil contains close to one gram of drug (purity may vary). Concentrations of between 25 and 75 mg/liter are effective in freshwater and marine species, and the results are comparable to MS-222, except that recovery may be prolonged.

After the fish loses its ability to maintain equilibrium, it is removed from the water, the required procedures performed, and it is then placed in a 'recovery' vessel containing clean aerated water. A coverslip, glass slide, or scalpel blade can be used to obtain the skin scraping sample. The coverslip (or other implement) should be firmly drawn across the area to be sampled, making sure that some mucus and epidermal tissue remain on the implement. Plastic coverslips are preferable to glass coverslips, which easily break. The tissue sample that is now on the tip of the scalpel blade, slide, or coverslip is placed on a slide that contains several drops of clean water. A coverslip is applied (unless one was used to obtain the sample) and the specimen is now ready for microscopic examination. A fin biopsy can be obtained using a pair of fine scissors. Slides prepared with drops of water should be close by before samples are taken. After deflecting the operculum, several small pieces of gill tissue can be safely cut away using small suture-removing scissors. Care must be taken to remove only a couple of millimeters of primary gill lamellae. There is usually some bleeding following this procedure, but it should quickly subside.

Blood collection

Obtaining blood samples from ornamental fish is challenging but not impossible. It is very difficult to do so in fish less than 7 cm (3 ins) long. A sterile blood sample is a useful way to culture for a suspected bacteremia or septicemia. Fresh whole mounted blood smears can be valuable in diagnosing protozoal blood parasites (e.g. trypanosomes) and, in an overwhelming septicemia, motile gram-negative rods can frequently be observed darting across the microscopic field of view. Stained blood smears will reveal numerous nucleated erythrocytes, leukocytes, and thrombocytes. Campbell and Ellis (2007) have published an excellent review of piscine hematology (see Bibliography section). Some people insert the needle just ventral to the lateral line of the caudal peduncle (tail stalk) of the fish, while others take a mid-ventral approach, entering the hemal arch from its ventral aspect. Once the needle touches the vertebral body, the needle can be gently 'walked' ventrally until it drops into the caudal venous sinus. Slight constant negative pressure on the plunger of the syringe will facilitate sample collection. Fish blood samples should usually be collected in heparinized syringes (EDTA may lyse the red cells in some species).

Fecal examination

Performing a fecal examination on a fish is a relatively easy and valuable test. If time is not a factor, the fish and some clean water can be placed in a plastic bag, clean jar, or small aquarium, and a fecal sample can be collected within a matter of hours in many cases. Many fish will defecate as they relax in an anesthetic solution.

Microbiology

One final and very important area of diagnostics involves the field of microbiology. Touch preparations of suspect lesions and acid-fast staining can help rule out mycobacteriosis.

Cultures of skin and gill tissues are not especially helpful due to the ubiquitous nature of aquatic bacterial pathogens. Cultures of clinically healthy fish and clean water will commonly reveal the presence of gram-negative bacteria. Clean blood samples are valuable in detecting and identifying septicemia. As with terrestrial animal medicine, every attempt must be made to procure sterile samples for microbiology. Buller (2004) has published a review of the subject (see Bibliography section). A popular culture site in fish is the caudal (tail) kidney. The kidneys of most fish run just ventral to the spinal column and are generally found the length of the body cavity. Culturing kidney tissue is a postmortem technique that is relatively easy to do. Culture samples may be processed in the clinic and antibiotic sensitivities run, although many companion animal clinics are not equipped to perform microbiology testing. Fish cultures can be sent 'out of house', since many veterinary schools and state agricultural diagnostic laboratories are familiar with fish bacteriology.

Radiology/imaging

Radiography is part of many pet fish diagnostic evaluations. Radiographic findings have been instrumental in diagnosing and treating a number of fish cases, and fish are relatively easy to radiograph. Most can be handled without anesthesia by simply removing the fish from a tank or bucket, placing it on a radiographic plate (protected by a plastic bag), and making the exposure. Fractious fish like koi should be tranquilized before radiography is performed. Fish will readily tolerate contrast studies, ultrasonography, computed tomography (CT) scans, and even bone scans.

Necropsy procedures

On some occasions, a full necropsy is the best way to arrive at an accurate diagnosis of a disease problem. Necropsies have some obvious advantages over biopsy procedures – tissues can be looked at thoroughly and completely and all tissues and organs are available for both gross and histopathologic inspection. Dead fish autolyze rapidly and as such are frequently not good necropsy specimens. If at all possible, the clinician should obtain a moribund fish and quickly kill it for examination. An overdose of tricaine methanesulfonate (over 400 mg/liter for 15 minutes) works well. A rapid cut with a scalpel at the base of the cervical spine will quickly dispatch a fish (this can be performed after heavy sedation). Once the fish is dead, the operculum can be removed to expose the gills. Samples can be taken for immediate inspection under the microscope and preserved in 10% neutrally buffered formalin for histopathology. Fish tissues can be preserved and handled like any mammalian sample. Once the abdominal organs are visible, they may be examined and removed. Small pieces of tissue may be excised, squashed on a slide under a coverslip, and examined under the microscope. This quick and easy procedure may be helpful in diagnosing a parasite problem or a condition such as hepatic lipidosis. One convenient aspect of tropical fish anatomy is that many of these animals are relatively small and entire organs or organ systems can be fixed in formalin.

Hospitalization

Hospitalizing fish patients can be a challenge, but will be necessary on occasion. A variety of aquarium support equipment and supplies, including tanks, pumps, filters, nets, siphons, heaters, and water conditioners, is required. In many situations the owner of the fish can provide some or all of the necessary materials, including conditioned biological filter substrate, for the hospitalized patient. A room or portion of a room dedicated to fish life support is ideal. The majority of the equipment and supplies listed below can be used in the hospital and in the field.

Equipment and supplies (not including most drugs and standard clinic supplies):
- Husbandry:
  - Air pumps.
  - Air tubing.
  - Assorted plastic storage boxes.
  - Assorted glass aquaria.
  - Assorted sizes of plastic 'fish bags'.
  - Assorted nets.
  - Commercial dechlorinator.
  - Rubber bands.
  - Sea salt.
  - Sponge filters.
  - Water test kit.
  - Water sample bottles (plastic, 250 ml).
  - 20 liter (5 gallon) bucket(s).

- Medical:
  - Centrifuge.
  - Complete dissecting kit.
  - Compound microscope.
  - Eugenol (clove oil) 1:9 with 95% ethanol (stock approx. 100 mg/ml).
  - Fish anesthesia machine.
  - Gram scale (to 1 kg).
  - Kilogram scale (to 10 kg).
  - MS-222 (10 mg/ml buffered stock solution).
  - Oxygen tank with regulator.
  - Plastic surgical drapes.
  - Refractometer.
  - Sterile surgical pack(s).

For the veterinarian interested in pursuing fish medicine, a list of informative textbooks and pertinent journals is given in the bibliography section.

Summary

Fish medicine is a growing and rewarding area of our profession. Many fish owners have strong emotional bonds to their fish and they seek state-of-the science care and support for their sick or injured pets. The fish medicine knowledge base is small compared with that of small domestic animals or even some of the other 'exotic' taxa. All fish practitioners are encouraged to contribute to this base of knowledge, either by publishing their findings or sharing information and discoveries with colleagues.

English and Latin names

Australian rainbowfish	*Melanotaenia fluviatilis*
Black grouper	*Myctopera bonaci*
Black tetra	*Gymnocorymbus ternetzi*
Blue-eyed plecostomus	*Panaque suttoni*
Bonnethead shark	*Sphyrna tiburo*
Brook trout	*Salvelinus fontinalis*
Carp (koi)	*Cyprinus carpio*
Cichlids	Family Cichlidae (>1,400 species)
Clown loach	*Botia macracanthus*
Clown triggerfish	*Balistoides conspicillum*
Corydoras catfish	*Corydoras* species
Discus	*Symphysodon discus*
Dog-faced puffer fish	*Arothron nigropunctatus*
Dwarf gourami	*Colisa lalia*
Electric eel	*Electrophorus electricus*
Emperor angelfish	*Pomacanthus imperator*
French angelfish	*Pomacanthus paru*
Freshwater angelfish	*Pterophyllum scalare*
Goldfish	*Carassius auratus*
Gouramis	Family Osphronemidae
Green terror cichlid	*Aequidens rivulatus*
Guppy	*Poecilia reticulata*
Jackknife fish	*Equetus lanceolatus*
Killifish	*Aphanius dispar*
Koi (carp)	*Cyprinus carpio*
Lemon shark	*Negaprion brevirostris*
Leopard shark	*Triakis semifasciata*
Lionfish	*Pterois volitans*
Melon butterflyfish	*Chaetodon trifasciatus*
Midas cichlid	*Amphilophus citrinellus*
Molly	*Poecilia latipinna*
Muskellunge	*Esox masquinongy*
Neon tetra	*Paracheirodon innesi*
Northern pike	*Esox lucius*
Oscar/red oscar	*Astronotus ocellatus*
Pearl cichlid	*Cichlasoma cyanoguttatum*
Pearci cichlid	*Cichlasoma pearsei*

Percula clownfish	*Amphiprion ocellaris*
Pictus catfish	*Pimelodus pictus*
Planehead filefish	*Stephanolepis hispidus*
Platy	*Xiphophorus maculatus*
Queen angelfish	*Holacanthus ciliaris*
Queensland grouper	*Epinephelus lanceolatus*
Red pacu	*Piaractus brachypomus*
Redtail catfish	*Phractocephalus hemioliopterus*
Sanke koi	*Tahuantinsuyoa macantzatza*
Scrawled filefish	*Aluterus scriptus*
Seahorses	*Hippocampus* species
Sharks	Order Selachii
Silver dollar	*Metynnis argentus*
Slippery dick	*Halichoeres bivittatus*
Snakehead	*Channa argus*
Squirrelfish	*Holocentrus adscensionis*
Stick catfish	*Farlowella acus*
Sunset thick-lipped gourami	*Colisa labiosa*
Upside-down catfish	*Synodontis nigriventris*
Weather loach	*Misgurnus angullicaudatus*
Yellow stingray	*Urolophus jamaicensis*

Case 302: **Ovarian prolapse in a tancho kohaku koi**

CLINICAL PRESENTATION. A mature female tancho kohaku koi from a 75,000-liters, well-maintained pond was presented because the owner had noticed that the fish was not eating and appeared swollen. On physical examination the skin was erythematous, the coelomic region was very enlarged, and there was a red amorphous protrusion from the vent (**302a**). A normal koi 'vent', with the cranial anus and caudal genital pore, is shown for comparison (**302b**) (photo courtesy LS Christian).

DIFFERENTIAL DIAGNOSES. Intestinal prolapse protruding from the vent; intestinal prolapse protruding from the genital pore; ovarian prolapse protruding from the genital pore.

INVESTIGATION. Physical examination can yield clues as to whether the prolapse is ovarian or intestinal in origin. Ovarian tissue is usually grainy in appearance with small white to yellow follicles incorporated in the vascular ovarian tissue. Intestinal tissue will usually have a smooth surface. Cytology can further help differentiate between organs: ovarian tissue will have immature ova; intestinal tissue impressions will yield epithelial cells and possibly fecal material.

DIAGNOSIS. Ovarian prolapse through the genital pore.

MANAGEMENT. Excision of the exteriorized ovarian tissue is recommended. This tissue is vascular and friable. Encircling ligatures can be placed and the distal tissue removed with a scalpel or scissors (**302b**). Depending on the fish's spawning condition, eggs can be manually stripped from the fish. To prevent further ovarian prolapse, a sterile syringe of appropriate size can be inserted into the genital pore and the eggs expressed by cranial–caudal milking pressure along the flanks to push the eggs around the syringe (**302c**). A purse-string suture can be placed around the genital pore while carefully avoiding the vent and allowing enough room for residual eggs to pass from the pore.

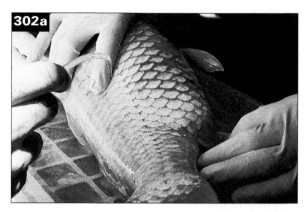

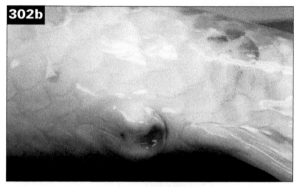

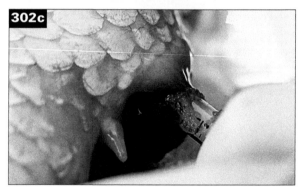

Case 303: **Spinal column lesion in a kohaku koi**

CLINICAL PRESENTATION. A five-year-old kohaku koi presented with anorexia and strange swimming behavior (**303a**).

INVESTIGATION. Radiography revealed a decreased intervertebral disc space and deviated vertebral body in the area of the spine just dorsal to the swim bladder (**303b**). A nuclear scan (**303c**) was made four hours after injection of technetium-labeled methylene diphosphonate (99mTc MDP) into the hemal arch to determine if this was an active or old lesion. Uptake of technetium may indicate

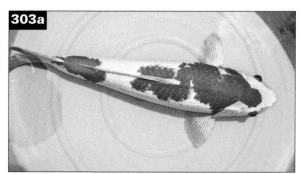

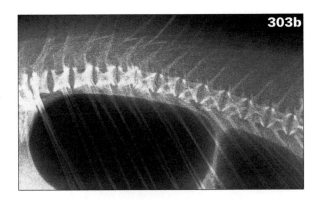

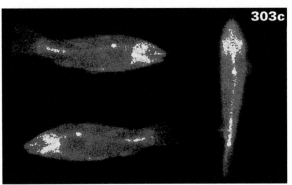

inflammation and increased osteoblast activity. Three areas of increased activity were identified:

- The ventral aspect of the caudal spine, probably caused by injection site extravasation.
- The opercular cavity. Because the gills are located in the opercular cavity, this area is highly vascular and technetium accumulates in pooled blood.
- The spinal column just dorsal to the swim bladder.

DIAGNOSIS. The radiograph indicates a lesion between trunk vertebrae 5 and 6. The nuclear bone scan confirmed the radiographic findings.

MANAGEMENT. The fish was treated initially with antibiotics and steroids and then conservatively with confinement, proper water quality, and proper nutrition. The fish recovered and regained 80% of its normal swimming ability.

Case 304: **Papilloma in a koi carp**

CLINICAL PRESENTATION. A koi carp presented with difficulty in eating. It was unable to eat, although it obviously wanted to. The food was taken into the buccal cavity but was soon ejected.

INVESTIGATION. Examination under anesthesia revealed a large, firm, round mass that was completely occluding the posterior buccal cavity (**304a**). There was a narrow stalk that was attached to the dorsal pharyngeal wall. The gross appearance was suggestive of a tumor.

DIAGNOSIS. Histopathology proved the mass to be a papilloma.

ETIOLOGY. Papillomas are common neoplasms and often do not require treatment. However, if these tumors affect vital areas such as the mouth or opercula, surgical removal is indicated. Many will periodically slough and leave a relatively normal but hyperplastic surface; however, the tumors may then spontaneously recur. Such events suggest that a virus may be involved, and other parts of the fish may also be affected.

MANAGEMENT. Because of the narrow area of attachment, it was felt that surgical removal was possible. This was achieved successfully with no postoperative complications.

PROGNOSIS. In this case the prognosis for full recovery was good. However, total excision is often not possible and regrowth of the tumor may occur.

DISCUSSION. Papillomas can also occur on the head. This koi carp (**304b**) presented with a large sessile mass on its head that had been present for three years.

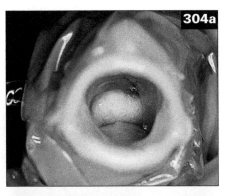

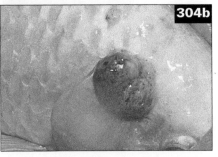

Case 305: **Carp pox in a koi**

CLINICAL PRESENTATION. A koi is presented with lesions, which resemble molten candlewax, on the dorsal fin (**305a**). Similar lesions may also be found on the body (**305b**).

DIAGNOSIS. Carp pox.

ETIOLOGY. Carp pox is caused by infection with *Herpesvirus cyprini*, also called cyprinid herpesvirus 1 (CHV1). The lesions are sometimes classified as neoplasia but are basically an epidermal hyperplasia.

MANAGEMENT. The disease is often seasonal and usually affects only a few fish in the pond. Lesions develop in low water temperatures (winter/spring) and regress when water temperatures increase. Treatment is seldom required because the disease is rarely fatal and is usually self-limiting. Lesions may recur the following year.

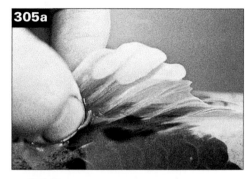

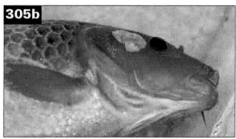

Case 306: **Skin ulcers in koi**

CLINICAL PRESENTATION. Skin ulceration in koi is a common problem (**306**).

ETIOLOGY. The cause of these ulcers is infection with *Pseudomonas* species and *Aeromonas* species bacteria, particularly *A. hydrophila* and atypical *A. salmonicida*.

MANAGEMENT. Treatment often depends on the severity of the lesions but frequently requires general anesthesia and local debridement. This should be followed by topical application of antiseptic/antibiotic and a protective waterproof paste. Improved water conditions with the addition of salt at 2–3 p.p.t. (2–3 g/l) and raising the water temperature often facilitates recovery. The use of systemic antibiotics by injection and/or inclusion into the feed is often recommended.

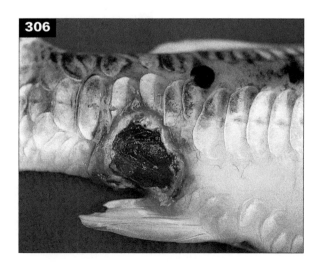

Case 307: **Chlorine/chloramine toxicity in a group of koi**

CLINICAL PRESENTATION. All nine of a group of prized koi are found one morning dead and floating in the pond (**307**). They were apparently normal the previous night and had good appetites for their evening feeding. The 2,500-liters pond is supplied with city water and has adequate biological and mechanical filtration as well as an aerating fountain. All the components were functioning normally, but the owner mentioned that the person who 'topped off' the pond last night with water had inadvertently left the hose running all night (the hose can be seen in the photograph).

DIFFERENTIAL DIAGNOSES. Chlorine/chloramine toxicity. Many toxic conditions will resemble chlorine poisoning (ammonia, copper, and organophosphates). An accurate history will usually rule these out. Hypoxia caused by overcrowding or poor aeration can also look like chlorine toxicity.

INVESTIGATION. The water was tested for chlorine levels. In this particular case, levels were recorded at 1.2 p.p.m. (several hours after the water sample was obtained). A bench-top chlorine titrimeter was used, although much simpler and less expensive colormetric tests are available.

DIAGNOSIS. Chlorine toxicity.

ETIOLOGY. Chlorine is highly toxic to fish. Concentrations of 0.2 p.p.m. can cause low-level mortality in a population, whereas concentrations of 0.4 p.p.m. can be 100% lethal. Chlorine reacts with living tissues and causes acute necrosis. Because the gills are vulnerable and exposed directly to the aquatic environment, this can lead to respiratory difficulty and asphyxiation. Fish experiencing chlorine toxicity will appear very stressed. Morbidity and mortality depends on chlorine levels in the water. High levels (greater than 1.0 p.p.m.) may cause fish to succumb in hours or even minutes. Affected fish may be piping at the surface and swimming abnormally, and they may appear pale and mucus covered. Most municipal water has been chlorinated to disinfect it for safe human consumption. Although relatively harmless to humans, chlorine can be deadly to fish. The amount of chlorine in tap water may fluctuate but is usually between 0.5 p.p.m. and 2.0 p.p.m. Chlorine can be 'bubbled' out of water by aerating for several days in a container with a large surface area. Another commonly used disinfectant is chloramine. This compound combines chlorine with ammonia, both of which are harmful to ornamental fish. Unlike chlorine, chloramine does not produce trihalomethanes, which are toxic to humans. Aerating water containing chloramaine may not be sufficient to remove the harmful chlorine component.

MANAGEMENT/PREVENTION. In cases where the fish are still alive, the contaminated water must be immediately neutralized or the fish removed to clean, chlorine-free water. A number of commercially available compounds quickly and safely remove chlorine from water. These products usually contain sodium thiosulfate, which inactivates chlorine through a chemical reaction in which sodium chloride is formed. Sodium thiosulfate is inexpensive, effective, and safe (just 7 g of sodium thiosulfate will remove the chlorine from 1,000 liters of municipal water with chlorine concentrations as high as 2.0 p.p.m.). Aeration must be maintained when sodium thiosulfate is introduced.

After the chlorine has been removed, the water containing the fish should be aerated well with room air or, preferably, 100% oxygen. Temperate species such as goldfish and koi will benefit from reducing the water temperature to increase dissolved oxygen levels. When possible or practical, administering dexamethasone intravenously or intracoelomically (2.0 mg/kg q12h) may improve the prognosis in debilitated fish.

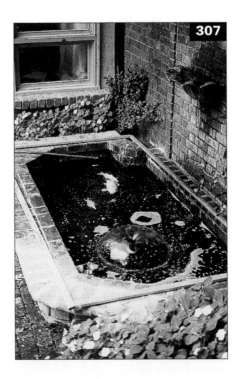

Case 308: **Koi herpesvirus**

CLINICAL PRESENTATION. Koi herpesvirus (KHV) is a recently described disease of koi that is frequently fatal. It is now an OIE reportable disease. The virus causes a severe branchitis and affected fish literally die of hypoxia (**308**) (photo courtesy B Szignarowitz). Since 1997, outbreaks of this disease have been reported in many European countries, Israel, Asia (including Japan), South Africa, and the US. Gross clinical signs include enophthalmia, mottled gills, excessive mucus production, and dermatitis. Mortality frequently exceeds 80% and is restricted to koi.

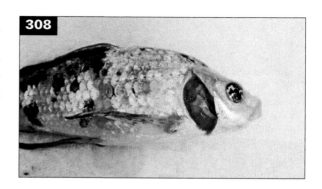

DIAGNOSIS. Diagnosis is made by virus isolation and confirmed by PCR of the viral isolates. Even without isolation of the virus, PCR can be used to detect the DNA of virus in fresh, infected tissues.

ETIOLOGY. The causative agent is a herpesvirus.

MANAGEMENT. There is a report with encouraging results that a live attenuated vaccine for this disease in koi may be practical (Ronen *et al.*, 2003). There is also anecdotal evidence that koi 'heated' to at least 30°C (86°F) may be resistant to an outbreak, since the virus appears restricted to environmental temperatures of 18–26°C (64.4–86°F). While this heat 'therapy' may save the fish, it could produce subclinical carriers of the disease. Since the KHV genome has been determined, other vaccination options are being explored (Waltzek *et al.*, 2005).

PREVENTION. One of the best ways to prevent the transmission of these two viral diseases is through adequate quarantine and biosecurity protocols. All new koi should be quarantined for a minimum of 30 days before introduction to an established population. Biosecurity, in the form of good hygiene and proper disinfection procedures, will greatly reduce the spread of these and other infectious diseases of koi.

Case 309: **Spinal defect in a koi**

CLINICAL PRESENTATION. A butterfly koi presented for slight asymmetry visible in the trunk area at the level of the cranial aspect of the dorsal fin (**309a**). The fish was behaving normally, but the owner wanted to know the source of the asymmetry.

DIFFERENTIAL DIAGNOSES. Scoliosis, neoplasia, ascites, and abscess or infection.

INVESTIGATION. Lateral and dorsoventral radiographs were taken.

DIAGNOSIS. This koi had a spinal defect, which was evident in the dorsoventral image (**309b**) but difficult to see in the lateral view (**309c**).

ETIOLOGY. This condition appears to be common in koi and may be nutritional (e.g. vitamin C deficiency), genetic, traumatic, or electrical in origin. Electrical surges, caused by lightning or a defective piece of equipment, have been implicated in causing vertebral luxation leading to scoliosis. Affected fish may remain stable or the condition may progress.

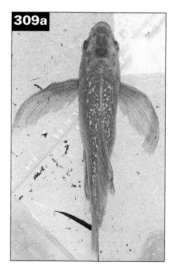

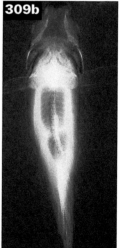

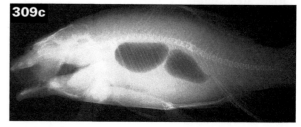

Case 310: **Blood parasites in a carp**

CLINICAL PRESENTATION. A carp presented because of a suspected blood parasite infection.

DIFFERENTIAL DIAGNOSES. *Sanguinicola inermis*, a digenean trematode; *Trypanosoma carassi*, a trypanosome; and *Trypanoplasma borreli*, a similar flagellate parasite.

INVESTIGATION. A blood sample should be obtained from the caudal vein (**310**).

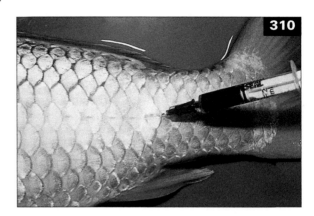

Case 311: **Pond medication for some outdoor koi**

CLINICAL PRESENTATION. Some outdoor koi have been diagnosed with a problem and the treatment involves medication of the pond.

MANAGEMENT. The volume of the pond must be calculated, ideally without draining and refilling it. The first method is to calculate the volume of the pond using the equation: volume = surface area x average depth. In order to calculate surface area, multiply the length by the width. For circular ponds, the equation for surface area is $3.14 \times \text{radius}^2$. For example, a rectangular pond 6 meters long × 4 meters wide would have a surface area of 24 square meters. A circular pond with a diameter (twice the radius) of 4 meters would have a surface area of

approximately 12.5 square meters. Calculating average depth can be difficult in a pond with a very uneven bottom. To keep things simple, assume that the average depth of both ponds is 1 meter. Applying the above formula, the rectangular pond has a volume of 24 cubic meters and the circular pond a volume of 12.5 cubic meters. Since each cubic meter equals 1,000 liters, the rectangular pond contains 24,000 liters and the circular pond 12,500 liters.

This equation can also be applied to aquaria. Length is multiplied by depth and width to arrive at the volume. For example, an aquarium with inside measurements of 0.6 × 0.3 × 0.25 meters would have a volume of 0.045 cubic meters. The aquarium contains 45 liters.

Case 312: *Dermocystidium koi* infection

CLINICAL PRESENTATION. A koi presented with an 8 mm skin lump.

INVESTIGATION. The lump was removed and histologic examination revealed many cystic structures full of spherical objects in the dermis (Periodic Acid-Schiff stain, ×400) (**312**). These large cystic structures are cross-section views through the fungal hyphae, which are packed with spores. The latter contain a large central vacuole or refractile body, with the cytoplasm and nucleus restricted to the narrow periphery. This gives the spores a characteristic 'signet-ring' appearance.

DIAGNOSIS. Infection with *Dermocystidium koi*.

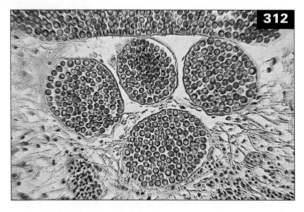

Case 313: **Branchiomycosis (gill rot) in a koi carp**

CLINICAL PRESENTATION. A koi carp recently imported into the UK from Japan presented with a discrete, oval, raised, plaque-like lesion on the gill (**313a**).

INVESTIGATION. Fresh scrapings taken from the lesion should be examined and these would be expected to yield branched aseptate hyphae. In this case, histopathology revealed large areas of necrosis containing fungal spores and hyphae (Gomori Methenamine Silver preparation) (**313b, c**).

DIAGNOSIS. These changes are consistent with a diagnosis of branchiomycosis (gill rot).

ETIOLOGY. Branchiomycosis is a disease of freshwater fish caused by the fungus *Branchiomyces*. It has been described in Europe, Japan, India, and parts of the US.

Spores attach to the gill surface and germinate to form hyphae. These hyphae proliferate, causing damage to the blood supply and necrosis. Sloughing of this necrotic tissue releases spores into the water, which then continue to develop on the floor of the pond or aquarium if conditions are favorable (i.e. temperatures of 25–32°C [77.0–89.6°F], high levels of organic material, low oxygen levels, and a low pH).

Fungal spores can be introduced directly by adding infected or carrier fish, or indirectly by birds or the use of raw fish products.

MANAGEMENT. Treatment is generally unrewarding, although 2-phenoxyethanol has been suggested. Control is achieved by good hygiene, avoiding the use of raw fish products, and adequate quarantine of all new fish to avoid introduction of the organism.

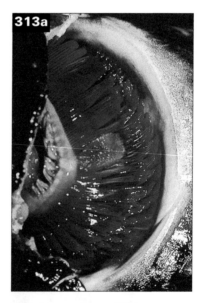

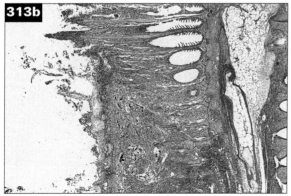

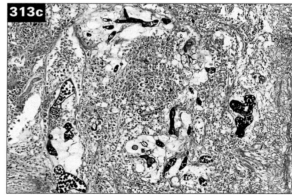

Case 314: **Fish louse (*Argulus* species) infestation in a koi**

CLINICAL PRESENTATION. A koi, one of 30 that were scratching and flashing in their 9,500-liters outdoor pond, was caught and presented for closer inspection. None of the fish had died as yet. The owner thought he could see small dark 'discs' moving across the skin of some of the fish. Six new fish purchased from a wholesaler had been added to the pond five weeks previously.

DIFFERENTIAL DIAGNOSES. An ectoparasitic infestation.

INVESTIGATION. A full diagnostic work up consisting of a thorough history, a complete water quality test, and skin, fin, and gill biopsies was carried out.

DIAGNOSIS. Infection with the crustacean parasite *Argulus* species. This parasite is commonly referred to as the 'fish louse'. A parasite can be seen on the dorsal surface of the head of the fish (**314**).

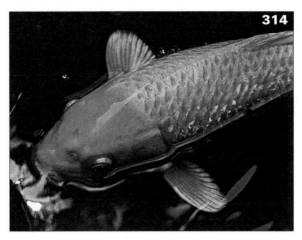

ETIOLOGY. Fish can become infested with crustaceans of the genus *Argulus* and other genera. Although a light infection is rarely fatal, the parasites irritate the skin, making the fish stressed and uncomfortable. The *Argulus* species 'louse' feeds by piercing the skin with its sharp stylet (visible along the ventral midline of the animal) and then sucking up body fluids with its mouth parts. A heavy fish louse infestation may allow opportunistic pathogens to infect the host, and fish lice are known to transmit bacterial and viral diseases.

Like most crustaceans, *Argulus* lays eggs and these hatch into a microscopic free-swimming larval form, which eventually finds a fish and completes its life cycle as a skin parasite. The eggs are usually deposited on plants, rocks, or other firm submerged surfaces. Fish infected with the early life stages will look normal and the parasites will not be visible to the naked eye until they mature.

MANAGEMENT. Once a pond is infected, the only way to eliminate the parasites, aside from draining the pond and removing the fish, is to treat the water with an organophosphate or a chitin synthesis inhibitor.

PREVENTION. The best way to prevent this condition is to quarantine all new fish for at least six weeks and monitor them closely for signs of ectoparasitic disease. If quarantine is not possible, new fish may be dipped in salt water (35 g/l) for 3–5 minutes in an effort to kill larval stages. This dip will not usually kill the adult parasites but it may force them off the fish.

Case 315: **'Pine cone' syndrome in a koi**

CLINICAL PRESENTATION. A koi presented with a condition affecting the skin (**315**).

DIAGNOSIS. Cutaneous edema and 'dropsy' (abdominal ascites) produces this characteristic 'pine cone' appearance.

ETIOLOGY. Dropsy is a clinical syndrome that can result from infection or neoplasia. The subsequent tissue damage in the skin, gills, heart, liver, or kidneys produces a failure of osmoregulation and development of edema and/or ascites. Retrobulbar accumulation of tissue fluid may or may not produce exophthalmia, which may be unilateral or bilateral. In this case the fish had a large hepatic tumor.

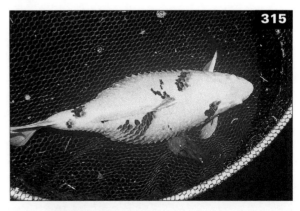

Case 316: **Swim bladder inflammation virus in a koi carp**

CLINICAL PRESENTATION. A koi carp is presented for postmortem examination.

INVESTIGATION. The left abdominal wall was removed (**316**). The surface of the bowel had a number of small petechial hemorrhages. Large hemorrhages were present on the posterior portion of the swim bladder. Sampling for bacteriology and histopathology would be necessary to make a specific diagnosis.

DIAGNOSIS. The postmortem findings are consistent with a generalized septicemia, viremia, or toxemia.

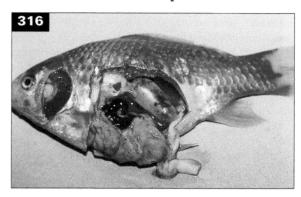

ETIOLOGY. One viral agent, swim bladder inflammation (SBI) virus, a rhabdovirus, specifically affects the swim bladder, causing degenerative changes with congestion, hemorrhage, and sloughing of the necrotic epithelium into the lumen. This particular virus usually affects cyprinids and is sometimes described as a component of the carp dropsy syndrome. It is very similar to spring viremia of carp (SVC) virus, although SVC virus is thought to be a distinct entity.

Case 317: **Wound management in a kohaku koi**

CLINICAL PRESENTATION. A kohaku koi presented for a laceration just caudal to the head. The owner suspected a bird strike (**317a**).

MANAGEMENT. Because the wound is obviously contaminated with dirt and debris, the tissues should be flushed with saline, clean water, or a dilute antiseptic. In this case the fish was anesthetized with MS-222 and the wound cleaned with dilute chlorhexidine solution. The skin flap was sutured with 4-0 absorbable suture material in a simple interrupted pattern (**317b**). The wound healed uneventfully with very little scarring.

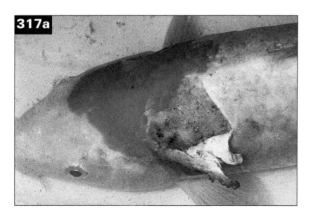

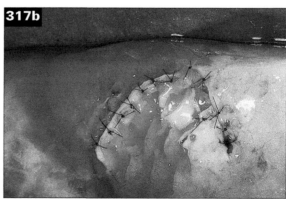

Case 318: **Pre-, peri-, and postoperative monitoring of a koi**

CLINICAL PROBLEM. A koi presented with an abdominal mass. An anesthetic protocol was determined and a midventral incision with the fish in dorsal recumbency was planned (**318a**).

MANAGEMENT.

- Anesthesia. The fish was monitored while under the anesthetic MS-222. Opercular movement is a good indicator of life, but in cases where the fish needs to be very deep, opercular movements may cease. Electrocardiography is an option, with leads placed at the base of each pectoral fin and one near the vent. The alligator clips can be attached to small needles placed in the skin.
- Surgery. The incision line was covered with a clear sterile surgical drape and the scales removed along the planned incision line (**318b**). The skin was treated carefully with a presurgical antiseptic, although this may not always be necessary. The mass turned out to be an ovarian granulosa-theca cell tumor and it was removed uneventfully (**318c**). The skin was closed with nonabsorbable nylon sutures and air was aspirated from the abdominal compartment following surgical closure (**318d**). An extra plastic tube was used to provide fresh water to the gills (two tubes providing water flow are in the mouth of the fish).
- Postoperatively. Enrofloxacin was administered (10 mg/kg i/m q48h for 10 days). The fish recovered and survived for over seven years before the condition recurred. During this time period the fish gained over four kilograms and was reported to be normal and active by the owner. Unfortunately, this fish died three days after extensive surgery to remove the tumor.

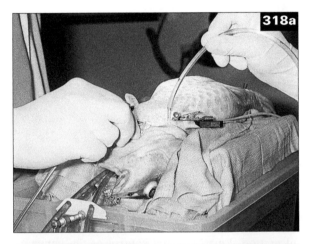

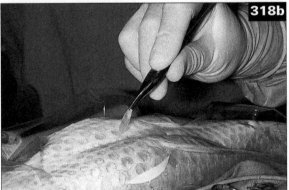

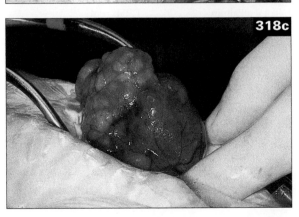

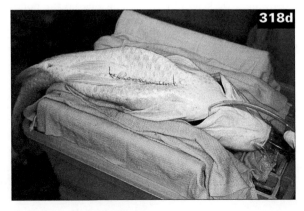

Case 319: Anchorworm (*Lernaea cyprinacea*) infestation in a koi and a goldfish

CLINICAL PRESENTATION. A koi presented with lesions on the skin (**319a**). The gross appearance of the skin revealed a number of discrete lesions showing an inflamed, hyperemic, raised rim with a central necrotic core. A similar condition was seen in a black Moor goldfish, which had several Y-shaped parasites attached to its skin (**319b**).

DIFFERENTIAL DIAGNOSES. An ulcerated tumor or granuloma, hypersensitivity reaction, or localized bacterial infection.

INVESTIGATION. Routine skin scrapings failed to reveal the presence of any parasites, and bacterial cultures failed to isolate any significant organisms. Clinically, the gross appearance was different from the typical bacterial ulcer in which the lesion appears as a crater with no raised rim. Under benzocaine anesthesia, a biopsy was taken and submitted for histopathology. The examination failed to indicate the presence of malignant cells, but showed cells typical of a hypersensitivity reaction.

DIAGNOSIS. The most probable cause of the lesions was a severe reaction to the anchor sites of the anchor worm *Lernaea cyprinacea*, a crustacean ectoparasite.

MANAGEMENT. Control of this parasite requires manual removal of these egg-laying adult stages, preferably under sedation or general anesthesia. The anchoring points on the fish's skin should be treated topically to avoid secondary bacterial or fungal infection and

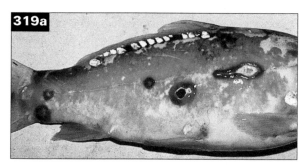

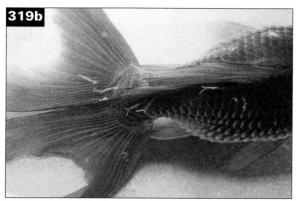

ulceration. Environmental control of the immature parasites will require the use of an organophosphate or a chitin synthesis inhibitor. The use of these products may be restricted in some areas.

Case 320: *Ichthyophthirius multifiliis* infestation in a koi pond

CLINICAL PROBLEM. A koi pond had been set up for approximately two years and no new fish had been introduced since it was initially stocked. Recently, the owner had been improving the aquascape by adding beautiful, flowering water lilies. On a Monday morning, following a weekend of planting new lilies in the pond, the fish were observed to be huddling near the bottom of the pond, refusing all food offered, and having an increased respiratory rate.

INVESTIGATION. Water quality was evaluated – the results are shown (right).
  Gill and fin biopsy (**320**) of an affected fish revealed numerous large, motile, ciliated organisms, some with a visible horseshoe-shaped macronucleus.

DIAGNOSIS. The clinical signs are suggestive of ectoparasitic disease, although the potential for systemic illness should be recognized. The organism observed on

Dissolved oxygen	7 p.p.m.
Total ammonia nitrogen	1 p.p.m.
Temperature	28°C (82.4°F)
pH	7.2
Total alkalinity	120 p.p.m.
Nitrite	0 p.p.m.
Total hardness	120 p.p.m.

the gill biopsy is *Ichthyophthirius multifiliis*. At water temperatures of 28°C (82.4°F), this parasite is capable of rapid replication and could cause serious disease within 3–4 days of introduction.

ETIOLOGY. Plants, nets, and other objects can serve as fomites for the encysted stage of *I. multifiliis*. In this case a probable source for the apparent recent introduction of the parasite to the fish population is the newly purchased lilies.

MANAGEMENT. To solve the immediate problem, either plants or fish should be removed from the pond, as chemical treatment may damage delicate lilies. Parasite control can be achieved using a number of chemical products. Formalin would be the treatment of choice in this case, as long as adequate aeration was available. Formalin is readily available through pharmacies, hospitals, chemical supply companies, and some pet stores. A concentration of 25 p.p.m. can be applied to the pond every other day for at least three treatments (with water changes between treatments) or until the problem is resolved.

PREVENTION. Plants can be quarantined for *I. multifiliis* by placing them in an aquarium that is not stocked with fish and maintaining the water temperature at 28°C (82.4°F) for at least seven days (2–4 weeks would be

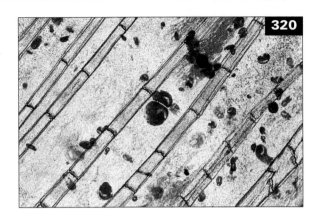

ideal). As individual cysts rupture, emerging tomites will not have access to a new host and therefore should not survive. Careful disinfection of inanimate objects such as nets (i.e. with 10–20 p.p.m. chlorine bleach for one hour followed by a thorough rinse) is important to avoid introduction of infectious agents during cleaning or movement of animals.

Case 321: **Abdominal sarcoma in a showa koi**

CLINICAL PRESENTATION. A very valuable showa koi presented with a swollen abdomen that the owner said has increased in size over the past several months.

INVESTIGATION. A standard clinical work up including fine-needle aspirate, radiographs, and ultrasonographic examination was performed.

DIAGNOSIS. A preliminary diagnosis of a large abdominal mass was made. Computed tomography (CT) was used to further characterize the size, shape, and location of the tumor. The fish was anesthetized with MS-222 at a concentration of 200 p.p.m. The fish was placed in the scanner in left lateral recumbency (**321a**) and a series of images obtained. This image clearly shows the large mass just ventral to the swim bladder, with most of the viscera displaced to the left (**321b**).

MANAGEMENT. Surgery was performed and a 215 gram sarcoma was successfully removed (**321c**). The fish was still doing well 18 months postoperatively, but succumbed with a number of other fish following an environmental problem (unrelated to the neoplasia).

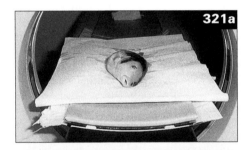

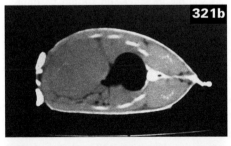

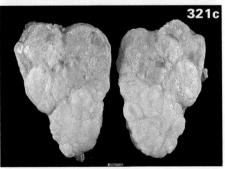

Case 322: **Algal dermatitis in a sanke koi**

CLINICAL PRESENTATION. A large sanke koi was presented with lesions on its trunk (**322a**). The fish had been lost when its pond flooded following a severe hurricane. It had found its way to a stream and then swam into a larger stream about a kilometer away, where it was located eight days later by a woman who noticed some teenagers throwing stones at the fish. The owner was contacted and the fish swam into a net. Several weeks later the owner noticed a number of green, raised lesions on various parts of the fish's body. The lesions ranged from 3–10 mm in diameter and were red at the margins.

INVESTIGATION. The water was tested and biopsies of the lesions were taken. The water quality parameters were unremarkable. Biopsies of the lesions revealed a mixed green and blue-green algal infection. Samples were saved for culture and histology.

DIAGNOSIS. Algal dermatitis.

ETIOLOGY. Algal dermatitis has been reported in fish but may not be common in koi.

MANAGEMENT. The fish was anesthetized with tricaine methanesulfonate (MS-222) (150 p.p.m.) and the wounds were carefully debrided and swabbed with povidone–iodine (**322b**). The fish was also placed on systemic antibiotics (enrofloxacin 10 mg/kg intra-coelomically q48h for 2 weeks) to reduce the possibility of septicemia. The fish recovered uneventfully.

DISCUSSION. A practical alternative to MS-222 is clove oil. Clove oil is available over the counter (OTC) at many pharmacies. Clove oil, also known as eugenol, is not completely soluble in water and should be diluted with ethanol at a rate of 1 part clove oil to 10 parts ethanol to yield a working stock solution of 100 mg/ml

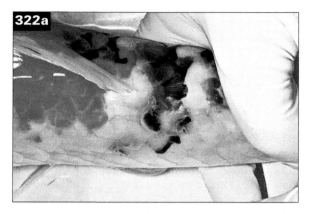

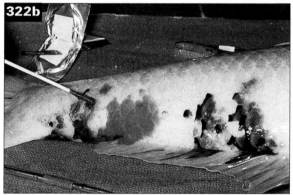

(each ml of clove oil contains approximately 1 g of drug [some OTC formulations may be less concentrated]). Concentrations of between 25 and 75 mg/l are effective in freshwater and marine species and results are comparable to MS-222. Although eugenol is a food additive in some situations, it is not approved for use in fish intended for human consumption in the US.

Case 323: **Lenticular cataract in a goldfish**

CLINICAL PRESENTATION. A mature goldfish presented with a problem in its right eye (**323**) (photo courtesy S Wada).

DIAGNOSIS. Lenticular cataract.

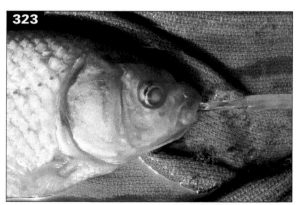

Case 324: **Suspected spring viremia of carp virus infection in a goldfish**

CLINICAL PRESENTATION. A goldfish presented with widespread hyperemia of the body surface and injection of the blood vessels of the fins (**324**). The abdomen was slightly swollen. These signs were nonspecific and were associated with generalized septicemia, toxemia, or viremia. Other signs might also have been evident such as exophthalmos and more obvious abdominal swelling with raised scales.

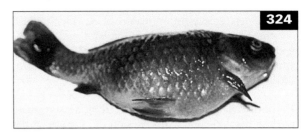

DIFFERENTIAL DIAGNOSES. The differential diagnoses include a wide range of bacterial, viral, and toxic agents. A careful history and examination of the environment might yield some important clues, but the definitive diagnosis is likely to be made at necropsy.

INVESTIGATION. At necropsy there was generalized erythema and hemorrhages of the visceral surfaces. Serosanguinous fluid was found in the abdomen. Peracute septicemias and viremias may occur in which there is mortality without prior clinical signs.

Bacterial sampling was taken from the posterior kidney, which is the optimum site. Smears were stained with Gram and Ziehl–Neelsen stains and the appropriate media chosen for culture. A selection of samples of the major organs (heart, liver, spleen, bowel, kidney, gill, and skin/muscle) was taken for histopathology.

DIAGNOSIS. Spring viremia of carp virus infection.

DISCUSSION. Special precautions should be taken if the history is consistent with the possibility of SVC virus infection, especially in the case of koi. The causative agent is *Rhabdovirus carpio*. In the UK this disease is 'notifiable' and requires specific samples to be sent to an approved Department for Environment, Food and Rural Affairs (DEFRA) laboratory for confirmation of the diagnosis. If a positive diagnosis is made, DEFRA has the power to impose restriction orders on the premises. This disease is also reportable in the US and was confirmed for the first time in North America in 2002. Details on this disease can be found on the World Organisation for Animal Health (OIE) web site.

Case 325: **Swim bladder torsion in a goldfish**

CLINICAL PRESENTATION. A goldfish presented that had been found swimming upside down at the surface of its pond.

INVESTIGATION. A radiographic image was taken (**325a**). The caudal sac of the swim bladder is ventral to the anterior sac. A radiograph of a normal goldfish swim bladder is shown (**325b**).

DIAGNOSIS. A swim bladder torsion was diagnosed at necropsy.

ETIOLOGY. Buoyancy disorders are very common in goldfish, especially those Asian varieties that have short, stout bodies. Some workers believe that because of these selected abnormal body conformations, the swim bladder tends to be unbalanced in these fish.

MANAGEMENT. Torsion of the swim bladder is not a common finding and supportive care in the form of clean water and good food is in order. Surgical correction is an option, but such a procedure is both risky and expensive. Aspiration of air from the caudal compartment might temporarily correct the problem.

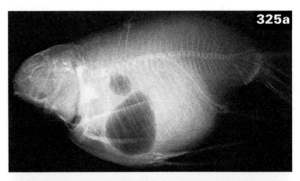

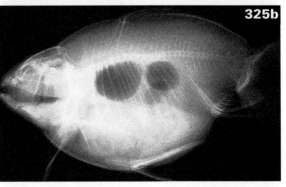

Case 326: **Nuptial tubercles in a Moor goldfish**

CLINICAL PRESENTATION. A mature black Moor goldfish presented because of pronounced, raised, 1 mm diameter nodules on the pectoral fins and opercula (**326**). The fish appeared otherwise healthy and the owner had not experienced any losses in his aquarium.

ETIOLOGY. During the spring breeding season, male goldfish develop nuptial tubercles on the surfaces of the opercula and pectoral fins. Grossly, these nodules can resemble the encysted stage of *Ichthyophthirius multifiliis.* This condition is normal.

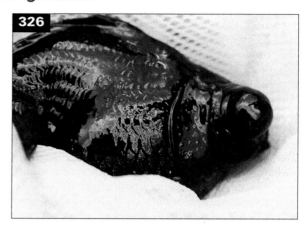

Case 327: **Fibrosarcoma in a goldfish**

CLINICAL PRESENTATION. A goldfish presented with a history of a slowly developing polypoid soft-tissue mass on the dorsum that sometimes is abraded and bleeds (**327a**).

DIFFERENTIAL DIAGNOSES. Neoplastic mass, granuloma, benign hyperplasia.

INVESTIGATION. Biopsy and histopathologic evalualtion.

DIAGNOSIS. Based on the history and gross appearance, the most likely diagnosis is a neoplastic mass. In this case the tumor is a fibrosarcoma (**327b**).

ETIOLOGY. In some fish, neoplasia has a viral etiology and may occur seasonally (i.e. appear and then regress spontaneously). There are several reports of sarcomas in goldfish but no etiology has been confirmed.

MANAGEMENT. If the mass does not impede the fish's movement it can be left, or it can be resected (after confirming the diagnosis by biopsy). Wide excision may be necessary to prevent recurrence. Laser surgery, combined with surgical debulking, may be a viable alternative as a treatment regimen for dermal tumors in goldfish. In addition to general anesthesia with MS–222, a local anesthetic such as 2% lidocaine is recommended. Postoperative care could include a topical antimicrobial agent and an injectable analgesic agent such as butorphanol or ketoprofen.

The result of using laser surgery to treat a goldfish with a dermal sarcoma located just caudal to the left dorsal operculum, which was initially debulked surgically with a scalpel blade, is shown (**327c**). Laser surgery was employed in an effort to destroy the remaining neoplastic cells. Note the mildly charred tissue associated with the lesion (**327d**). Silver sulfadiazine cream was applied topically (**327e**). The tumor did not recur, but within a year the fish had lost all grossly visible skin pigmentation (**327f**). The stress/physical impact of anesthesia and surgery may have precipitated this pigment change, and this potential side-effect should be discussed with owners/aquarists.

DISCUSSION. In some cases an alternative to surgical removal of the mass and histopathologic evaluation is preferable. Radiography was performed in an oranda goldfish that presented with a large mass just dorsal to the lateral line and ventral to the dorsal fin (**327g**). A lateral radiograph showed the mass to be well isolated above the vertebral column, with no apparent metastasis to deeper tissues (**327h**). Other features to note in this radiograph are the otoliths (ear stones), the pharyngeal teeth, the bilobed swim bladder, and the caudal kidney that can be seen just dorsal to the center of the swim bladder and ventral to the spine.

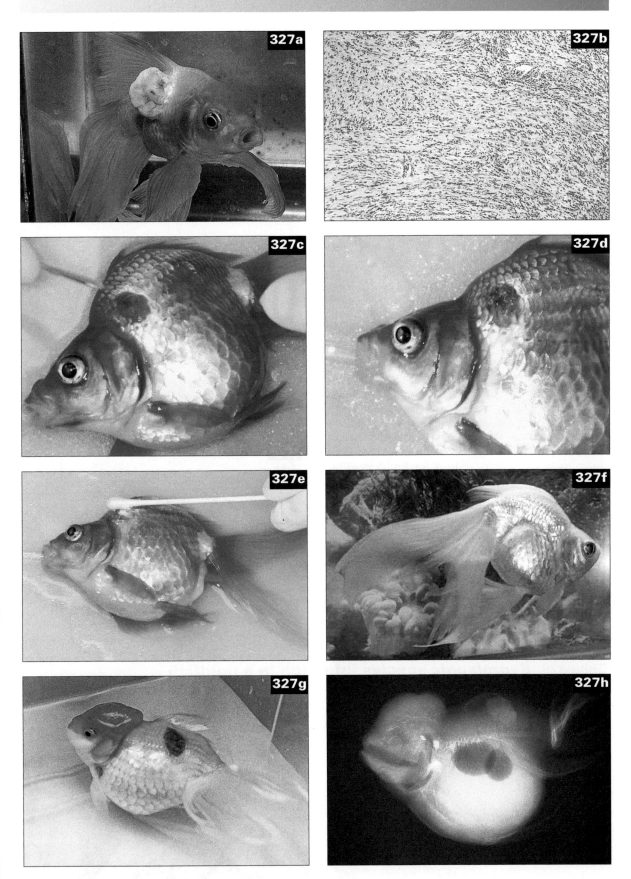

Case 328: **Zinc toxicity in a group of goldfish**

CLINICAL PRESENTATION. A fish that had just died was brought in for necropsy. The fish was from a group of goldfish that had been purchased but, because construction of their pond had not been completed, they were housed in galvanized steel tanks as a temporary measure. After three days the fish began to die.

INVESTIGATION. Water quality parameters were evaluated with the following results:
- Dissolved oxygen: 7.0 p.p.m.
- Total ammonia nitrogen: 3.0 p.p.m.
- Temperature: 26°C (78.8°F).
- Nitrite: 0.5 p.p.m.
- Total alkalinity: 51 p.p.m.
- pH: 8.2.
- Total hardness: 68 p.p.m.
- Chloride: 155 p.p.m.

Gill and skin biopsies were negative. A bacterial culture taken from the posterior kidney showed no growth after 48 hours at 25°C (77°F).

A toxin was suspected and efforts were made to confirm the presence of the suspect contaminant in the environment and in tissue of affected fish. State veterinary diagnostic laboratories are usually able to perform these assays at a reasonable cost. In the situation described, a water sample from the tank should be frozen in an inert plastic bottle. A few freshly dead fish should be frozen in a plastic bag. These samples should then be submitted to the appropriate laboratory for analysis.

DIAGNOSIS. Zinc toxicity, which is commonly associated with fish mortality after housing in a galvanized steel tank.

ETIOLOGY. The toxicity of zinc to fish varies dramatically between different species of fish and water quality parameters. A number of studies have reported 96-h LC50 data in the range of 0.87–40.90 p.p.m. Zn^{2+} in water. In general, zinc toxicity increases as water temperature and pH increase, and total hardness decreases.

DISCUSSION. While zinc toxicity is likely to come from the metal being dissolved in the water, ingested coins may also lead to systemic zinc toxicity. A dead, anemic brook trout is shown that had ingested a penny introduced into its exhibit (**328a, b**).

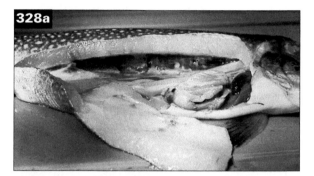

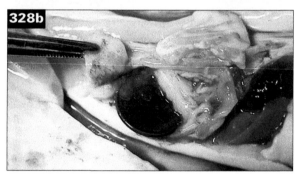

Case 329: *Saprolegnia* **species infection in a goldfish**

CLINICAL PRESENTATION. A goldfish presented with a skin infection.

INVESTIGATION/DIAGNOSIS. A skin scraping was taken, which demonstrated long branched aseptate hyphae characteristic of *Saprolegnia* species (**329**) (×80 magnification).

ETIOLOGY. This water mold (fungus) is widespread in fresh and brackish water but does not occur in the marine environment.

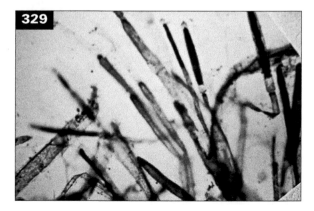

MANAGEMENT. The recommended treatments include salt or formalin dips or more prolonged water treatments using mixtures of formalin and malachite green. Focal lesions can be debrided and the underlying tissue treated with a topical antimicrobial agent such as povidone–iodine or triple antibiotic ointment.

DISCUSSION. Infection is generally regarded as secondary to other underlying factors such as poor management or chronic parasitic infestation. A complete investigation of the problem is therefore essential before initiating treatment. The chemicals used for treatment are potentially toxic, so their use in the presence of substandard water quality conditions might at best be unsuccessful and at worse cause death of the fish.

Case 330: **Red gill in a goldfish**

CLINICAL PRESENTATION. A recently purchased fancy goldfish presented because of what the owner described as a very red right gill (**330a**). The condition had not been noticed at the time the fish was purchased.

INVESTIGATION. The left operculum was examined and found to be normal (**330b**). Part of the right operculum was missing but the underlying gill tissue appeared grossly unremarkable.

DISCUSSION. This condition is likely to be either congenital or caused by trauma, perhaps at an early age. Cultured ornamental fish with congenital/developmental deformities are normally 'culled' at the fish farm or wholesaler.

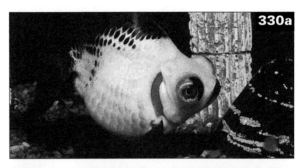

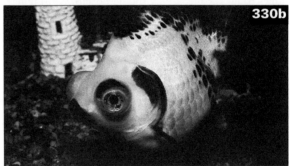

Case 331: **Anorexia in a comet goldfish due to poor water quality**

CLINICAL PRESENTATION. An 11-year-old comet goldfish presented with anorexia of one-week duration and areas of petechiation at the base of the dorsal fin and along the back. The fish lived alone in a 75-liters aquarium with undergravel filtration (**331**). The owner rarely changed the water (only replaced water lost due to evaporation). The fish had lived alone for five years and was fed flake food and some pellets.

INVESTIGATION. Water quality evaluation showed the pH to be 4.0 and the total ammonia nitrogen to be 2.0 p.p.m.

DIAGNOSIS. Although the ammonia is not toxic at this pH, the extremely low pH of the water is certainly a stress to the fish. Gradual water changes are in order.

MANAGEMENT. Ten to twenty percent of the water should be changed every day for 10–14 days until the pH returns to between 7.0 and 7.5. In this case the fish improved dramatically after several days and the owner was instructed to continue regular water changes at a rate of 30% per month.

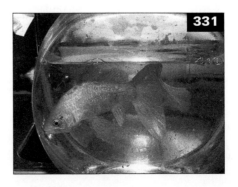

Case 332: **Corneal ulcer or abrasion in a synodontid catfish**

CLINICAL PRESENTATION. A synodontid (upside down) catfish presented because the fish's left eye appeared cloudy. On examination it was noted that the affected eye was cloudy and possibly ulcerated. The fish was in a quarantine tank with several other fish, some driftwood, and a sponge filter. The right eye appeared normal.

DIFFERENTIAL DIAGNOSES. Corneal ulcer or abrasion.

INVESTIGATION. Fluorescein staining of the eye was performed.

DIAGNOSIS. The eye retained the stain after flushing, which confirmed the presence of a significant corneal defect (**332**).

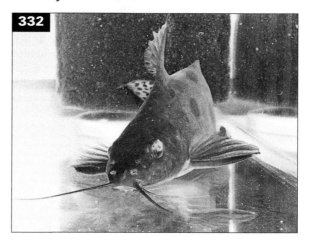

MANAGEMENT. There are generally two ways to manage this condition. If the fish is easy to catch and owner compliance is adequate, topical antibacterial ophthalmic ointment or drops can be applied directly to the eye 2–4 times daily. The medication should be allowed to remain on the eye for at least 30 seconds before returning the fish to the aquarium.

If this course is not practical, a broad-spectrum antibiotic can be added to the water in a hospital aquarium and the fish treated for 5–7 days or until the cornea heals. This fish responded well to daily, five-hour bath treatments of 20 p.p.m. nitrofurazone.

Case 333: **Nitrite toxicity in a redtail catfish**

CLINICAL PRESENTATION. A four-year-old redtail catfish presented after it was found lying on its back with a swollen abdomen (**333a**). The fish had been kept in a 530-liters tank and had begun to develop mild fin necrosis about six weeks ago. It had been treated with antibiotics by the owner, first with a two-week course of tetracycline added to the water at 400 p.p.m. and then a kanamycin water treatment for the entire tank at 100 p.p.m. The fish was found on its back a day after the kanamycin treatment.

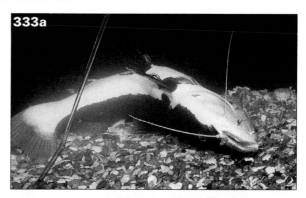

INVESTIGATION. Water analysis of the tank was carried out. Total ammonia was found to be 1.0 p.p.m. and nitrite exceeded the limits of the test kit, which was 4.0 p.p.m.

DIAGNOSIS. Nitrite toxicity, probably secondary to destruction of the biological filter by the administration of antibiotics directly into the tank water.

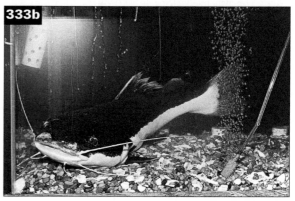

MANAGEMENT. Daily 50% water changes were instituted immediately. Sodium chloride was added to the water to achieve 100 p.p.m. in order to reduce the uptake of nitrite. A 23 gauge butterfly catheter was used to remove 160 cm^3 of air from the swim bladder and the fish was able to right itself (**333b**). It is not known what caused this swim bladder condition.

Case 334: **Copper toxicity in two pictus catfish**

CLINICAL PRESENTATION. Two pictus catfish presented because they had died within 12 hours of being received from a local wholesaler (**334a**). Numerous other species of freshwater tropical fish (tetras, cichlids, and other catfish species) had also died in the same circumstances. The fish had been truck-shipped and had spent six hours in their packing bags. They were allowed to acclimatize to tank temperature and pH before being carefully placed in the aquaria. Over one hundred 75-liters aquaria shared a common water supply, with adequate aeration and biological and mechanical filtration.

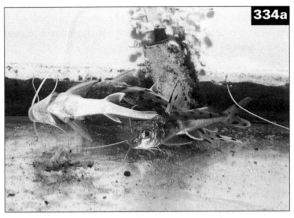

DIFFERENTIAL DIAGNOSES. A toxicity of some kind is almost surely the cause of this problem. It would be extremely unlikely that a pathogen could act this quickly against such a broad range of species. Potential toxins would include copper, other heavy metals, pesticides, and chemotherapeutics. Supersaturation (gas-bubble disease) could cause this, but the fish displayed no clinical signs of this disease.

INVESTIGATION. Standard water quality parameters were tested (ammonia, nitrite, nitrate, total alkalinity, pH, dissolved oxygen, and temperature) and all were within acceptable limits. The water was tested for copper, and the levels were found to be 0.8 p.p.m.

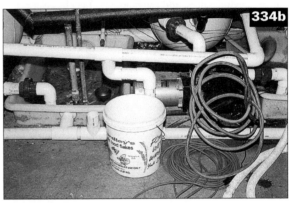

DIAGNOSIS. Copper toxicity. The history helps to rule out any water quality shock and in any case the standard water quality values were normal.

ETIOLOGY. The copper level in the water is very high and certainly toxic for freshwater fish, especially in soft, acidic water. Several weeks before, six meters of fresh copper tubing had been installed in the sump as a heating coil to warm the water (**334b**). The copper in the system had been leaching into the water from the tubing.

MANAGEMENT. The tubing was removed, water changes were initiated, and a copper chelating agent was added to the system.

Case 335: **Upside-down catfish**

CLINICAL PRESENTATION. A catfish spent most of its time swimming upside down at the water's surface (**335**). People seeing the fish commented that they thought it was sick.

DISCUSSION. This is an upside-down catfish belonging to the genus *Synodontis*. Many species belonging to this genus and related genera utilize this swimming pattern to obtain food floating at the surface. The condition is normal.

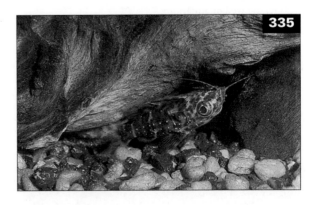

Case 336: **Leech (hirudinean) infestation in a stick catfish**

CLINICAL PRESENTATION. A recently imported stick catfish presented with a parasite visible near the oral cavity (**336a**).

INVESTIGATION/DIAGNOSIS. Low-power magnification of the parasite demonstrated the presence of an anterior and posterior sucker, characteristics unique to leeches (*Hirudo* species) (**336b**). Digenean trematodes, by contrast, have an anterior and ventral sucker, and are not segmented.

ETIOLOGY. Leeches are uncommon in aquarium fish because they are relatively large parasites that are easy to remove. Most are detected and removed by tropical fish farmers, wholesalers, and transhippers. Leeches can act as vectors for a variety of viral, bacterial, and parasitic diseases, as well as causing a mild to moderate anemia. Leeches are annelids (segmented worms) and, while most are parasitic, some are free living.

MANAGEMENT. If the fish can be caught, the leeches should be manually removed and disposed of. The organophosphate trichlorfon has proven to be effective in a pond or larger aquarium.

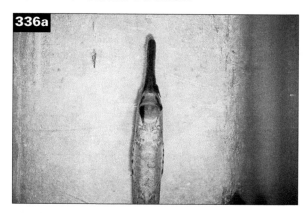

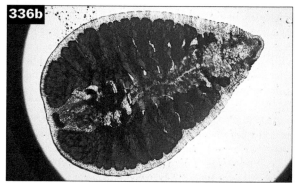

Case 337: **Yellow or white 'grub' disease (*Clinostomum* species infestation) in a corydoras catfish**

CLINICAL PRESENTATION. A sick corydoras catfish presented with distinct, pale white to yellow, subcutaneous nodules visible in all areas of the body (**337**). The fish was one of five that had been recently purchased from a pet store and placed in a 200-liters community aquarium. The fish were behaving normally and the rest of the fish in the tank were fine. The owner had not noticed the nodules in the pet store, but remembered seeing them shortly after introducing the fish to the well lit aquarium.

INVESTIGATION. A nodule was examined more closely and found to be an encysted metacercaria. Using a scalpel, forceps, and fine scissors, the metacercaria was teased from its cyst and examined under the microscope. The presence of an oral and ventral sucker confirmed its identity as a digenean trematode.

DIAGNOSIS. The nodules are encysted metacercaria of a digenetic trematode, most likely belonging to the genus *Clinostomum*.

ETIOLOGY. This condition is common in wild-caught or pond-raised corydoras catfish, Australian rainbowfish, and pond-reared live-bearers such as guppies, mollies, and platys. Aquarists and aquaculturists frequently call

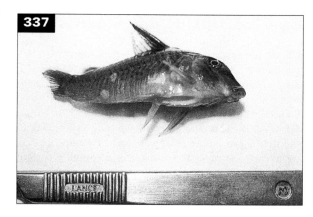

this condition yellow or white 'grub' disease. The fish is actually an intermediate host for this parasite. The definitive host is usually a fish-eating bird or other higher vertebrate, and a molluscan invertebrate, usually a snail, is the first intermediate host.

This condition is usually not harmful to fish and cannot be transmitted to other fish in the aquarium without the definitive and first intermediate hosts being present. In severe cases, where the metacercaria are very numerous or involve internal organs, clinical signs including general debilitation and weight loss can be observed.

MANAGEMENT. There is evidence that treatment using parasiticides that target trematodes (e.g. praziquantel, 5–10 p.p.m. for 24 hours as a bath immersion) will kill the metacercaria.

Case 338: **Lymphosarcoma in a cichlid**

CLINICAL PRESENTATION. A male *Pseudotropheus* species cichlid presented with an asymmetric swelling of the frontal dome, with a bleeding ulcer measuring 3 mm in diameter.

INVESTIGATION. A punch biopsy of the lesion was obtained. The fish is shown after the biopsy had been taken (**338a**). An impression smear (**338b**) and histology (**338c**) of the biopsy are also shown. Aerobic microbial culture of the swelling yielded no bacterial growth.

DIAGNOSIS. Lymphosarcoma.

ETIOLOGY. Lymphosarcomas in northern pike and muskellunge are suspected to be of retroviral origin; a similar cause in other species has not been determined.

MANAGEMENT. The cichlid died before therapy could be initiated. No metastases were detected.

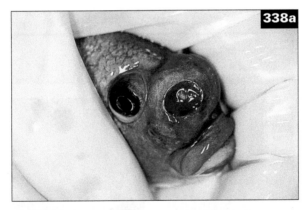

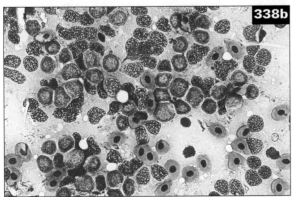

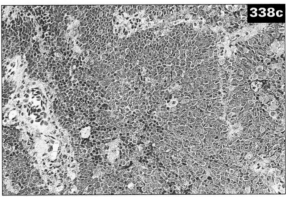

Case 339: **Normal swim bladder of a Midas cichlid**

INVESTIGATION. A lateral radiograph of a Midas cichlid is shown (**339**). The radioluscent area is a normal swim bladder. Careful inspection of the radiograph reveals a thin septum located in the caudal aspect of the swim bladder. This is normal for Midas cichlids and related species.

ETIOLOGY. Cichlids and many fish with spiny fin rays are physoclistous (i.e. they regulate gases in the swim bladder by a rete mirabile, which allows for vascular diffusion of gases). Most adult physoclistous fish do not have a patent pneumatic duct, a tube that connects the esophagus and the swim bladder.

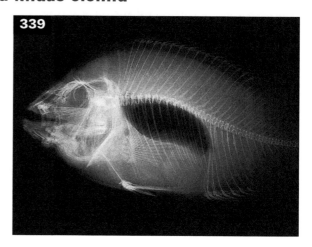

Case 340: **Contrast radiography in a Pearci cichlid**

CLINICAL PRESENTATION. A 2-kg Pearci cichlid presented with a three-week history of anorexia and failure to produce feces (**340a**). The fish broke a submersible aquarium heater one month ago.

DIFFERENTIAL DIAGNOSES. Gastrointestinal obstruction is high on the differential list.

INVESTIGATION. Contrast radiography was carried out. After tranquilizing the fish with 150 p.p.m. MS-222, a flexible rubber catheter was used to introduce 5 ml/kg (10 ml) of iohexol-300 into the stomach. Iohexol is a low osmolar, nonionic water soluble contrast media that is safe when administered i/v, intrathecally, or p/o. Serial radiographs are then made until the contrast media is excreted. Radiographs were made at time zero (**340b**) and 10 minutes (**340c**). After 10 minutes the iohexol had already filled the stomach and proximal intestine, and a small amount can be seen in the lower intestine.

DISCUSSION. This fish did not have an impaction, but it took nearly five days for the contrast to clear the GI tract. Times for contrast clearance vary widely between species. Iohexol was selected due to a demonstrated decrease in transit time in other species (bird, dog, and cat). Factors such as gut motility, length of GI tract, and metabolic rate can all affect contrast clearance.

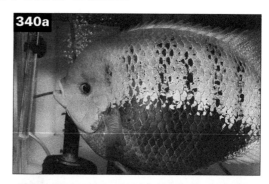

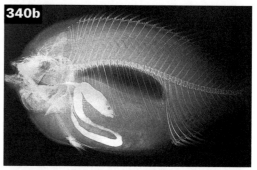

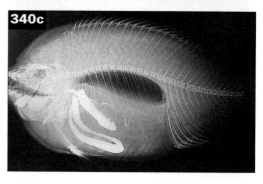

Case 341: **Head and lateral line erosion in a pearl cichlid**

CLINICAL PRESENTATION. A pearl cichlid presented for multiple erosions of the head, which were visible ventral to the eye and dorsal to the mouth (**341**).

INVESTIGATION. A thorough evaluation of the water quality parameters, as well as lesion scrapings and culture, was undertaken.

DIAGNOSIS. Freshwater 'hole in the head' disease or head and lateral line erosion (HLLE). The syndrome differs between freshwater and marine species.

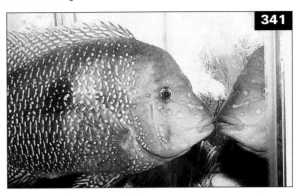

ETIOLOGY. HLLE has been linked to poor water quality, inadequate nutrition, protozoal ectoparasites (*Hexamita* species or *Spironucleus* species), and a variety of bacterial pathogens.

MANAGEMENT. Treatment should progress according to diagnostic findings. This fish had a history of improving slightly after metronidazole was administered to the water (6 p.p.m.) by the owners. The fish lived for several years with the lesions and was finally killed painlessly when it became debilitated and stopped eating at the age of nine years. Necropsy findings included systemic mycobacteriosis and mycobacterial involvement of the erosive lesions.

Case 342: **Swim bladder surgery in a cichlid**

CLINICAL PRESENTATION. A six-year-old cichlid presented because it required surgery to repair an apparent deformity of its swim bladder. The estimated time for the surgery was two hours. Tricaine methanesulfonate was the only anesthetic agent available and the surgeon had to consider how best to deliver the anesthetic to the fish during surgery.

MANAGEMENT. Because of the length of the procedure, continuous delivery of the anesthetic agent is required. This can be achieved in the following two ways:
• A large syringe may be used to force water manually through the mouth and over the gills of the fish. Using this method, water leaving the fish should trickle down into a pan to be readministered; otherwise, a sufficient volume of anesthetic-containing water should be available for the surgery and the collecting pan should be periodically drained.
• Alternatively, an automated system can be assembled in which a small pump delivers anesthetic-containing water, via tubes, through the fish's mouth and over its gills (**342**). The water then trickles into a catch pan and flows back to a reservoir to be readministered to the fish. Flow rates may be adjusted by use of in-line valves. Drug concentrations may be changed by the addition of water or anesthetic to the reservoir.

A complication of these methods is that water flows across the surgical field, along the ventral abdomen. To solve this problem without reducing the flow rate, the anesthetic-containing water can be delivered from the opercular cavity into the buccal cavity (reversing the direction of water flow). Although less efficient, it will provide the fish with adequate oxygen and help prevent water entering the surgical field.

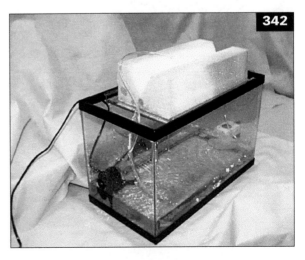

Case 343: *Trichodina* species infection in African cichlids

CLINICAL PROBLEM. An African cichlid breeder has experienced chronic, low-level mortality in certain groups of fish. The fish are housed in 950-liters vats on a flow-through system. Water exchange occurs every 60–90 minutes and stocking densities are moderate to heavy. Severe infestations with *Trichodina* species are frequently found on gills or skin of unthrifty and dying fish (**343a, b**). Repeated treatment with formalin at 25 p.p.m. has slowed mortality but has not eliminated the problem.

INVESTIGATION. Water quality parameters from a representative vat were evaluated with the following results:
- Dissolved oxygen: 6 p.p.m.
- Total ammonia: 2 p.p.m.
- Temperature: 30°C (86°F).
- pH: 8.2.
- Total alkalinity: 220 p.p.m.
- Toxic ammonia: 0.2 p.p.m.
- Total hardness: 280 p.p.m.
- Nitrite: 0.5 p.p.m.

A skin scrape was prepared by obtaining a small quantity of mucus from the skin surface of an anesthetized fish (**343c**). Rapidly spinning ciliated protozoal organisms were seen on a skin scrape examined under a microscope (**343d**) (×100). Gill, fin, and skin biopsies were also prepared (**343e**).

DIAGNOSIS. *Trichodina* species infection, a common cause of skin and gill disease in ornamental fish.

ETIOLOGY. *Trichodina* species is a motile, ciliated protozoan and a common gill and skin parasite on fish. This parasite thrives under conditions of crowding, heavy feeding, and high organic load. Warm temperatures may also exacerbate *Trichodina* problems.

MANAGEMENT. In general, any of the chemicals that are effective against external protozoans should be efficacious against *Trichodina*. The parasite's direct life cycle dictates that one treatment should be adequate.

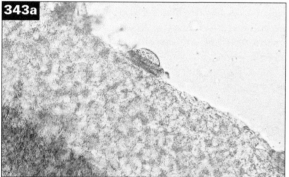

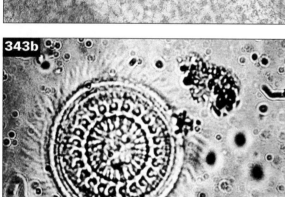

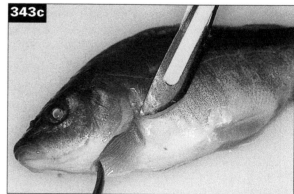

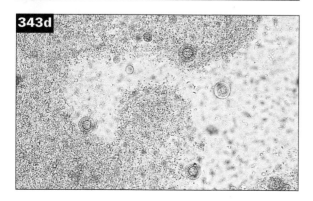

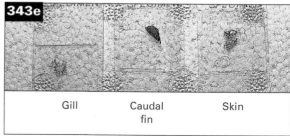

Gill   Caudal   Skin
fin

Examples of efficacious chemicals include formalin, copper sulfate, potassium permanganate, or salt.

In the situation described above, thorough cleaning of the environment will be necessary, including removal of all organic debris. Stocking rate, feeding rate, and water exchange rate may need to be adjusted to avoid accumulation of excessive organic debris in the future. Once the environment is clean, a single treatment with one of the chemicals listed above should result in decreased mortality and improved condition of the fish.

DISCUSSION. Areas of predilection for skin parasites are those adjacent to the fins, and it is a good approach to obtain material from these sites. The mucus is suspended in a small quantity of water on a microscope slide (preferably pond or tank water from which the fish was taken; tap or distilled water may destroy the parasites), a cover slip applied, and the preparation examined under the microscope (×400 total magnification should be sufficient to visualize most parasites).

Case 344: **Fish hook in a bonnethead shark**

CLINICAL PRESENTATION. A recently acquired male bonnethead shark presented dead (**344a**). The shark came from a 155,000-liters aquarium that housed several species of elasmobranchs, including several bonnethead sharks. Examination of the shark revealed a large hemorrhagic cutaneous lesion just caudal to the right commissure of the mouth. The shark appeared thin and probably had not eaten well. It died shortly after capture for examination. External examination of the shark revealed a large fish hook in the mouth that penetrated into the gills on the right side (**344b**).

MANAGEMENT/PREVENTION. Sharks recently captured from the wild should be closely examined for the presence of fish hooks and other foreign objects. Fish hooks are often found in the oral cavity, esophagus, and stomach. Fish hooks and other ingested foreign material can lodge in the stomach and be present in sharks that have been in captivity for many years. They have the potential to migrate into or through the stomach wall, creating a coelomitis and septicemia. Fish hooks and other radiodense foreign objects can be detected by radiographic examination. Esophageal and gastric foreign objects can also be detected by endoscopy. Whenever possible, foreign objects with the potential of harming the shark should be retrieved from the animal to prevent future complications.

Gastric foreign bodies can be retrieved from the esophagus and stomach of large sharks by inserting a PVC pipe into the mouth. The pipe should be large enough in diameter to facilitate passage of a well-lubricated hand and arm. The pipe shields the hand and arm from contact with the sharp teeth. Obviously, proper attention to restraint of the animal is important. The shark can be restrained in a vinyl stretcher that is tied around the shark, leaving the head exposed.

Once a hand is in the stomach, the foreign object can be grasped. If necessary, the stomach lining can be gathered using the fingers to bring the objects that are out of reach closer to the hand. The gastric fluids of sharks are highly irritating to human skin. It is advisable to wear protective sleeves or heavy lubrication to minimize exposure of the skin to the gastric fluids when performing this procedure. Gastric foreign objects can also be retrieved from small and large sharks using endoscopy and grasping instruments. Gastrotomy can be considered if other methods of gastric foreign body retrieval have failed and the shark is suffering from complications associated with the foreign body. In this case the bonnethead shark apparently died of septicemia as a result of secondary bacterial infection associated with the wound created by the fish hook in the gills.

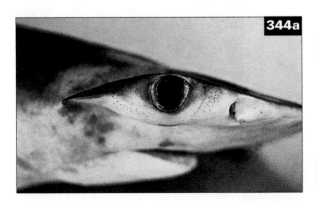

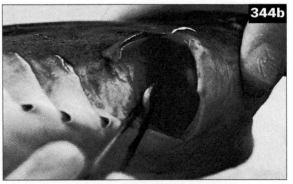

Case 345: *Fusarium solani* mycosis in a bonnethead shark and a scrawled filefish

CLINICAL PRESENTATION. A bonnethead shark died shortly after its removal from a 150,000-liters aquarium that housed bonnethead sharks as well as other species of elasmobranchs (**345a**). The majority of the bonnethead sharks in the aquarium exhibited varying degrees of similar cutaneous lesions. The other animals appeared normal. The affected sharks were lethargic and ate poorly. They exhibited cutaneous papules, ulcerations, and erosions on the dorsal and ventral aspects of the head.

The aquarium contained artificial sea water that shared the rapid sand filtration and ozonation with a much larger (2,500,000 liters) aquarium containing many large elasmobranchs and bony fishes. The water quality parameters included temperature of 22–23°C (71.6–73.4°F), pH of 8.0–8.4, and a salinity of 32 p.p.t. The fish in the larger aquarium appeared healthy.

In a separate case, a scrawled filefish was found to be near death and was killed painlessly. It lived in a 38,000-liters marine aquarium with a variety of other marine fish species. No other fish were affected and water quality parameters were within normal limits. The fish had a necrotic, pale-white to yellow, friable lesion that involved a large portion of the ventral musculature of the fish (**345b**).

INVESTIGATION. Gross necropsy of the bonnethead shark revealed a severe liquefaction necrosis of the tissue on the head. The pattern of the lesions suggested involvement of the ampullae of Larenzini. Histopathology and cytology indicated a fungal cause.

Fungal hyphae were found throughout the lesions in both the bonnethead shark and the scrawled filefish. Microbial culture demonstrated the classic canoe-shaped or banana-shaped microconidia of *Fusarium solani* (**345c**). *Fusarium* cultures usually display a lavender color (**345d**).

Vibrio species was cultured from the kidney of the filefish, indicating a bacteremia in addition to the mycosis.

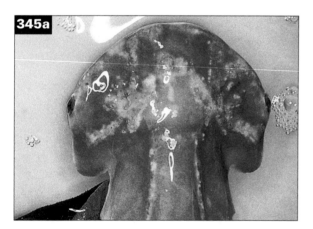

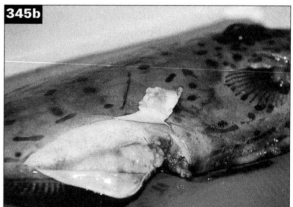

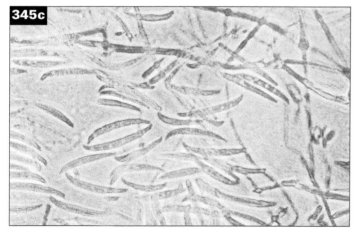

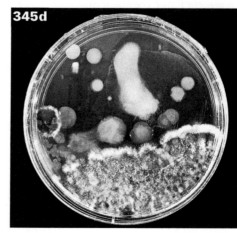

DIAGNOSIS. Both the bonnethead shark and the scrawled filefish had a mycosis caused by *F. solani*.

ETIOLOGY. *Fusarium* infections have been reported in a number of wild and domestic animals, including humans and several species of fish. The organism is a ubiquitous opportunistic pathogen that rarely presents a problem to the uncompromised fish. Although it could not be proved, it is likely that the filefish sustained some type of trauma near the infected area, allowing for colonization by *Fusarium*.

MANAGEMENT/HUSBANDRY. Bonnethead sharks with similar lesions failed to respond to treatment with antifungal drugs, including itraconazole and ketoconazole. Bonnethead sharks live in slightly warmer waters than those provided in this case, therefore the aquarium temperature was raised to 24.5–25.5°C (76.1–77.9°F). After only a few months with the increased water temperature, the lesions disappeared from the affected sharks and no new cases occurred. It was concluded that water temperatures below 24.5°C (76.1°F) are immunosuppressive to bonnethead sharks and predispose them to opportunistic pathogens, such as *Fusarium* species, that are present in the aquatic environment.

Case 346: **Bufotoxin ingestion in a leopard shark**

CLINICAL PRESENTATION. A leopard shark was found dead in a 150,000-liters outdoor aquarium in the southeastern US (**346**). The aquarium consisted of a round concrete pool buried in the ground, with the water surface approximately 30 cm below the ground level. Other sharks and bony fish in the aquarium appeared healthy.

INVESTIGATION. Gross necropsy revealed a hemorrhagic gastritis and a large intact toad was found in the stomach.

DIAGNOSIS. Bufotoxin ingestion.

ETIOLOGY. Apparently, the toad fell into the open aquarium, where it had easy access, and was eaten by the shark. The giant tropical toad (*Bufo marinus*) was introduced into the southeastern US in the early 1970s as a method of controlling undesirable insects. All toads, and especially this species, produce a toxic substance from their parotid glands. The thick, cream-colored toxic secretion is easily expressed from pinhole openings on the skin overlying the parotid glands. Mortality rates of dogs in the southeastern US exposed to oral contact with the toxins from *B. marinus* approach 100%. The bufotoxins secreted from the parotid glands have a digitalis-like effect, resulting in ventricular fibrillation in mammals. Other compounds found in the toxic secretions include epinephrine, cholesterol, ergosterol, and 5-hydroxytryptamine. Orally ingested bufotoxins in sharks can result in acute death and a hemorrhagic gastritis.

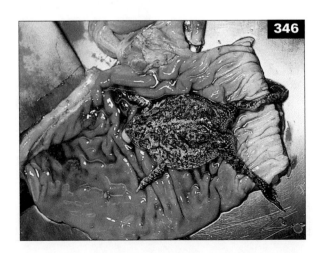

Case 347: **Blood loss anemia in a lemon shark**

CLINICAL PRESENTATION. A captive male lemon shark, measuring 44.1 kg in weight and 190 cm in length, presented with a two-day-old deep bite wound on the caudal one-third of its caudal fin. The deep wound involved the caudal vertebrae and the tail was unstable.

INVESTIGATION. Blood was taken for a complete blood cell count (day 2). Four days later the wound was observed to be filling with a red colored tissue. A blood sample was taken for a blood profile (day 6) and a systemic antibiotic (amikacin, 3.0 mg/kg i/m q72h) was initiated for a total of seven treatments. Twenty-four days after the initiation of the antibiotic therapy the shark was evaluated and a third blood profile was obtained (day 30). A fourth blood profile was obtained at day 56 following healing of the surgery to remove the caudal tip of the shark's tail. The profiles (partial) are shown below. Smears were made of the peripheral blood (**347a–c**).

DIAGNOSIS. The changes in the RBC, PCV, and Hb values between day 2 and days 6 and 30 are suggestive of a blood loss anemia.

ETIOLOGY. Lemon sharks have three types of granulocytes in the peripheral blood, along with two types of mononuclear leukocytes, lymphocytes, and monocytes. They also have nucleated erythrocytes and thrombocytes.

347a demonstrates a G1 granulocyte, a lymphocyte, and mature nucleated erythrocytes. The normal G1 granulocytes typically resemble avian heterophils, except that they tend not to have a lobated nucleus. Normal G1 granulocytes have prominent round to oval eosinophilic cytoplasmic granules and a colorless cytoplasm.

347b demonstrates a G2 granulocyte, two thrombocytes (adjacent to the G2 granulocyte), and mature nucleated erythrocytes. There is a small, mature lymphocyte with a scant amount of blue cytoplasm below the G2 granulocyte. The cytoplasm of the thrombocytes is colorless in contrast to the blue cytoplasm of the lymphocyte. The G2 granulocytes of sharks often have a lobed nucleus and a colorless cytoplasm (when stained with Wright's stain). They lack the distinct eosinophilic cytoplasmic granules observed in G1 and G3 granulocytes.

347c demonstrates a G3 granulocyte, a thrombocyte, a lymphocyte, and mature nucleated erythrocytes. The G3 granulocyte of sharks resembles the avian eosinophil, except that they tend not to have a lobed nucleus. They have distinct eosinophilic cytoplasmic granules that are round and have tinctorial properties that differ from the G1

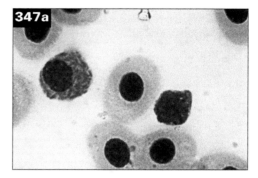

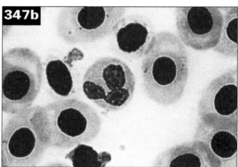

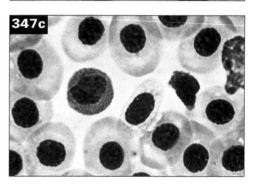

Day:		2		6		30		56	
RBCs (10^{12}/l)	(10^6/µl)	0.50		0.31		0.27		0.37	
PCV (l/l)	(%)	0.21	(21)	0.12	(12)	0.10	(10)	0.16	(16)
Hb (g/l)	(g/dl)	61	(6.1)	30	(3.0)	17	(1.7)	30	(3.0)
WBCs (10^9/l)	(10^3/µl)	19.8		32.6		25.1		12.3	
Lymphocytes (0/0)		36		14		30		49	
G:L ratio		1.7		5.4		2.3		1.0	
BUN (mmol/l)	(mg/dl)	–		257	(720)	228	(638)	191	(535)
Total protein (g/l)	(g/dl)	–		30	(3.0)	21	(2.1)	22	(2.2)
AST (u/l)		–		35		8		8	
GGT (u/l)		–		12		1		2	
CK (u/l)		–		735		599		157	

granulocytes. In general, G3 granulocytes have brighter eosinophilic granules and a blue cytoplasm when compared with G1 granulocytes. **347c** demonstrates the difference between a thrombocyte with a colorless cytoplasm and a lymphocyte with a blue cytoplasm.

MANAGEMENT. The wounded tail remained unstable and did not appear to be healing. The caudal tip of the tail did not appear viable and was surgically removed just cranial to the original bite wound. The tissue was allowed to granulate closed. After 26 days, the wound had nearly healed by establishment of a healthy granulation bed that was being covered by normal appearing epithelium.

DISCUSSION. The improvement in the RBC parameters on day 56 indicate that the shark is responding to his anemia. The leukogram changes reflect a leukocytosis, with slight improvement between days 6 and 30. This could reflect a favorable response to the antibiotic therapy; however, a significant inflammatory response still exists on day 30. The granulocyte to lymphocyte (G:L) ratio shows a significant increase between day 2 and day 6. This, along with the increase in the total leukocyte count, is indicative of a severe inflammatory response. The improvement in the G:L ratio on day 30 supports a favorable response to therapy. The return of the G:L ratio to normal (1.0–1.5) by day 56 is a positive sign. The blood biochemistries indicate high BUN values typical of sharks. Sharks utilize urea nitrogen to maintain their normal plasma oncotic pressure. The significant changes in the biochemical profile include elevations in AST, GGT, and CK enzymes on day 6 that show decreases on day 30 and a return to normal by day 56. This is suggestive of a recovery from the severe skeletal muscle damage that resulted from the bite wound to the tail. Removal of the necrotic tissue helped return the blood profile to normal parameters.

Case 348: *Cryptocaryon* species infection in some marine fish

CLINICAL PRESENTATION. A hobbyist with a dedicated quarantine tank for his marine fish recently purchased some fish that had 'broken' (become infected) with *Cryptocaryon* species.

MANAGEMENT. Copper sulfate administered properly is a very effective treatment against marine ectoparasitic protozoans. Most experts in the field consider 0.15–0.25 p.p.m. as free copper ion to be the effective treatment concentration. A target of 0.20 p.p.m. may be the best way to ensure that levels do not fall too low to be effective or so high as to severely stress or even kill the fish. Treatment levels must be maintained for enough time to ensure that the vulnerable stage of the parasite's life cycle (the free swimming, or tomite, stage) is killed or disabled to the point of not being able to reinfect the fish. Measuring for copper levels daily with a reliable test kit is essential, and additions of copper sulfate must be done as needed. If levels fall below 0.15 p.p.m., there is a chance that a fish can become reinfected. Once the parasite burrows into the fish's integument, it will not be killed by copper, and the cycle of infection may continue. The hobbyist should maintain a treatment level for at least 10 days; however, 15–21-day treatments are recommended to ensure eradication of the parasite. An elevated temperature (27–29°C [81–84°F]) is also recommended to accelerate parasite life cycles. This will greatly reduce the chances that parasites will be encysted during the treatment period and increase the probability that the tomite stage is exposed to the copper sulfate. Fish should be watched carefully for signs of copper toxicity; these may include stress coloration, diminished appetite or refusal to eat, excessive mucus production, and/or respiratory distress. If fish react in such a way and it seems that the copper sulfate is the cause, water changes or removal of copper sulfate with activated carbon should be done immediately.

HUSBANDRY/PREVENTION. There are many ways to set up a life support system for a marine fish tank, but a quarantine tank is a special consideration. Because fish will not be in these tanks for very long, lighting becomes less crucial. In fact, subdued lighting may be preferable or even critical if using light sensitive chemotherapeutics. Esthetic considerations regarding tank decorations should not interfere with medical treatments. For example, copper adsorbs to decorative corals or crushed coral substrates. A bare floor is recommended, except when it seems to benefit the fish to have some sort of substrate (i.e. flounders, wrasses, or other fish that use substrate partially or completely to bury themselves), in which case a silica or quartz sand can be used. PVC piping or other inert plastic items can be used as cover and hiding places for fish. Maintaining good water quality may be the single most important stress reducer for fish in a quarantine system. Careful management is required to ensure an active filter capable of maintaining proper water quality parameters when new fish are introduced to the tank. Filters must be kept active during times when the quarantine tank is not being used. This can be done artificially by using ammonium chloride to 'feed' the tank bacteria that are responsible for the metabolism and removal of ammonia and nitrites from the fish tank. Using a live fish as a permanent resident is not recommended, as this fish can act as a reservoir for parasites. Using live invertebrates is also not recommended, because many prophylactic quarantine treatments are lethal to marine invertebrates.

Case 349: *Amyloodinium* species infestation in marine fish

CLINICAL PRESENTATION. A pet store owner sought advice because he had lost 30% of his marine fish in the past five days and the surviving fish were extremely lethargic. Some had been seen 'coughing' (backflushing water across the gills) and rubbing their opercula along objects in the tank. Some had a shimmering golden appearance along the dorsal body surface. None were eating very well. All the marine fish were housed in a 5,700-liters recirculating system. There was no ozonation or ultraviolet sterilization of the system water. A moribund percula clownfish was submitted for examination.

INVESTIGATION/DIAGNOSIS. Gill biopsy revealed massive numbers of *Amyloodinium* species on the lamellae (**349a**). Moderate numbers were present on skin scrapings. A micrograph of infected gill tissue from a sand tiger shark is shown (**349b**) (photo courtesy A van Weltere).

MANAGEMENT. Given the situation presented – 30% mortality rate over a five-day period, and examined fish heavily infested with *Amyloodinium* species – salvaging the fish remaining in the store may be difficult. In the author's experience, the treatment of choice would be chloroquine at 10.0 p.p.m. The chemical can be added to the entire 5,700-liters system and fish should begin to improve almost immediately. The other option would be to add 0.2 p.p.m. copper ion (Cu^{2+}) to the system for three weeks. Any invertebrates would need to be removed from the system before copper addition.

The main disadvantage of chloroquine treatment is that it is not approved for use in any aquatic species in the US. The compound is an antimalarial and, under experimental conditions, has provided excellent control of *Amyloodinium* species in red drum. Copper has been used as a parasiticide in marine systems for many years. An important disadvantage to using copper in the situation described is that the fish are severely compromised (i.e. fish that are very sick and heavily infected with *Amyloodinium* do not tolerate copper well). In addition, maintaining active copper (Cu^{2+}) concentrations of 0.2 p.p.m. can be labor intensive. Copper concentration should be checked several times a day and additional copper may need to be added to the system.

PREVENTION. The occasional introduction of undesirable infectious agents into a pet store is not completely preventable. At the very least, incoming fish should be dipped in freshwater (marine fish) or sea water (freshwater fish) for 3–10 minutes. Additionally, a system such as the one described should have some means of sanitizing water before it recirculates back to the tanks. A properly installed and maintained ultraviolet light unit can do a reasonable job of preventing the transmission of infectious agents from one tank to another.

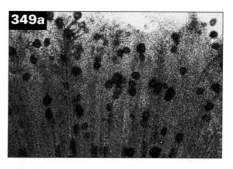

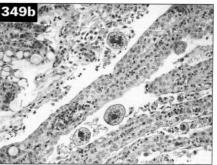

Case 350: Osmoregulation in marine fish

CLINICAL PROBLEM. Marine fish face particular problems with regard to their osmoregulation.

ETIOLOGY. The body fluids of marine fish are hypotonic to their environment, the concentrations being about 25–30% of seawater. As a result of diffusion and osmosis, there is a tendency for water to leave the fish's body and for salts to enter. It is essential for the normal physiologic processes of the fish that the concentrations of body fluids are controlled within narrow limits.

Various physiologic mechanisms are in place to address this problem. The factors involved in the control of the concentrations of the body fluids of marine fish are:
• Limitation of the overall permeable surface area. The structure of the normal skin, with its mucus layer, ensures that the skin surface remains impermeable. Thus, the surface area available for the exchange of water is reduced to that of the gill and, to a lesser extent, the bowel. This factor is important in those diseases in which the skin surface becomes ulcerated.

- The uptake of water from the gastrointestinal tract. Marine fish continually drink saltwater at a rate of about 0.5% of body weight per hour. This in turn results in the absorption of sodium and chloride ions through the bowel.
- Excretory processes within the kidney. The urine of marine fish is more concentrated than that of freshwater fish. The maximum concentration achieved can only be that of the body fluids, so this does not

represent a net excretion of salts. Magnesium and sulfate ions are excreted in the urine.
- Excretory processes in the gill. The principal agents of salt excretion are the chloride cells situated within the gill epithelium. This is an active process in which sodium and chloride ions are excreted, producing localized areas of a high concentration of salt with resultant local diffusion gradients.

Case 351: **Space-occupying mass in the posterior chamber of the left eye of a Queensland grouper**

CLINICAL PRESENTATION. An adult Queensland grouper (aged 25 years old and weighing about 180 kg) presented with trauma to its lower jaw and some abrasions over its left operculum. The fish had been eating well and its respiratory rate was within normal limits. Two other groupers in this exhibit appeared normal. The aquarist reported that for the past several months this fish had been swimming around the tank, predominantly to the left, and would not accept food presented on its left side.

INVESTIGATION. The fish's visual capabilities were evaluated. Most fish react to even a dim light beam shown into their eyes. If no reaction is evident, a close physical examination is warranted. In this case a diver entered the animal's tank with a pressurized garden sprayer containing a solution of concentrated MS-222 (25 g/l). A small amount of dye such as methylene blue can be added to the solution to aid in visualizing the stream of anesthetic. The solution is then sprayed into the animal's mouth, which is 'inhaled' by the fish and passes over the gills. Induction usually occurs within five minutes. The cornea and lens of both eyes appeared normal and there were no other signs of abnormalities.

Ultrasonographic examination is particularly useful in evaluating the fish patient provided that the scales are not too thick.

DIAGNOSIS. In this case, ultrasonography revealed a large space-occupying mass in the posterior chamber of the left eye (**351a**). The right eye is apparently normal (**351b**).

ETIOLOGY. The etiology of this problem is unknown.

PROGNOSIS. The animal continued to be blind in the left eye but was otherwise normal.

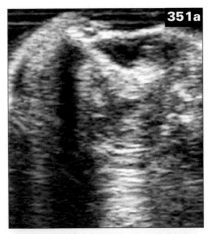

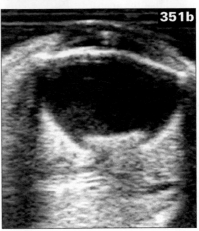

Case 352: **Spinal fracture and subluxation in a black grouper**

CLINICAL PRESENTATION. A juvenile black grouper, approximately six years old, presented with acute anorexia, lethargy, and a slight skin darkening over the caudal one-third of its body. The fish was a three-year resident of a 240,000-liters community Atlantic coral reef tank. The tank contained hundreds of other bony fish as well as elasmobranchs. This fish was the only representative of its species in this exhibit and it was introduced directly from the wild. Its medical and husbandry histories to date were unremarkable. The fish was being fed previously frozen fish and invertebrates, with no vitamin supplementation. Capture of the fish and examination was made easily because the animal was resting upright on the bottom of the tank.

INVESTIGATION. External examination revealed a slight abrasion on the most rostral portion of the lower jaw and a relatively darkened integument over the caudal one-third of the body. Skin scrape and gill biopsy revealed no parasites but some excess mucus covering the respiratory epithelium. On neurologic examination it appeared that the animal could not sense noxious stimuli on its tail and it appeared to be paralyzed in the caudal one-third of the body. Radiography revealed a spinal fracture and subluxation (**352a**).

DIAGNOSIS. It appeared that the animal had made contact with some object in the tank and subsequently fractured its spine.

MANAGEMENT. A surgical reduction was attempted with an external fixator (**352b**). A lateral approach was used and two pins were placed cranial and caudal to the lesion site. It was necessary to balance the stainless steel hardware with small amounts of closed-cell foam floatation to allow the animal to maintain an upright position. The animal began to eat and show signs of improvement; however, it was found dead about two weeks after surgery.

DISCUSSION. Gross pathologic examination revealed a black cottony mass in the dorsocaudal region of the swim bladder. It has been reported that uncomplicated spinal fractures have healed with tank rest. Electrical surges from electric pumps and lightning strike have been implicated in causing this condition in pond fish such as koi.

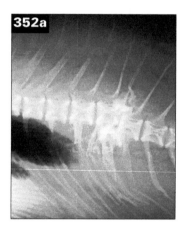

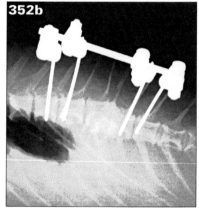

Case 353: **Attacked French angelfish in an aquarium of marine fish**

CLINICAL PRESENTATION. A 5 cm long French angelfish, that had been introduced into a 200-liters aquarium seven days previously, presented after being found in the corner of the aquarium and nearly dead. The owner had held a stable population of marine aquarium fish in the aquarium for the past several months (**353a** [photo courtesy C Goldwaithe], **b**). This included four 5 cm blue damselfish, six 5 cm percula clownfish, and a 12 cm emperor angelfish. There was no history of any morbidity or mortality in the aquarium during this time. All the other fish appeared clinically normal.

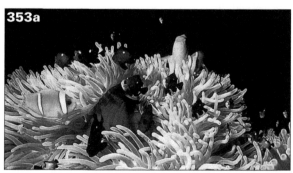

INVESTIGATION. Water quality examination revealed a temperature of 26°C (78.8°F) (obtained from history), total ammonia nitrogen of 0 p.p.m., nitrite of <0.1 p.p.m., and a pH of 8.1. Physical examination of the moribund angelfish showed frayed fins and several foci of depigmentation on the flanks. No pathogens were visible in wet mounts of skin or gills. Necropsy results were within normal limits. No bacteria were recovered from kidney culture.

DIAGNOSIS. The absence of any pathogens in the skin wounds and lack of any discernible infectious agent on necropsy strongly indicated that the fish was the target of aggression by its tankmates. The owner was queried thoroughly to see if there was any evidence of this event. The larger emperor angelfish was probably the most significant source of this aggression, but the other fish may have contributed to attacks.

MANAGEMENT. An attacked fish should be immediately placed into a separate isolation tank to allow it to recover from its wounds. Prophylactic antibiotics may be used to prevent secondary bacterial infections if lesions are very deep or extensive.

PREVENTION. Many marine reef fish are highly territorial. This territoriality is usually displayed most aggressively against members of their same species. For solitary species such as angelfish, it is best not to have more than one individual of the same species in the tank. It is often inadvisable even to have more than one individual of the same family. Fish that naturally school together, such as damselfish, can be kept as a group, but it is important to have at least three or four members of this group to avoid one dominant individual from constantly harassing

only one other member of the group. When introducing any new individual into a tank with a well-established dominance hierarchy, it is best to acclimatize the newcomer gradually into the population. This can be done by placing the newly introduced fish into a clear container that is suspended into the tank. The fish should be kept in this container for at least several days before releasing it into the aquarium.

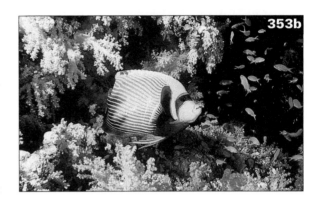

Case 354: **Angelfish fibroma**

CLINICAL PRESENTATION. A freshwater angelfish presented because of a mass on its maxilla (354a).

INVESTIGATION. A biopsy was taken and the histologic appearance of the tumor is shown (354b). Note the presence of teeth embedded in the fibrous mass. Some workers have referred to these masses as odontogenic hamartomas.

DIAGNOSIS. Angelfish fibroma.

ETIOLOGY. Angelfish fibroma is not uncommon in freshwater angelfish and it is believed to be associated with a retrovirus.

MANAGEMENT. Treatment involves anesthetizing the patient and debulking the mass, as was done in this

particular case with dramatic cosmetic improvement (354c). Affected fish should remain isolated from other angelfish.

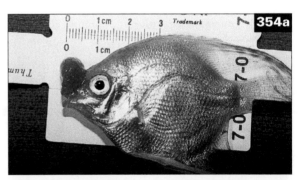

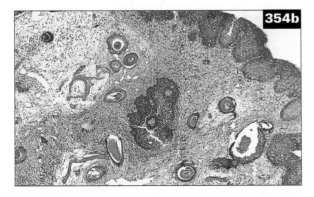

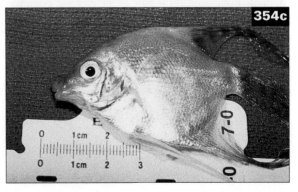

Case 355: *Spironucleus* species infection in freshwater angelfish

CLINICAL PRESENTATION. A freshwater angelfish breeder was experiencing difficulty raising fry. The number of eggs laid by his broodstock had decreased over the past few months, with only a 70% hatching success. Of the fry that did hatch, only about 40% survived to the swim-up stage.

INVESTIGATION. Water quality evaluation of a typical hatching jar revealed:
- Dissolved oxygen: 7.5 p.p.m.
- Total ammonia nitrogen: 1.4 p.p.m.
- Temperature: 26°C (78.8°F).
- pH: 7.2.
- Total alkalinity: 140 p.p.m.
- Nitrite: 0 p.p.m.
- Total hardness: 120 p.p.m.

Examination of broodstock revealed small numbers of motile flagellates in the intestinal tract. Examination of eggs and fry with light microscopy revealed large numbers of flagellated protozoans on the external surface of the eggs, and internally and externally in the fry.

DIAGNOSIS. The most likely cause of poor egg quality, hatch rate, and fry survival is *Spironucleus* species infection.

ETIOLOGY. *Spironucleus* species is a diplomonad flagellate (10–20 mm) that is frequently found in the intestinal tract of angelfish (**355**). Flagellates are occasionally found in the intestine of dying fry. Whether or not they are present on the external surface of fry is uncertain. The flagellates are so small that a slide could be easily contaminated with gut contents, giving the impression of external infection.

The most likely source of *Spironucleus* in fry is infected broodstock. The apparent level of infection in adults may not be indicative of the level of infection on eggs or in fry. Poor sanitation appears to exacerbate the problem in eggs and fry.

MANAGEMENT. Broodstock of species that are highly susceptible to *Spironucleus* should be treated prophylactically with a metronidazole-medicated food (50 mg/kg fish) every 2–4 months. Species of particular concern include angelfish, discus, oscars, African cichlids, and gouramis. Infected eggs or fry can be treated with a metronidazole bath (at 6 p.p.m.) every other day for three treatments. Particular attention should be paid to sanitation. Dead eggs, fry, and uneaten food should be removed from the environment promptly.

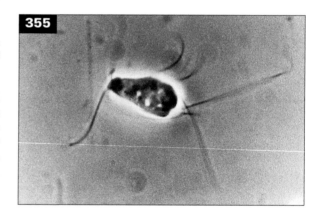

Case 356: Thyroid hyperplasia (goiter) in an emperor angelfish

CLINICAL PRESENTATION. An emperor angelfish selected randomly from a large marine exhibit aquarium presented for routine health screening. A large bilateral nodular swelling was noticed at the base of the gills and extending upward along the lower gill arches (**356a, b**).

INVESTIGATION. A biopsy of the lesion was taken and a histologic section prepared (**356c**). Eosinophilic colloid fills thyroid follicles of varying size and shape. Secondary lamellae of the gill are present at upper right quarter of the section.

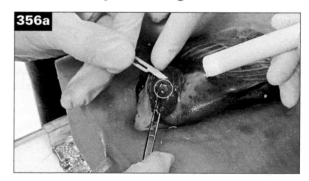

DIAGNOSIS. A diagnosis of thyroid hyperplasia was made.

ETIOLOGY. The thyroid of most fish is a diffuse organ located along the floor of the gill chamber, but thyroid tissue can also be found in the spleen, heart, and cranial kidney. Goiter may be difficult to distinguish from thyroid carcinoma, and was mistakenly described as such when initially found in salmonids on iodine deficient diets.

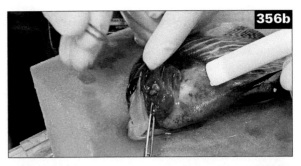

MANAGEMENT. Iodine deficiency goiter responds to iodine replacement therapy. A primary iodine deficiency is unlikely in marine fish. It is important to search for and eliminate goitrogenic substances in the feed. A similar syndrome in sharks responds to thyroxine therapy, presumably by restoring the negative feedback loop on thyroid-releasing hormone and thyroid-stimulating hormone production.

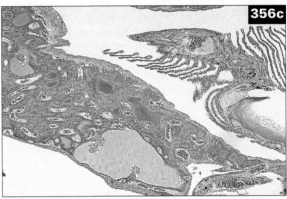

Case 357: *Amyloodinium ocellatum* infestation in a planehead filefish

CLINICAL PRESENTATION. A planehead filefish was presented because it was anorectic, severely emaciated, and had multifocal white blotches on the skin (**357a**). It began to experience equilibrium problems and was euthanatized for diagnostic work-up to determine the risk to and the potential prophylactic treatment for its tankmates.

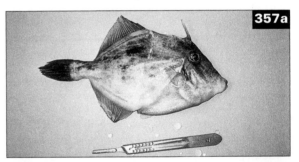

INVESTIGATION. A skin scraping was easily obtained (in contrast to a normal filefish with the rough and abrasive skin for which they are named). The scraping revealed several nonmotile, pear-shaped organisms of varying diameter. These organisms contained multiple small golden-yellow spherules, and had basal rhizoids. A histologic section of the same organism on the gills is shown (×250) (**357b**).

DIAGNOSIS. *Amyloodinium ocellatum* infestation.

ETIOLOGY. *A. ocellatum* is a parasitic dinoflagellate. Trophonts attach to gills and skin by rhizoids, causing severe tissue damage at the sites of attachment. Natural infection with *A. ocellatum* is rare in elasmobranches.

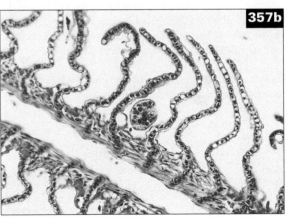

MANAGEMENT. Treatment is complicated by a life cycle that includes resistant tomonts. Copper at a free divalent ion concentration of 0.2 p.p.m. as a continuous bath is the current treatment of choice. Chloroquine has also been recommended. Treatment must continue long enough for resistant stages to form susceptible dinospores. Latent infections are common. Monitoring for reinfestation following treatment is important.

Case 358: **Gas-bubble (supersaturation) disease in a lionfish**

CLINICAL PRESENTATION. A lionfish was one of several fish found dead in a quarantine facility. The fish died acutely with few premonitory signs.

INVESTIGATION. Necropsy was performed and the only lesions observed grossly were air bubbles in the tissues of the fins (**358a**).

DIAGNOSIS. Gas-bubble disease. Diagnosis of this condition is based primarily on the presence of gas emboli in the vessels of the fins and periorbital tissues. This has been shown in a Moorish idol with marked exophthalmia, which, on close inspection, had a large air bubble behind the globe (**358b**). Microscopic air bubbles can often be found in the gills when examining fresh branchial samples.

ETIOLOGY. Gas-bubble disease (or supersaturation) is a condition that occurs in fish as a result of supersaturation of the water with nitrogen, oxygen, or other gases. The most common cause of this problem is a cavitating pump that literally supersaturates the water with atmospheric air (meaning the majority of the gas will be nitrogen). This results when air is allowed to leak into the water intake side of the pump. The condition is usually associated with pumps of 0.5 horse power (about 350 W) or greater in closed systems without excessive algal growth. Excessive oxygen production by algae and other plants is a less frequent cause. Overaerating an aquarium with air bubbles from an air stone can, but rarely does, lead to supersaturation disease.

MANAGEMENT. Generally, by the time the problem is discovered, many fish have already died. Locating and correcting the pump problem will prevent this situation in the future. Treatment usually involves finding the source of the excessive gas and eliminating it. In the case of a cavitating pump, filling the sump or reservoir or locating a leak in the system usually solves the problem. Air bubbles under the skin and within the fins will usually resolve within a day or two. Air bubbles in the circulatory system, especially in the branchial vasculature, can be acutely fatal (**358c**).

DISCUSSION. Exophthalmia in fish can also be caused by trauma, ammonia toxicity, ocular parasites, septicemia, or neoplasia.

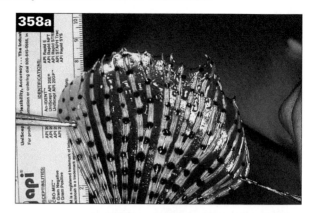

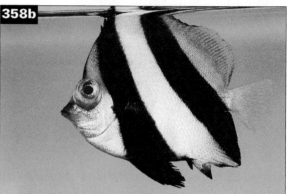

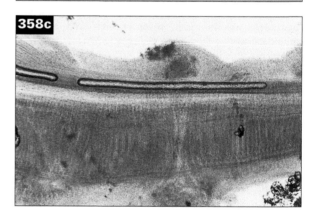

Case 359: **Lymphocystis disease in a jackknife fish**

CLINICAL PRESENTATION. A jackknife fish that was being held in a marine quarantine tank was presented with a cutaneous lesion on its body. The lesion had a raised, gray, cauliflower-like appearance. The fish was eating and exhibited normal behavior. The water quality parameters were within acceptable limits and the other jackknife fish in the aquarium appeared normal.

A similar condition was observed in a green terror cichlid that was presented with pale white to gray nodular lesions on the pectoral fins, opercula, and caudal fin (**359a**). The fish was eating and appeared to be strong, the water quality parameters were within normal limits, and no other fish were affected.

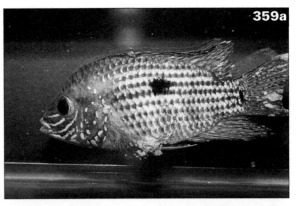

DIFFERENTIAL DIAGNOSES. Lymphocystis disease, neoplasia (chlamydial epitheliomas, dermal sarcomas), fungal infection, protozoal disease (e.g. *Heteropolaria*), and clusters of trematode cysts.

INVESTIGATION. A small biopsy of the lesion was obtained and examined directly under the microscope. Microscopic examination of the excised tissue (×10 objective) (**359b**) revealed the dermal cells (fibroblasts) to be greatly enlarged.

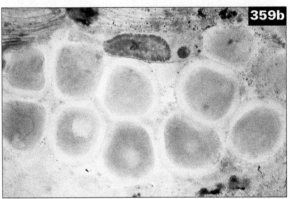

DIAGNOSIS. This was indicative of lymphocystis disease. Note that the photomicrograph also includes a trematode. Diagnosis can be confirmed with histology and/or electron microscopy.

ETIOLOGY. Lymphocystis is the most common viral disease of ornamental fish. The disease is caused by lymphocystis disease virus, a member of the the iridovirus family, and it has been identified in over 100 species of fish. The infection causes a marked hypertrophy of the dermal connective tissue cells. Individual cells are frequently visible to the naked eye. Clusters of round cells of various size (hypertrophied fibroblasts) will indicate a diagnosis of lymphocystis disease (**359c**).

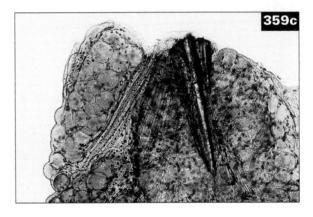

Transmission is probably horizontal, although not all fish exposed will contract the disease. Viral particles can survive for at least several days in the water and subclinical carriers probably exist. The disease is typically self-limiting and lesions frequently disappear within a few weeks.

MANAGEMENT. Environmental stresses should be removed. In order to prevent spread of the disease, affected fish should be isolated from other fish for at least six weeks or until the lesions have disappeared. If practical, lesions can be surgically removed and the fish monitored for secondary bacterial infections.

Case 360: *Brooklynella hostilis* infestation in a seahorse

CLINICAL PRESENTATION. A seahorse presented because of abnormal pale areas on its body (**360a**). An external protozoal infestation was suspected.

DIFFERENTIAL DIAGNOSES. *Brooklynella hostilis* or *Uronema marinum* infestation.

INVESTIGATION. Wet mounts of skin and fin biopsies were examined immediately, since many protozoal organisms die quickly and lose their characteristic morphology.

DIAGNOSIS. This seahorse had a severe *B. hostilis* infestation. Living parasites are ciliated, heart-shaped, and measure approximately 50 microns in diameter. A dried and stained parasite is shown (**360b**).

ETIOLOGY. *B. hostilis* affects many species of marine fish, especially clownfish. Infections occur in crowded conditions and/or in debilitated fish.

MANAGEMENT/PREVENTION. Prevention of the disease is directed at identification and treatment during quarantine. Short baths in freshwater (five minutes) will kill the parasites. Combinations of formaldehyde and malachite green have been used for aquarium treatments at a final concentration of 15–25 p.p.m. formalin and 0.05 p.p.m. malachite green.

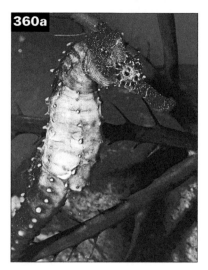

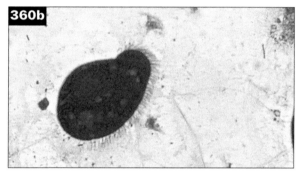

Case 361: Columnaris disease in a tank of platys

CLINICAL PRESENTATION. Mortalities were being experienced in a tank of platys at a local wholesaler (**361a**). Many of the fish hung listless in the water near the surface. A few seemed to have a white ring around their mouth and/or whitened areas on their back and along the borders of their fins. Some of these areas were hemorrhagic.

DIAGNOSIS. Skin and fin biopsies confirmed the presence of columnaris disease (*Flavobacterium columnare*). The 'haystack' appearance of the bacteria is characteristic of this organism (**361b**).

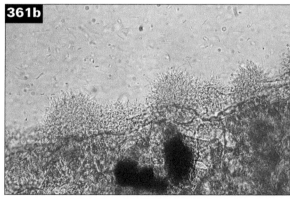

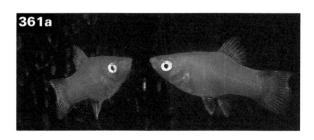

Case 362: **Malachite green toxicity in a group of clown loaches**

CLINICAL PRESENTATION. A group of clown loaches were treated prophylactically for *Ichthyophthirius multifiliis* infection with 0.1 p.p.m. malachite green. The treatment was repeated two days later but now fish are dying.

INVESTIGATION. The water quality parameters tested were within normal limits. A gill biopsy was performed and a photomicrograph taken (**362**).

DIAGNOSIS. Malachite green toxicity.

ETIOLOGY. Scaleless fish, including clown loaches and catfish, are extremely sensitive to malachite green. The second treatment compounded the damage done by the first chemical application, and significant destruction of secondary gill lamellae has resulted (**63**). Mortalities are probably secondary to inappropriate chemical treatment.

MANAGEMENT. The surviving fish should be maintained in clean water and not exposed to further chemical stress. Clown loaches are best treated for *I. multifiliis* by

temperature manipulation. In the clown loaches presented, there is no evidence that the fish actually had an *I. multifiliis* problem. Owners should be educated on proper chemical use and quarantine protocols.

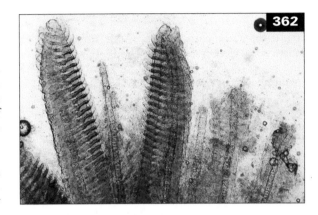

Case 363: *Uronema marinum* infestation in a melon butterflyfish

CLINICAL PRESENTATION. A melon butterflyfish presented with obvious skin lesions in the form of multifocal ulcerations (**363a**) (photo courtesy G Blasiola). It appeared that the lesions were being caused by an external protozoal parasite.

DIFFERENTIAL DIAGNOSES. *Brooklynella hostilis* or *Uronema marinum* infestation.

INVESTIGATION. Wet mounts of skin and a fin biopsy were taken. Living parasites, which were ciliated, pear-shaped, and measured approximately 25 microns in diameter, were seen (**363b**). The wet mount from this fish was teeming with parasitic organisms. Bacterial culture of the lesion produced *Pseudomonas* species.

DIAGNOSIS. *Uronema marinum* infestation.

MANAGEMENT. Antibiotic therapy by injection is suggested.

PREVENTION. Prevention of the disease is directed at identification and treatment during quarantine. This parasite is very difficult to kill with chemotherapeutic agents since it burrows into the musculature of the fish.

PROGNOSIS. The prognosis for recovery is guarded with this condition since the parasite is very invasive and produces a portal of entry for bacterial pathogens like *Pseudomonas* species and *Vibrio* species.

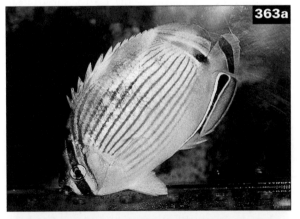

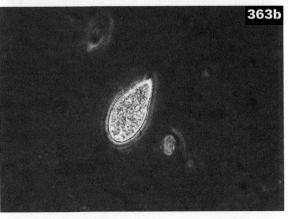

Case 364: **Nematode and cestode infection in a group of snakeheads**

CLINICAL PRESENTATION. A recently imported group of snakeheads presented because they were losing weight and appeared generally unthrifty.

INVESTIGATION. Water quality parameters were within normal limits and gill, skin, and fin biopsies were unremarkable. A direct fecal examination revealed the presence of nematode as well as cestode eggs (**364a**).

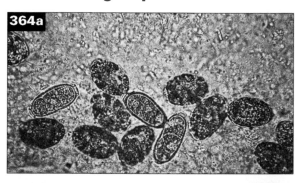

DIAGNOSIS. Nematode and cestode infection. The microscopic view of the cestode clearly shows the scolex and proglottids (**364b**). This cestode probably belongs in the genus *Circumonocobothrium*.

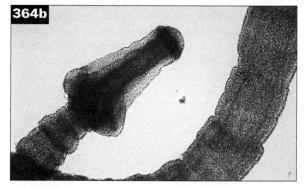

MANAGEMENT. Praziquantel treatment (2.0 p.p.m. for 3 hours) will cause the fish to expel many intact, mature cestodes. A mature cestode can be seen trailing from the vent of this snakehead (**364c**). In general, most ornamental fish will tolerate a praziquantel bath of between 2.0 p.p.m. and 10.0 p.p.m. for up to six hours. The nematode infection can be treated with a levamisole bath (2.0 p.p.m. for 24 hours). Both of these treatments should be repeated in 14–21 days.

DISCUSSION. Snakeheads are aggressive, freshwater tropical fish, native to Asia. At least one species has received a lot of publicity in the US for surviving in natural aquatic systems after inappropriate introduction. Non-native fishes should never be introduced to ponds, lakes, rivers, streams, or the ocean.

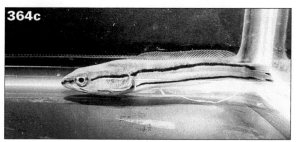

Case 365: **Exophthalmia in a squirrelfish**

CLINICAL PRESENTATION. A squirrelfish presented with unilateral exophthalmia that had slowly evolved over the last week (**365a**).

DIFFERENTIAL DIAGNOSES. A retrobulbar mass (neoplasia, bacterial, or fungal granuloma), retrobulbar or intraocular gas, and pseudobranch pathophysiology.

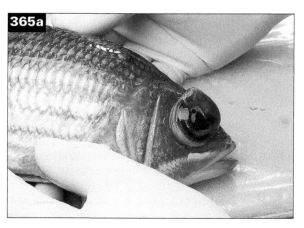

INVESTIGATION. The eye should be examined thoroughly using a slit lamp device (**365b**) or other suitable ophthalmic instrument. Intraocular gas in the anterior chamber can help differentiate whether the problem is intraocular or retrobulbar. A transcorneal intraocular aspirate can be taken at the limbus using a 27 gauge needle attached to a tuberculin syringe. This technique not only relieves intraocular pressure, but it also produces a sterile sample for microbiologic culture. Aspiration of the retrobulbar chamber can be performed for cytology or culture and can be handled in a similar manner to the intraocular technique. A small amount of sterile saline can be introduced into the chamber through the periocular skin and collected with the same needle by inverting the fish and aspirating at the most dependent portion of the conjunctiva.

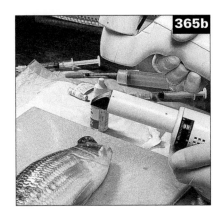

DIAGNOSIS. The layman's name for this syndrome is 'pop eye disease.'

Case 366: *Rickettsia*-like organisms in a blue-eyed plecostomus

CLINICAL PRESENTATION. A blue-eyed plecostomus (pleco) presented after several leeches had been removed by the owner. Several fish from a population of 20 had already died and another six were debilitated.

DIFFERENTIAL DIAGNOSES. *Rickettsia*-like organisms, intracellular hemoparasites, intracellular bacteria.

INVESTIGATION. A Giemsa-stained blood film showed a monocyte containing numerous basophilic granules in the cytoplasm (366a). On necropsy, histopathology revealed similar large accumulations of obligate intracytoplasmic organisms in the spleen (366b), kidney, and heart (epicardium) (366c). A transmission electron micrograph revealed the ultrastructure of these granules (366d) and showed organisms with the characteristic features of a *Rickettsia*.

DISCUSSION. The shape, size, and triple membrane are consistent with *Rickettsia*-like organisms found in blue-eyed plecos and other fish, including salmonids. Several reports have linked rickettsia-like organisms with clinical disease in fish. Proper quarantine practices combined with antibiotic therapy appropriate for rickettsia is warranted.

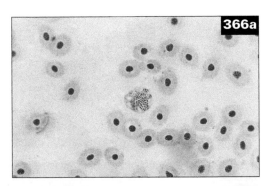

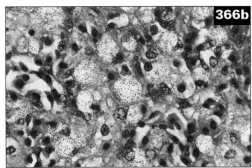

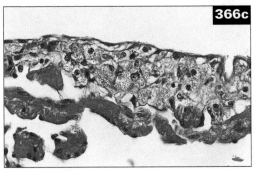

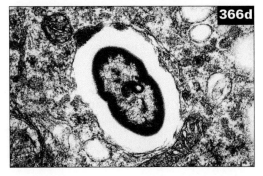

Case 367: Trematode (*Neascus* species) infestation in a silver dollar

CLINICAL PRESENTATION. A silver dollar presented with distinct, raised, black spots on its skin that looked like poppy seeds (367). This fish, together with four other silver dollars that had similar spots on their skin, had been recently purchased from a pet store and placed in a 200-liters community aquarium. The fish were behaving normally and the rest of the fish in the tank were fine. The owner had not noticed the spots in the pet store but remembered seeing them shortly after introducing the fish to her well lit aquarium.

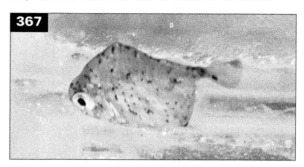

DIAGNOSIS. These spots represent the encysted metacercaria of a digenetic trematode, most likely belonging to the genus *Neascus*.

ETIOLOGY. This condition is common in wild-caught silver dollars and related characins. The fish is an intermediate host for this parasite. The definitive host is usually a fish-eating bird; a molluscan invertebrate, usually a snail, is the first intermediate host. In most cases the black color of the cysts is caused by a host reaction to the parasite, and melanin is deposited around the encysted metacercaria.

MANAGEMENT. There is evidence that treatment using a parasiticide that targets trematodes (e.g. praziquantel, 5–10 p.p.m. for 24 hours as a bath immersion) will kill the metacercaria; however, the pigmented cysts will likely remain for some time.

DISCUSSION. This condition is not detrimental to the fish and cannot be transmitted to other fish in the aquarium without the definitive and first intermediate hosts being present. Many pet store owners call this condition 'salt and pepper' and will commonly advise customers that the condition is not harmful to the fish.

Case 368: Chronic alkalosis in an electric eel

CLINICAL PRESENTATION. An electric eel presented with a dramatic swelling that had suddenly developed behind its head. (368a) The eel has been maintained uneventfully in a 1,100-liters display tank for the past six months.

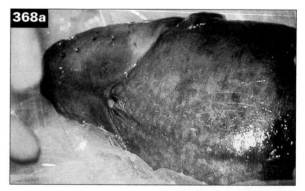

INVESTIGATION. The eel was anesthetized and a radiograph taken (368b). This showed dramatic abdominal distension caused by accumulation of coelomic fluid, compatible with a diagnosis of ascites. Coeliocentesis was performed, removing several milliliters of a clear sterile transudate. The coelom refilled with fluid within 24 hours. Evaluation of the water quality of the tank was unremarkable, with the exception of a pH of 7.8.

DIAGNOSIS. A diagnosis of chronic alkalosis, resulting in an inability of the eel to compensate for water balance through the exchange of hydrogen ions at the gill, was made.

ETIOLOGY. The normal habitat of this fish is in mud streams and pools of northern South America and Central America where the pH is routinely below 6.0.

MANAGEMENT. Adjusting the pH to 6.5 will result in rapid resolution of the ascites, which should not recur.

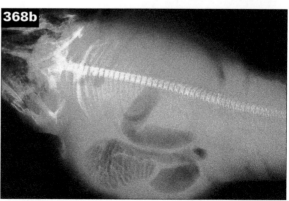

Case 369: **Pregnancy/parturition in a yellow stingray**

CLINICAL PRESENTATION. Advice was sought because a pregnant yellow stingray was several weeks past its expected parturition date.

INVESTIGATION. Visual examination and palpation of the distended coelomic wall was carried out to indicate the health status of the ray pup(s). If fetal movement is not seen, palpation of the mother can stimulate the pups to move or ultrasonographic examination can be performed to search for fetal heartbeats.

ETIOLOGY. Some ray species easily conceive in captivity, but dystocias are common. Healthy mature pups are generally lively and can be observed swimming inside the uterus by closely examining the body wall of the mother for their characteristic fluttering swimming motion. As the fetuses mature past term, they can die in the uterus, where they are either absorbed or mummified. The mother may become sick if the fetuses putrefy.

MANAGEMENT. If the fetus(es) are alive and the known parturition date is past, the female can be anesthetized, placed on a soft moist substrate, and the cloaca examined (**369a**). In this case a smooth syringe case was used as a speculum, allowing access to the 'cervix.' A small blunt catheter can be introduced into the cervix, which is dilated by rotating the catheter in a slowly expanding circular motion. Clear to cloudy uterine fluid evacuates once the cervix is expanded, and a gloved finger can be introduced to continue dilating the cervix. Once the cervix is adequately dilated, the tail of the pup can be exteriorized and gentle but steady pressure is placed on the mother's body wall, thereby expelling the pup (**369b**). If the pup cannot be extricated in this manner, the fetus can be removed by placing careful but steady traction on the venomous spine using a pair of forceps or hemostats.

Another option is chemical induction of parturition. A 100 µg tablet (or half a 200 µg tablet) of misoprostol (a synthetic prostaglandin E1 analog) can be crushed and made into a suspension with sterile water (2.5 µg/ml). This suspension (0.2 ml) is then added to about 1.0 ml of lubricating jelly. The jelly is then injected into the cloaca and the animal observed for parturition. If successful, the cloaca should be gavaged liberally with sterile saline to remove any residual drug. (Information courtesy Dr. C Harms).

If cervical dilatation and chemical induction are unsuccessful, the pups can be removed surgically. Yellow ray pups are miniatures of the adults (**369c**). This particular ray produced four healthy young.

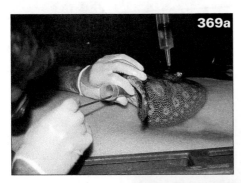

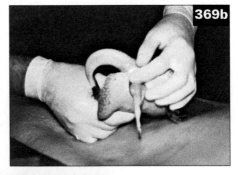

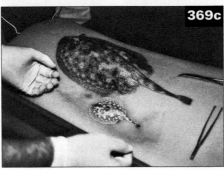

Case 370: *Ichthyobodo* species infestation in a group of discus

CLINICAL PRESENTATION. A group of five medium sized discus presented because they had recently darkened in color, some appearing gray along the dorsal body wall. The fish were housed in a 280-liters circular tank. Their respiratory rates were increased and the fish were not eating very well.

INVESTIGATION. The results of water quality evaluation are shown (next column).

Scanning electron micrographs of a gill biopsy of one fish revealed moderate numbers of *Ichthyobodo* species (**370a, b**; ×200 and ×2,000, respectively). A skin scraping from the cloudy area along the dorsal body wall revealed very high numbers of the flagellate.

DIAGNOSIS. *Ichthyobodo* species infestation.

MANAGEMENT. A formalin bath (25 p.p.m.) applied directly to the display tank is the easiest management strategy. For fish that can be removed from an infected system, a 10 minute 150 p.p.m. bath is frequently appropriate and effective. In this case the water quality parameters were excellent. Owners should be reminded to maintain vigorous aeration during the treatment period. Water changes following the formalin bath are recommended but not necessary. One application of formalin should be adequate to control *Ichthyobodo* species.

Other treatment options include potassium permanganate, copper sulfate, and salt. Potassium permanganate could be used at 2 p.p.m. as a prolonged bath; however, it imparts a purple, then brown, color to the water. The discoloration of the water is highly undesirable in a display or exhibit tank; therefore, potassium permanganate baths should usually be done in a treatment or quarantine tank. Copper sulfate (0.15–0.20 p.p.m.) is an excellent treatment for *Ichthyobodo* species, but it is contraindicated given the low alkalinity of the water. Salt is also effective against many protozoal agents, including *Ichthyobodo* species. Discus will tolerate only short-term salt treatments.

Most clinicians believe that *Ichthyobodo* is an opportunistic pathogen and is normal when present in low

Dissolved oxygen	7.8 p.p.m.
Total ammonia	0 p.p.m.
Temperature	29°C (84.2°F)
Nitrite	0 p.p.m.
Total alkalinity	51 p.p.m.
pH	6.8
Total hardness	51 p.p.m.

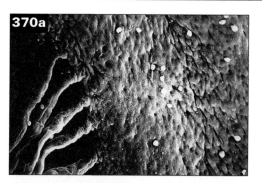

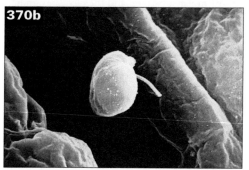

numbers. In fact this organism may be beneficial in cleaning up sloughing tissue/cells. The best way to prevent *Ichthyobodo* species infestation is to minimize stress to the fish, screen newly acquired fish (with gill/skin biopsies), and implement a sound quarantine program.

Case 371: Fight trauma in a red pacu

CLINICAL PRESENTATION. A red pacu presented that had been severely ravaged by a tankmate. When found it had bilateral deep ulcerative lesions that coalesced at the lateral midline (**371a**).

INVESTIGATION. A skin scraping revealed numerous *Tetrahymena* species as well as some fungal hyphae consistent with *Saprolegnia* species.

DIAGNOSIS. The protozoal and fungal infections are secondary to the trauma sustained during the fish fight.

MANAGEMENT. Pacu are very hardy fish, so the major concern should be secondary bacterial infection and a loss of osmotic equilibrium, in addition to the parasite and fungal problems. Daily saltwater dips (35 p.p.t. for 5 minutes) combined with an antibiotic in the water

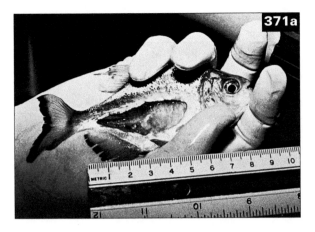

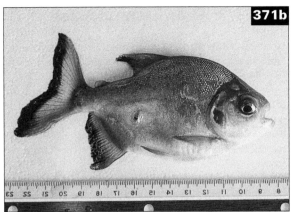

(nitrofurazone at 20 p.p.m. in this case) for 5–7 days would be an acceptable course of treatment. Freshwater fish thus affected may benefit from salt in their water (1-2 p.p.t.) during the healing period. This particular fish responded well to the treatment and survived, although a permanent scar remained. The fish is shown three months after the trauma (**371b**).

Case 372: **Cachexia plus trematode infection in a clown triggerfish**

CLINICAL PRESENTATION. A clown triggerfish presented because of cachexia and an inability to gain weight (**372**). The fish weighed 200 g and lived in an 800-liters marine aquarium with a dozen other reef fish. The fish was eating a commercially prepared frozen marine fish food as well as some marine flake food. The other fish in the tank also ate this food. The owner was concerned that the fish had liver disease secondary to being captured with the aid of cyanide (there was no evidence to support this claim).

INVESTIGATION. Water quality was evaluated and the results were within normal limits. A direct fecal examination revealed the presence of digenean trematode eggs. Serum chemistry values showed no gross abnormalities (although reference ranges do not exist in this species) and radiographs were unremarkable.

DIAGNOSIS. This fish had two identifiable problems: although the fish was eating, it might not have been getting enough food; and it had a trematode infection.

MANAGEMENT. The fish was given an intracoelomic injection of praziquantel (6 mg/kg) and it was isolated and fed between 5% and 7% of its body weight per day of a balanced gelatinized food diet. Subsequent fecal examination was negative for parasitic ova and the fish steadily gained weight and body mass. Six months after treatment, the fish weighed 250 g and was strong, healthy, and in normal body condition.

DISCUSSION. Because both the parasite treatment and the diet correction were applied at the same time, it is not possible to be sure which management practice contributed most to the fish's improvement. It is likely that both problems had some effect on the fish.

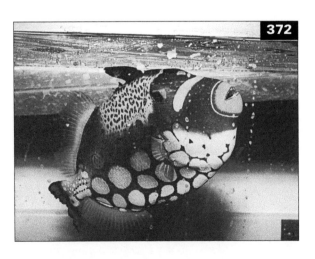

Case 373: **Neon tetra disease**

CLINICAL PRESENTATION. A neon tetra from a community tank presented with muscle wasting and focal color loss (**373a**).

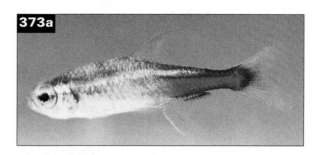

DIAGNOSIS. Neon tetra disease caused by the microsporidian *Pleistophora hyphessobryconis*. The diagnosis is confirmed by identifying the characteristic spores, which are present in 'packets' (sporophorous vesicles) (**373b**).

ETIOLOGY. *P. hyphessobryconis* infects muscle fibers, causing wasting and focal color loss. In heavy infections the disease may spread to the connective tissue of the intestine, ovary, or skin.

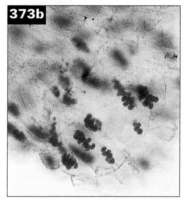

MANAGEMENT. There is no proven treatment for any microsporidian parasite. A toltrazuril bath (20 p.p.m. for 1 hour every other day 3 times) has shown experimental efficacy against the vegetative stages, but not the spores, of another microsporidian, *Glugea* species.

PREVENTION. The best method of control is destruction of infected stocks and disinfection of facilities.

Case 374: **Ulcerative mycobacteriosis in a dwarf gourami and other fish**

CLINICAL PRESENTATION. This ulcerative lesion developed in a dwarf gourami that had not been eating well and was slightly emaciated (**374a**).

DIFFERENTIAL DIAGNOSES. With a history of wasting and debilitation, an important differential to consider, especially in pet fish, is mycobacteriosis (ulcerative bacterial disease). Neoplasia would be another differential.

INVESTIGATION. Histopathology revealed numerous dermal and visceral granulomata (**374b**). An acid-fast stain can help support the diagnosis. Culture on specific media such as Loweinstein–Jensen agar and identification are required for a definitive diagnosis. PCR techniques are also used to identify *Mycobacterium* species.

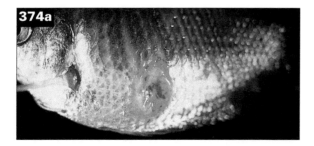

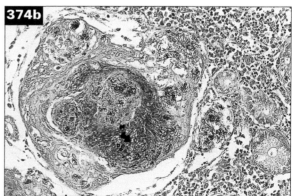

DIAGNOSIS. Ulcerative mycobacteriosis.

ETIOLOGY. Besides *Mycobacterium* species, other acid-fast bacteria such as *Nocardia* species have also been reported in fish. Most of the mycobacteria isolated from fish are atypical, with *M. fortuitum* and *M. marinum* being the most common.

MANAGEMENT. Ulcerative bacterial disease is generally considered to be untreatable; however, there are empirical accounts of of fish improving on long-term oral or injectable antibiotic therapy.

DISCUSSION. Other examples of ulcerative mycobacteriosis have been seen. For example, this mature black tetra presented for an erosive lesion of the maxilla and mandible (**374c**). The owner had noticed the lesion several weeks previously and it had progressed to the point that the fish had difficulty eating. Biopsy and subsequent histologic examination confirmed this to be a case of mycobacteriosis. Because of the severity of the lesion, the fish was humanely destroyed.

This queen angelfish had multiple ulcerative lesions on its body (**374d**). Culture and biopsy of the lesions confirmed this as a case of ulcerative mycobacteriosis.

This weather loach presented with deep cutaneuous ulcerative disease (**374e**). An *Aeromonas* species was cultured, but the fish did not respond to immersion antibiotic therapy in a hospital tank. Histopathology confirmed a diagnosis of acid-fast bacterial disease. A section of kidney is shown (**374f**). During the initial work up, a touch preparation was made of the ulcer but, interestingly, it did not reveal any acid-fast organisms. Touch preparation cytology and acid-fast staining can be of great diagnostic value as the procedure is fast, inexpensive, and provides information promptly.

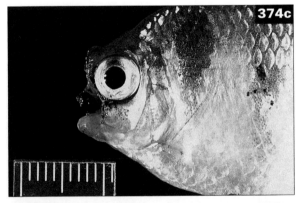

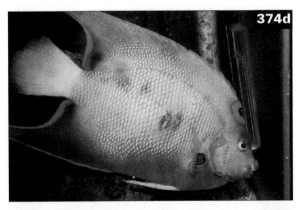

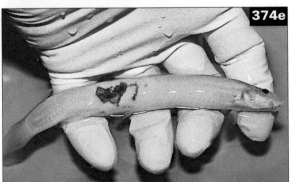

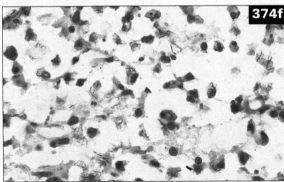

Case 375: **Overgrown puffer teeth in a dog-faced puffer**

CLINICAL PRESENTATION. A mature dog-faced puffer fish presented with a history of probable weight loss and apparent difficulty eating.

DIAGNOSIS. The fish was anesthetized with MS-222 (100 p.p.m.) and examined. It was soon evident that the maxillary incisors were overgrown (**375a**), making it nearly impossible for the fish to prehend its food (puffers typically have four teeth: two maxillary and two mandibular).

ETIOLOGY. Captive puffers fed a 'soft' diet may be prone to this condition. Wild puffers (members of the family Tetradontidae) feed on fish and invertebrates that likely help keep the teeth 'trimmed'.

MANAGEMENT. In this case the fish was anesthetized and placed on an anesthesia machine. A Dremel® drill (**375b**) was used to trim the overgrown teeth until there was a space between the mandibular and maxillary teeth when the jaws were opened (**375c**).

PREVENTION. Feed a mixed diet including whole crustaceans and whole fresh fish (not live), or fish chunks with skin, scales, and bones.

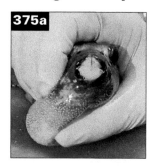
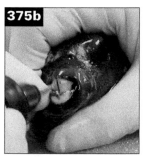
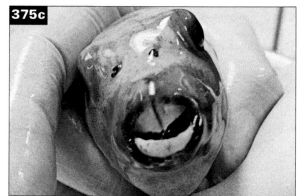

Case 376: **Hematoma in a gourami**

CLINICAL PRESENTATION. A sunset thick-lipped gourami weighing 8 g presented because of a 5 mm diameter midventral abdominal swelling.

DIFFERENTIAL DIAGNOSES. Differentials include neoplasia (e.g. carcinoma of epithelial origin, fibrosarcoma, hepatic tumor), abscess, hernia (without intestinal involvement), parasitic cyst, and hematoma.

INVESTIGATION. A fine-needle aspirate revealed only red blood cells and thrombocytes. A barium gastrointestinal study was performed to help determine visceral involvement in the swelling (**376a**). The cranial radiolucent area is the labyrinth organ. Fish of the family Anabantidae use this organ to extract atmospheric oxygen, supplementing oxygen absorbed by the gills. The caudal radiolucent area is the swim bladder. On excisional biopsy the mass had a sessile base communicating with the coelomic cavity.

DIAGNOSIS. Histopathology of a cross-section of the entire mass demonstrated a consolidated hematoma of undetermined origin (**376b**).

MANAGEMENT. The mass was removed for the biopsy and it did not recur.

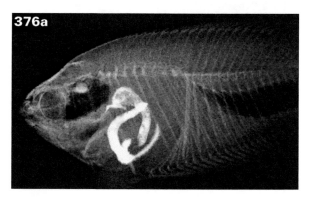
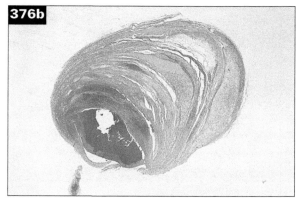

Case 377: **Acid rain**

ETIOLOGY. Acid rain occurs when acidic emissions from industrial processes, car exhausts, and power stations enter the atmosphere and dissolve in the rain falling in affected areas. The acidified water enters fish ponds directly or through water sources used to replenish ponds, and it causes a significant fall in pH. Acid water can also dissolve metals (particularly aluminum) as it travels through water courses.

DISCUSSION. Acid water is irritating to fish and can directly damage the epithelium of the skin and gills and/or cause acid-base and electrolyte imbalances. Dissolved metals can be acutely harmful to fish. Aluminum is in its most toxic form at pH levels around 5.0. It may also cause long-term damage. Fish are in particular danger following a thaw of accumulated acid snow, when a flush of acid water and dissolved metals may enter fish ponds and cause acute mortalities.

Case 378: **Melanomacrophage center**

CLINICAL PRESENTATION. Brown–black discrete foci consisting of large, round to polyhedral cells containing intracytoplasmic pigment within their foamy cytoplasm are shown in this histopathology slide (**378**).

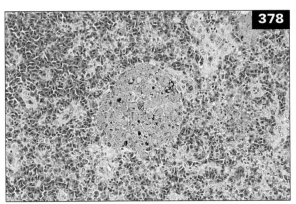

DIAGNOSIS. This is a melanomacrophage center (MMC), which is a normal lymphomyeloid feature of fishes and is found in the spleen, liver, and kidney.

ETIOLOGY. Although MMC numbers and size have been loosely correlated with environmental contamination, infection, and injuries, the presence of MMCs reveals little about cause of death, and should be expected. The exact role of MMCs is uncertain, but they may represent homologs of germinal centers of mammals and birds and are involved in antigen processing. Pigments in melanomacrophages include lipofuscin from oxidation of unsaturated fatty acids, hemosiderin from hemoglobin degradation, and melanin as a free-radical scavenger.

Case 379: **De-icers**

CLINICAL PRESENTATION. A pond owner lives in a geographical area where the temperature is below freezing for an average of 18 days per season. The owner wants to know if it would be advisable to purchase a de-icer.

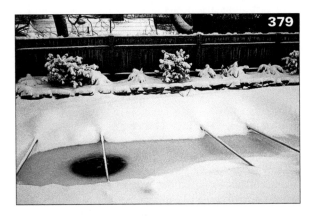

MANAGEMENT. Brief periods of icing are not harmful to temperate pond fish if the pond is of sufficient depth. It is recommended that a section of the pond should have a depth of at least 120 cm. In a location where the pond is frozen for a majority of the winter, a de-icer may be necessary to provide a water–air interface for gas exchange (**379**). If an external filtration system is run throughout the winter, this may agitate a section of the water surface enough to prevent icing, and the filter itself will facilitate gas exchange.

Case 380: **Bacterial septicemia**

ETIOLOGY. Bacterial septicemias are common in fish. The kidney is a major filtering organ and any systemic bacterial infection should be found here.

DISCUSSION. The kidney can usually be exposed aseptically by carefully displacing the abdominal organs and swim bladder, allowing a bacteriological loop or swab to be conveniently and easily inserted (**380**). Bacteriological samples are occasionally obtained from external lesions, particularly if it is not intended to sacrifice the fish under examination. However, these are frequently contaminated with insignificant environmental organisms, and care must be exercised in the interpretation of results.

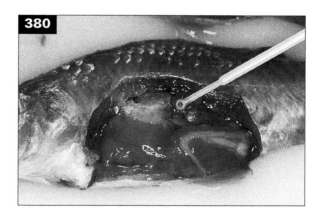

Case 381: **Fish heart**

DISCUSSION. The fish heart has four chambers (**381**), the sinus venosus (1), the atrium (2), the ventricle (3), and the bulbus arteriosus (also referred to as the conus) (4), which differ histologically.

The wall of the sinus venosus is very thin and almost completely devoid of cardiac muscle. It consists of an epicardium and an inner layer of endothelium, the endocardium. A few isolated cardiomyocytes and a little melanin are present between the epicardium and the endocardium.

The atrium is anterior to the sinus venosus. This thin-walled chamber is thicker than the sinus venosus and consists of cardiac muscle covered by epicardium and an inner portion of endothelium-lined cardiomyocytes, arranged in a widely spaced network bathed by blood.

The ventricle is the most muscular chamber, consisting of an outer compact layer and a thicker, inner, spongy layer of anastomosing cardiomyocytes lined by endothelium. The outer layer is supplied by the coronary vessel and is lined on the outer surface by epicardium.

The bulbus arteriosus lacks cardiac muscle and is composed of elastic connective tissue and smooth muscle. This structure helps to provide consistent blood flow and pressure to the gills.

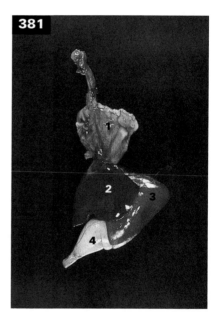

Case 382: **Blood flow**

DISCUSSION. Mammals and fish have different blood flow systems. Fish have a single-pass system. Deoxygenated venous blood is received by the heart and pumped to the gills to be reoxygenated and then distributed to the rest of the body before returning to the heart. Mammals have a double-pass system with deoxygenated blood being received by the right atrium and pumped by the right ventricle to the lungs for oxygenation. The reoxygenated blood returns to the left atrium and is redistributed to the body by the left ventricle.

Case 383: **Normal fish kidney histology**

DISCUSSION. The piscine kidney is not separated into the medulla and cortex as in the mammalian kidney. The trunk kidney is composed of identical nephrons (which are the functional excretory units of the kidney) mildly separated by small amounts of hematopoietic elements (**383**).

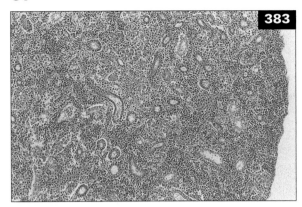

Case 384: **'Dropsy'**

CLINICAL PRESENTATION. A fish presented with symmetrical swelling of the abdomen and elevation of the scales, which gave the fish a 'pine cone' appearance (**384**). Bilateral exophthalmos was also present.

ETIOLOGY. The changes seen are typical of 'dropsy' in which there is an upset in the fluid balance mechanisms, with retention of fluid within the abdominal cavity and tissues. Tissue edema results in retrobulbar swelling, which in turn produces the exophthalmos. Edema in other tissues may be apparent, as well as swelling of the vent or of bowel loops when examined at necropsy. While the term 'dropsy' is common in the vernacular, ascites would be more clinically accurate.

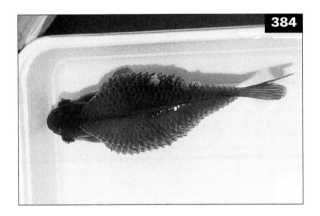

Case 385: **Anesthetic agents for exploratory coeliotomy**

CLINICAL PROBLEM. A red oscar presented because it required an exploratory coeliotomy.

MANAGEMENT. There are several anesthetic agents that should be considered in fish:
- Carbon dioxide: can be used to achieve anesthesia in fish. As with isoflurane, the amount delivered to the fish can be difficult to control. Carbon dioxide also affords little or no muscle relaxation, which is desirable when performing a coeliotomy.
- Isoflurane: is an effective anesthetic agent in mammals; however, it is difficult to control the concentration delivered to fish. Also, human exposure to isoflurane gas that escapes from the water can cause concern.

- Ketamine hydrochloride: has been used effectively as a fish anesthetic; however, it is difficult to maintain a surgical anesthetic plane for prolonged periods with injectable anesthetic agents.
- Quinaldine sulfate: can be administered in a very controlled fashion to the piscine patient. Quinaldine is superior to tricaine in that it is less expensive and has a wider margin of safety. Unfortunately, quinaldine sulfate does not suppress reflex motion and fish anesthetized with this compound often move in response to touch.
- Tricaine methanesulfonate (MS-222): is the best choice for the procedure specified. This drug is readily available, has a high margin of safety with a variety of freshwater and marine species, and is approved for use in fish intended for human consumption in the US and Canada.

Case 386: **Postmortem examination.**

DISCUSSION. The clinical examination of live fish is limited by their aquatic environment and by the relatively narrow range and nonspecificity of clinical signs. Postmortem and laboratory investigations are therefore essential in the diagnosis of fish disease and it is often necessary to sacrifice an affected individual in a population to carry out these investigations.

After obtaining a detailed clinical history, affected individuals should be examined for external abnormalities (e.g. scale loss and ulcers, hemorrhage, fin and tail erosion, eye abnormalities, gill damage, abdominal swellings, grossly visible parasites or fungal infection). Changes in pigmentation and overproduction of mucus are often more noticeable while the fish is in the water. Skin scrapes and gill biopsies should be examined for the presence of parasites and other disease processes.

The abdomen of the fish should be opened along the ventral midline, taking care not to puncture the gastrointestinal tract (**386**). The presence of abdominal fluid, hemorrhage, or both, should be noted.

The abdominal organs should be examined for abnormalities and the presence of grossly visible parasites. At this point the kidney can be exposed aseptically and a sample of kidney tissue obtained for bacteriological examination.

Tissue samples can be taken for histopathologic examination and the gut and stomach opened and examined for the presence of parasites.

If a toxic insult or viral infection is suspected, a specialized laboratory should be contacted to discuss the most appropriate diagnostic procedures.

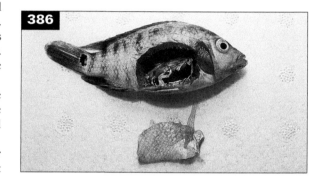

Case 387: **Abnormally inflated swim bladder**

CLINICAL PRESENTATION. A fish presented because of a buoyancy problem (**387a**).

INVESTIGATION/DIAGNOSIS. Radiography (**387b**) revealed an abnormally inflated swim bladder.

ETIOLOGY. This is a common disorder of Asian fancy goldfish and is frequently difficult to resolve. Because the swim bladder has a patent connection to the esophagus by the pneumatic duct in goldfish and other cyprinids, it has been suggested that there may be a nutritional component to the problem. Another possibility is that many of these varieties of goldfish have been bred for abnormal conformation and thus are prone to be 'off balance.'

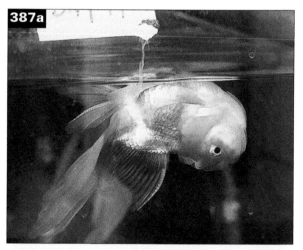

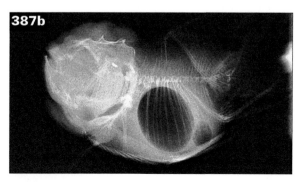

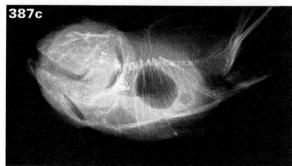

MANAGEMENT. Air should be aspirated from the overfilled compartment. The second radiograph and gross picture were taken after 3.0 cm³ of air was removed from the swim bladder (**387c**). After this procedure, which was performed with a 25-gauge needle, the fish became negatively buoyant but was able to eat and appeared to be more comfortable (**387d**).

Anecdotal reports of fish improving after being fed fresh or cooked peas have been confirmed by the author, although no controlled studies have been performed regarding this 'treatment'.

In recent years some clinicians have tried using surgical implants (small crystals or stones) to help 'balance' the fish. As more of these surgeries are attempted and the results published, surgical intervention may become commonplace for this disorder.

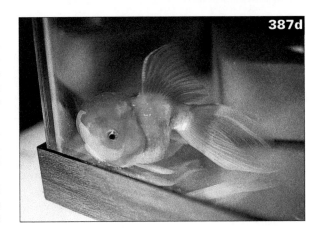

387d

Case 388: **Euthanasia**

DISCUSSION. Veterinarians often must recommend to a client that a fish be euthanatized. Several methods of fish euthanasia have been approved including:
- Cranial concussion followed by decapitation.
- Cervical dislocation followed by double pithing (both the brain and spinal cord).
- Chemical overdose.

If available, tricaine methanesulfonate (MS-222) at a dose of 300–500 p.p.m. for 15 minutes will kill most fish. Since most hobbyists and many veterinary clinics do not have MS-222 on hand, alternatives include benzocaine hydrochloride, oil of cloves, and even carbon dioxide in the form of antacid tablets (2–3 tablets/liter of water). Injectable sodium pentobarbital (60 mg/kg) given i/v or intracoelomically is another chemical alternative for larger fish. As a last resort, a client in a remote location can use ethanol at a final concentration of 10%. Veterinarians should consider offering a euthanasia service since many clients are attached to their piscine pets.

Case 389: **Water quality**

CLINICAL PROBLEM. A pond owner called in the autumn because several fish had died in the last three days in a pond that had been trouble free since its installation in the spring. The pond was roughly 10,000 liters, 120 cm deep at its maximum, moderately stocked, and situated close to the house under a large maple tree. A large number of leaves were floating on the surface. Filtration was accomplished by two submersible box filters attached to pumps, each running at 3,000 liters/hour. Filter pads were rinsed in pond water every other week.

INVESTIGATION. Water quality evaluation revealed:
- Temperature: 17°C (62.6°F)
- Total ammonia nitrogen: 1.7 p.p.m.
- Nitrite: 1.2 p.p.m.
- Dissolved oxygen: 8.0 p.p.m.

DIAGNOSIS. A large quantity of leaves decaying on the pond bottom can be a source of water quality problems.

MANAGEMENT/PREVENTION. Immediate treatment should include daily water changes until the unionized ammonia concentration is below 0.1 p.p.m., removal of the decaying plant matter from the pond bottom, and treatment of opportunistic infections as indicated.

Prevention of this problem can be accomplished by covering the pond in the autumn with fine netting or a commercial pond cover, daily skimming of leaves from the pond surface, and/or more frequent water changes.

Case 390: **Skin fluke infection**

ETIOLOGY. *Gyrodactylus* species is a freshwater monogenean skin fluke (**390a**) (photo courtesy R Vogt). The characteristic features enabling it to be recognized from *Dactylogyrus* species (the gill fluke) are the paired hooks with which it anchors to the skin and the lack of eye spots characteristic of *Dactylogyrus*.

Gyrodactylus has a direct ovoviviparous life cycle. Careful microscopic examination may reveal the presence of an embryonated larva with its own set of hooks. This allows for rapid, temperature-dependent reproduction. Fluke eggs are shown in **390b** (photo courtesy LS Christian).

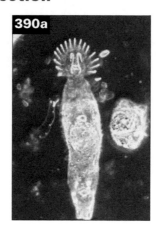

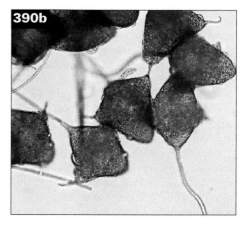

The nature of the life cycle means that a single treatment may be sufficient to control the infestation. This is different from the oviparous species in which the eggs are resistant to treatment, allowing reinfestation to occur. In the latter case, several parasiticide treatments may be required.

Case 391: **Handling of fish**

DISCUSSION. Latex or plastic gloves should always be worn when handling a fish (**391**) because fish can carry zoonotic organisms such as mycobacteria. Moistened latex gloves also protect the fish by decreasing the disruption of the protective mucus layer, which is important in osmoregulation and immune function. Eye protection can protect the fish handler from splashing water.

Fish should only be handled when absolutely necessary and handling time should always be minimized. All work done with the animal should be carefully planned and thought out. If one has never worked with a particular species of fish, it is very important to learn as much as possible about that species before handling the animal. Potentially dangerous animals should never be handled alone.

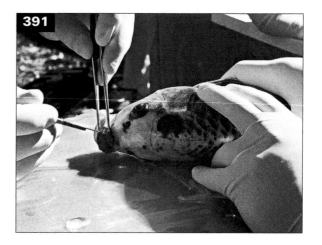

Case 392: **Administration of chemotherapeutic agents**

MANAGEMENT. A variety of routes of administration are used to treat pet fish with chemotherapeutic agents. It is important that the protocol for each route is properly understood.

- Bath: usually refers to a treatment in which the drug is dissolved in the water in which the fish are swimming. The treatment usually lasts for a minimum of 15 minutes and not more than 24 hours. Dosage is usually based on volume of water and not fish biomass.

- Dip: refers to a treatment in which the fish is submerged in a particular solution for between one second and 15 minutes. Water volumes are usually smaller than those for bath treatments.

- Flush or flow-through: this requires constant water flow and is most frequently used in raceways or narrow vats. Medicant is added to the inflow area and the fish are exposed to the drug as it passes over them with the water current. It is similar to the dip procedure except that the fish may not have to be removed from their normal holding area.

- Indefinite bath: self-explanatory. Medication is added to the tank or pond and usually there is no water change or immediate retreatment.
- Injectable: medication that is given by injection into the body of the fish with the aid of a hypodermic needle and syringe. Routes may be subcutaneous, intradermal, intramuscular, intravenous, and intraperitoneal (intracoelomic).
- Oral: medication is mixed with the food in order to treat the fish. It is usually done by incorporating the drug into a food mixture. For larger fish patients, medication can be placed in a chunk of food and then fed or force-fed to the sick fish.
- Topical: medication is applied directly to the lesion or parasite.

DISCUSSION.
- Before using any drug in the water, any chemical (e.g. carbon) filtration must be discontinued as this will inactivate the medicant. Adequate aeration is also important during any water treatment.
- When antibiotics are used as bath treatments, ideally they should be used daily for at least 7–10 days. Water changes (at least 50%) should take place between treatments. This protocol is much easier to follow in a home or hospital tank than in a pet store or wholesale facility.
- A biotest with one or two fish should always be performed when working with unfamiliar drugs, water, or species to determine if the fish will tolerate the treatment.

Case 393: **Ultraviolet light treatment of water**

DISCUSSION. Ultraviolet (UV) light sterilization of aquarium water is very helpful under the right conditions. Three UV sterilizers are shown adjacent to a wet/dry trickle filter (**393**).

UV sterilizers consist of a UV light bulb housed within a quartz tube, which allows water to flow freely around the UV light source. UV light inactivates viruses, bacteria, protozoal parasites, and a variety of pathogenic spores by disorienting the structure of cellular DNA. For UV sterilization to be effective, enough energy must be delivered to kill the largest of the biological targets such as protozoans and the eggs of trematodes and other helminths. It has been determined that 180 microwatts per square centimeter is needed to kill *Ichthyophthirius* species. To remain efficient and effective, UV systems require prefiltered water, a clean quartz tube, periodic tube replacement, and a sufficient number/size of bulbs to obtain the required energy level.

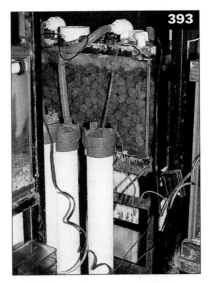

Case 394: **Parasiticide treatment regimens**

CLINICAL PROBLEM. An ectoparasitic monogenean problem was diagnosed in a group of fish. The fish were quite sick and in need of immediate treatment. The water quality was being managed adequately.

MANAGEMENT. Three parasiticide treatment regimens should be considered:
- Praziquantel: 5–10 p.p.m. as a 3–6-hour bath, repeated in seven days. The fish should be placed in a treatment tank, if possible, and the water must be well aerated. Some marine species may be sensitive to praziquantel.

The aquarium may still be contaminated, so treated fish should ideally be moved to a new aquarium. Praziquantel may not kill all species of monogeneans. This treatment will kill most internal cestodes.
- Saltwater/freshwater dips: these may be effective against some parasites. Marine fish can be placed in a freshwater dip for 4–5 minutes and freshwater fish placed in saltwater (35 p.p.t salt) for 4–5 minutes.
- Acetic acid: 2 ml glacial acetic acid/liter of water as a 30–45-second dip is safe for goldfish, but smaller tropical fish may not tolerate this treatment.

Case 395: **Bird predation**

CLINICAL PROBLEM. Piscivorous birds such as herons (**395a**) and cormorants can be serious predators of ornamental pond fish, causing loss, damage, and stress.

MANAGEMENT. Several measures can be taken to reduce the risk of bird predation:
- Ensure that the pond is deep enough and provide plants and structures within the pond to allow the fish to seek refuge.
- Ensure that pond sides are steep enough not to allow birds to land and stand at the pond edges. Wires or monofilament line over the pond can be used to prevent access, but these must be high enough not to allow birds to use the wires as perches to obtain fish. Monofilament fishing line has been used for this purpose (**395b**).
- Artificial predatory birds and other decoys may act as deterrents.

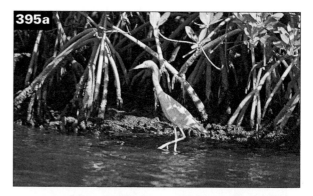

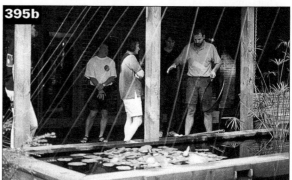

Case 396: **Gill function**

DISCUSSION. The normal microscopic structure of a gill is shown (**396**). The gill has several functions:
- Respiration. The gill is the site of gas exchange, where dissolved oxygen in the aquatic environment diffuses into the blood, and carbon dioxide diffuses out.
- Nitrogenous excretion. Unlike mammals, where nitrogenous waste is excreted in the form of urea in the urine, this route accounts for only about 10% of nitrogenous waste excretion in fish. The majority is excreted through the gill in the form of ammonia. Ammonia is very soluble in water, forming ammonium and hydroxyl ions. The ammonia and ammonium ions are then either washed away or metabolized by bacteria to nitrite and then nitrate as part of the nitrogen cycle.
- Fluid balance. To maintain the correct fluid balance, there are active transport mechanisms in the gill to regulate sodium and chloride concentrations. In freshwater fish this involves the uptake of sodium ions (in exchange for ammonium and hydrogen ions) and chloride ions (in exchange for bicarbonate ions). In marine fish the problem is reversed and sodium and chloride ions are actively excreted.

The anatomic structure of the gills aids the functions listed above in the following ways:

- To perform these functions, the blood and the water must be separated by only a very thin layer of tissue. The gill surface available for exchange must also be as large as possible. This is achieved by the anatomic arrangement of the gill filaments, which are divided into multiple finger-like processes, the primary lamellae, which in turn are subdivided into secondary lamellae. The membrane covering the secondary lamellae provides the exchange surface. Under normal circumstances there is very little mucus produced at the gill lamellar surfaces.

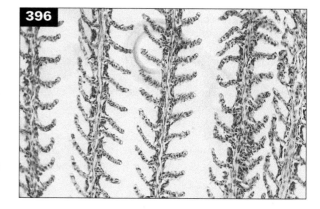

- Gill function is additionally facilitated by the continuous passage of water over the gill surface resulting from the unidirectional pumping action of the buccal cavity and opercula.

Hyperplasia results in shortening and rounding of the secondary lamellae, and this affects the structure and function of the gills. As the condition progresses, adjacent secondary lamellae fuse, resulting in clubbing. This greatly reduces the surface area available for exchange. The irritants causing hyperplasia also stimulate excessive mucus production, which further compromises gill function.

Case 397: **Ozonation**

CLINICAL PROBLEM. A hobbyist client, who raises a variety of killifish, has sought advice because of a recurrent problem with mixed protozoal infections. Several outbreaks had been treated previously, each apparently caused by a different mixture of organisms. The client shows her fish regularly and cannot pass up new and exciting specimens she finds at the shows. She has been encouraged to set up strict quarantine procedures, but she is reluctant to keep her short-lived new fish isolated for a prolonged period. Instead, she has decided that she wants to install an ozonation chamber on her main system, which recycles water through 50 tanks containing a total of approximately 5,000 liters. Unfortunately, there are dozens of different ozonation systems, all touting different strengths and amounts, but all of the literature refers to bacterial infections.

MANAGEMENT/DISCUSSION. Ozonation is becoming more popular for dedicated hobbyists with multiple tank systems. Hobbyists should be advised of the risk of ozone to human lungs and encouraged to use systems that have a sealed contact chamber. Ozone can cause permanent lung scarring at levels that cannot be detected by the human nose. Hobbyists should also be made aware of the effects of ozone on plastic and rubber. Systems must be checked frequently for deterioration of polymer parts. The contact chamber or countercurrent system should provide for a minimum of five minutes contact time and preferably 10 minutes. This will reduce the risk of free ozone reaching the tanks. Attempts to solve problems caused by organisms that colonize tanks by ozonating side streams of water are rarely successful. Only the organisms that reach the contact chamber are affected by the ozone. Protozoa are less susceptible to ozone than most bacteria and require a higher dose.

Case 398: **Secondary gill lamellar hyperplasia**

DISCUSSION. Secondary gill lamellar hyperplasia can occur due to an environmental toxin or bacterial pathogen. In this photomicrograph of a primary gill lamella (398a) there are numerous secondary lamellae that are partially fused with one another.

A histologic section of normal healthy gill tissue is shown (398b). Note the even, parallel, unfused secondary lamellae extending nearly perpendicular from the primary gill lamella. The fresh whole mount shows even, secondary gill lamellae (398c). Note the lack of mucus or parasites.

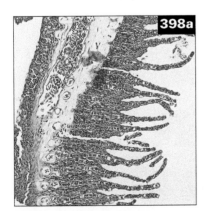
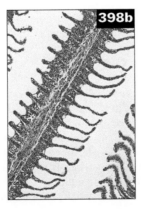
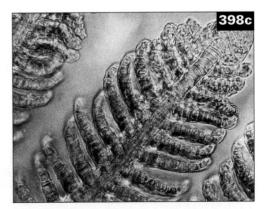

Case 399: **Anesthesia**

DISCUSSION. A fish has been anesthetized (**399**). There are four stages of anesthesia in fish, as described below, and the following can be observed when using tricaine methanesulfonate (MS-222):

- **Stage 1.** Sedation. This is observed as coordinated excitatory behavior with increased respiratory rate. This often appears to be a short stage of anesthesia in a fish that is induced with water-borne anesthetic agents such as MS-222. It is often difficult to determine where stage 1 ends and stage 2 begins.
- **Stage 2.** Excitement. This is recognized by thrashing and jumping, sometimes violent. A loss of coordination accompanies these behaviors. It is important to prevent the fish from injuring itself or jumping from its container during this time. Eventually the thrashing will subside, the fish will lose its equilibrium, and fin movements will cease. Reflex motion and response to tactile stimuli are maintained.
- **Stage 3.** Surgical. This stage is divided into four planes:
  - Plane 1. The fish no longer responds to tactile stimulation. Respiration remains strong and the fish will respond to painful stimuli.
  - Plane 2. Respiratory rate slows and there is a loss of response to painful stimuli. This is the most desirable depth of anesthesia for surgical procedures.
  - Plane 3. Respiration is severely depressed.
  - Plane 4. Further respiratory depression. Careful observation is required to observe any opercular/gill movement. Surgical planes 3 and 4 may be required for procedures requiring absolutely no movement. These procedures should only be attempted by persons experienced in fish anesthesia.
- **Stage 4.** Cardiovascular collapse. All gill/opercular movements cease. Hypoxia may become evident as blanching of color from the fins. Death follows shortly.

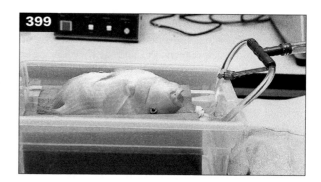

Case 400: **Hematopoietic organs of fish**

DISCUSSION. The main hematopoietic organs of fish are the thymus, head kidney (**400**) (and to a much lesser extent the trunk kidney), and spleen. However, hematopoiesis can occur anywhere along the reticuloendothelial stroma of the vascular system and its associated organs.

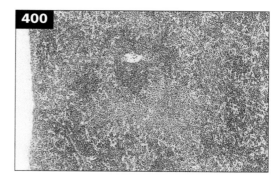

Case 401: **Routine water quality testing**

CLINICAL PROBLEM. Advice is sought on what tests should be performed routinely to check water quality in an ornamental pond and in fish tanks that are housed indoors.

HUSBANDRY. The basic tests to run would be pH, temperature, total ammonia nitrogen (to calculate un-ionized ammonia), nitrite, nitrate, alkalinity, and total hardness. Although it would be helpful to know dissolved oxygen levels, the test can be difficult to perform and might soon discourage further testing. Tests such as alkalinity, hardness, nitrate, and nitrite are more likely to be needed when a tank or pond is first established, whereas pH, ammonia, temperature, and possibly nitrite should be tested on a regular basis. For marine systems, salinity or SG testing is essential.

Summary questions and answers

Q1. What is the most commonly used immersion anesthetic in fish? It is the only approved anesthetic in the US for fish intended for human consumption.

Q2. What is the most important component of any preventive medicine program for captive fish?

Q3. How would you deal with a case of nitrite toxicity in a freshwater aquarium?

Q4. What is the primary organ of hematopoiesis in fish?

Q5. Water quality abnormalities and imbalances are a common predisposing factor to fish morbidity and mortality. What parameters should be tested as part of a routine screening of water quality?

Q6. What is gas bubble disease, and how is it managed?

Q7. What type of swim bladder do cichlids have?

Q8. Compare and contrast 'carp pox' and 'koi herpesvirus'.

Q9. Discuss the proper way to handle fish and include aspects of fish and human health.

Q10. What are the standard primary level (can be implemented in the field or examination room) diagnostic procedures, listed in order, utilized to diagnose a problem in a population of aquarium or pond fishes?

Q11. What is gill (branchial) lamellar hyperplasia, and what is its clinical significance?

Q12. What is the cause of 'grub disease'? Discuss its clinical significance.

Q13. What are the important components to a successful treatment protocol for external protozoal infestations of fish such as *Ichthyophthirius multifiliis* ('Ich'), *Cryptocaryon irritans* (white spot disease), or *Ichthyobodo* species?

Q14. Discuss buoyancy disorders in goldfish and include etiology and management.

Q15. What are some general recommendations regarding nutrition and feeding for pet fish?

A1. Tricaine methanesulfonate (MS-222). This sodium channel blocker is readily available, has a high margin of safety with most freshwater and marine species, and is approved for use in fish intended for human consumption in the US and Canada.

A2. An appropriate quarantine period. Pet fish owners and professional aquarists should be educated on the importance of quarantine and isolation of any new animals, plants, and ornaments before introduction to an established system. While duration of quarantine and treatment of fish during this period varies with species, numbers, environmental parameters, etc., a generally accepted guideline is a 30-day period of isolation and observation.

A3. Daily 50% water changes and the addition of sodium chloride to compete with and reduce nitrite uptake by the branchial epithelial tissue. The water should also be well aerated and the cause of the elevated nitrite levels addressed and corrected.

A4. The cranial or head kidney (fish lack bone marrow). Hematopoiesis can occur in other organs as well, including the thymus, spleen, and caudal (tail, trunk) kidney.

A5. Temperature, pH, dissolved oxygen (when appropriate), total ammonia nitrogen (to calculate un-ionized ammonia), nitrite, nitrate, alkalinity, and total hardness. For marine systems, salinity or SG testing is essential.

A6. Gas-bubble disease (or supersaturation) is a condition that occurs in fish as a result of supersaturation of the water with nitrogen, oxygen, or other gases. The most common cause of this problem is a cavitating pump that leads to supersaturation of the water with nitrogen from atmospheric air. Excessive oxygen production by algae and other plants, leading to oxygen supersaturation, is a less frequent cause.

In many cases a large number of the fish have already died by the time the problem is discovered. Locating and correcting the pump problem will prevent this situation in the future. Treatment usually involves finding and eliminating the source of the excessive gas. Air bubbles under the skin and within the fins will usually resolve within a day or two. Air bubbles in the circulatory system, especially in the branchial vasculature, can be fatal.

A7. Cichlids and many fish with spiny fin rays have a physoclistous swim bladder (gas in the swim bladder is regulated by a rete mirabile, which allows for vascular diffusion of gases). Most adult physoclistous fishes do not have a patent pneumatic duct, a tube that connects the esophagus and the swim bladder. Adult fish (e.g. goldfish, koi, and other cyprinids) with a functional pneumatic duct possess a physostomous swim bladder.

A8. 'Carp pox' is caused by infection with *Herpesvirus cyprini*, also called cyprinid herpesvirus 1 (CHV1). The lesions are sometimes classified as neoplasia, but they are really an epidermal hyperplasia. The disease is typically seasonal (periods of low water temperature) and usually affects only a few fish in a pond. Treatment is seldom required because the disease is rarely fatal and is usually self-limiting (lesions resolve when water temperature rise). Lesions may recur the following year.

Koi herpesvirus (KHV) is a disease of koi that is frequently fatal (mortality commonly exceeds 80%). The virus causes a severe branchitis and affected fish literally die of hypoxia. Outbreaks of this disease have been reported in many European countries, Israel, Asia (including Japan), South Africa, and the US. Gross clinical signs include enophthalmia, mottled gills, excessive mucus production, and dermatitis. Diagnosis is made by virus isolation and confirmed by PCR testing of the viral isolates (even without isolation of the virus, PCR testing can be used to detect viral DNA in fresh, infected tissues.) There are reports that a live attenuated vaccine for this disease in koi has been produced. There is also anecdotal evidence that koi 'warmed' to at least 30°C (86°F) may be resistant to an outbreak, since the virus appears restricted to environmental temperatures of 18–26°C (64.4–86°F); however, this 'heat therapy' could produce subclinical carriers of the disease. Since the KHV genome has been determined, other vaccination options are being explored.

One of the best ways to prevent the transmission of these two viral diseases is through adequate quarantine and biosecurity protocols. All new koi should be quarantined for a minimum of 30 days before introduction to an established population.

A9. Latex or plastic gloves should always be worn when handling fish, because fish can carry zoonotic organisms such as *Mycobacterium* species (mycobacteriosis is one of the most common and important zoonotic diseases linked to pet and display fishes). Moistened latex gloves also protect the fish by decreasing the disruption of the protective mucus and epidermal layers, which are important in osmoregulation and immune function. Eye protection can protect the fish handler from splashing water.

Fish should only be handled when absolutely necessary and handling time should be minimized. All work done with the animal should be carefully planned before the fish is captured or restrained. The use of mesh nets should be minimized, and innovative ways to corral and capture fish using clear plastic bags or specialized plastic nets are preferred. Potentially dangerous animals should never be handled alone.

A10. History taking; water testing; hands-off physical examination; hands-on (usually with anesthesia/sedation) physical examination; gill, skin and/or fin biopsies; blood collection; feces collection; fine needle aspiration/fluid collection. Once these data/samples have been collected and recorded, secondary procedures such as radiography, ultrasonography, computed tomography, surgical biopsy, and microbiological culture/sensitivity may be employed.

A11. There are two types of lamellar hyperplasia, primary and secondary. In both cases an insult to the lamellar tissue (toxin, pathogen, water quality imbalance) causes an inflammatory response that leads to lamellar hyperplasia. In mild to moderate cases the secondary lamellae will appear mucus covered and may fuse with adjacent secondary lamellae. In severe cases the primary lamellae (of gill filaments) can become hyperplastic and fused. Lamellar hyperplasia results in gills that are inefficient, or worse, dysfunctional. Since the gills are important for respiration and waste removal, compromised gill tissue, depending on severity, can lead to morbidity and eventually mortality.

A12. This condition is common in wild-caught or pond-raised fishes, both in the aquarium industry and in food fish aquaculture. Aquarists and aquaculturists frequently call this condition yellow or white 'grub' disease. The fish is actually an intermediate host for these parasites, which are digenean trematodes. The definitive host is usually a fish-eating bird or other higher vertebrate, and a molluscan invertebrate, usually a snail, is the first intermediate host.

This condition is usually not harmful to fish and it cannot be transmitted to other fish in the aquarium without the definitive and first intermediate hosts being present. In severe cases, where the metacercaria (grubs) are very numerous or involve internal organs, clinical signs including general debilitation and weight loss can be observed.

There is evidence that treatment using parasiticides that target trematodes (e.g. praziquantel as a bath immersion) will kill the metacercaria.

A13.
- Thorough knowledge of the parasite's life cycle and hosts.
- Selection of an appropriate chemotherapeutant(s) such as formaldehyde.
- Proper environmental management, including temperature, water quality, and fish density.
- Appropriate duration of treatment and frequent water changes.
- Post-treatment diagnostic sampling to determine successful treatment.

A14. Buoyancy disorders of Asian fancy goldfish are common and frequently difficult to resolve. Since the swim bladder has a patent connection to the esophagus (via the pneumatic duct) in goldfish and other cyprinids, it has been suggested that there may be a nutritional component to the problem. Another possibility is that many of these goldfish varieties have been bred for abnormal conformation and thus are prone to be 'off balance'. A clinical work-up, including radiographs and ultrasonography, will usually help define the specific problem, which is commonly associated with an abnormal swim bladder (torsion, overinflated, underinflated, fluid filled, etc.). Buoyancy problems may also be linked to gas in the GI tract, skeletal deformities/fractures, or neurologic problems.

In cases of positive buoyancy due to an overinflated/large swim bladder, air should be aspirated from the overfilled compartment with a needle and syringe. Butterfly catheters can be employed and in most cases the patient should be sedated. The author has confirmed anecdotal reports of fish improving after being fed fresh or cooked peas, although no controlled studies have been performed regarding this 'treatment'. Other conservative therapies include elevating the water temperature, changing the diet (usually from a floating to a sinking food), and adding salt to the water.

In recent years some clinicians have tried using surgical implants (small crystals or stones) to help 'balance' the fish. As more of these surgeries are attempted, and the results published, surgical intervention may become commonplace for this disorder.

A15.
- Store food appropriately between feedings. Generally this means in the refrigerator or freezer for commercially prepared flakes, pellets, and frozen foods.
- Discard any commercial food preparation that is older than six months.
- Only feed live prey when absolutely necessary.
- When having someone who is not familiar with the particular animal(s) or exhibit care for fish, leave clear instructions and contact information, and in some cases provide pre-packaged and labeled meals.

Bibliography

References

Hartman KH, Yanong RPE, Harms CA, Lewbart GA (2006) The future of training for aquatic animal health veterinarians. *Journal of Veterinary Medical Education* **33**, 389–393.

Reimschuessel R, Stewart L, Squibb E, Hirokawa K, Brady T, Brooks D, Shaik B, Hodson C (2005) Fish drug analysis—phish-pharm: a searchable database of pharmacokinetics data in fish. *American Association of Pharmaceutical Scientists Journal* **07(02)**, E288–E327.

Ronen A, Perelberg A, Abramowitz J, Hutoran M, Tinman S, Bejerano L, Steinitz M, Kotler M (2003) Efficient vaccine against the virus causing a lethal disease in cultured *Cyprinus carpio*. *Vaccine* **21**, 4677–4684.

Waltzek TB, Kelley GO, Stone DM, Way K, Hanson L, Fukuda H, Hirono I, Aoli T, Davison AJ, Hedrick RP (2005) Koi herpesvirus represents a third cyprinid herpesvirus (CyHV-3) in the family Herpesviridae. *Journal of General Virology* **86**, 1659–1667.

Wise JK, Heathcott BL, Gonzalez ML (2002) Results of the AVMA survey on companion animal ownership in US pet-owning households. *Journal of the American Veterinary Medical Association* **221(11)**, 1572–1573.

Textbooks

Brown L (1993) *Aquaculture for Veterinarians*. Pergamon Press, Oxford.

Buller NB (2004) *Bacteria from Fish and Other Aquatic Animals: A Practical Identification Manual*. Cabi Publishing, Cambridge, MA.

Campbell TW, Ellis CK (2007) (eds) *Avian and Exotic Animal Hematology and Cytology* (3rd edn) Blackwell Publishing, Ames.

Gratzek JB, Matthews JR (1992) *Aquariology: The Science of Fish Health Management*. Tetra Press, New York.

Johnson EJ (1997) *Koi Health and Disease*. Johnson Veterinary Services, 3805 Robinson Road, Marietta.

Lewbart GA (1998) *Self-Assessment Color Review of Ornamental Fish*. Iowa State University Press, Ames.

Lewbart GA (2005) Fish. In *Exotic Animal Formulary* (3rd edn). (ed JW Carpenter) Elsevier Saunders, St Louis, pp. 5–29.

Noga EJ (2000) *Fish Disease: Diagnosis and Treatment*. Iowa State University Press, Ames.

Saint-Erne N (2002) *Advanced Koi Care*. Erne Enterprises, Glendale.

Stoskopf MK (1993) *Fish Medicine*. WB Saunders, Philadelphia.

Treves-Brown KM (2000) *Applied Fish Pharmacology*. Kluwer Academic Publishers, Dodrecht.

Wildgoose WH (2001) (ed) *Manual of Ornamental Fish* (2nd edn). British Small Animal Veterinary Association, Gloucester.

Journals

Diseases of Aquatic Organisms
Exotic DVM Veterinary Magazine
Journal of Aquatic Animal Health
Journal of Fish Diseases
Journal of the American Veterinary Medical Association
Journal of Zoo and Wildlife Medicine
Journal of Exotic Pet Medicine (Elsevier) (Formerly Seminars in Avian and Exotic Pet Medicine [WB Saunders])
Veterinary Clinics of North America: Exotic Animal Practice (WB Saunders)
Veterinary Record

Industry resources

American Cichlid Association. www.cichlid.org

American Pet Products Manufacturers Association, Inc. www.appma.org

Associated Koi Clubs of America. www.akca.org

Florida Tropical Fish Farms Association (FTFFA). www.ftffa.com

National Ornamental Goldfish Growers Association (NOGGA), 6916 Black's Mill Road, Thurmont, MD 21788 PH: (301)271-7475

Ornamental Fish International (OFI). www.ofish.org

Pet Industry Joint Advisory Council (PIJAC). www.pijac.org

University of Florida Tropical Aquaculture Laboratory. www.fishweb.ifas.ufl.edu/Facilities/RuskinLabPics/RuskinLab.htm

APPENDIX

Conversion factors for converting SI units to Old units

	SI units	Conversion factor	Old units
Hematology			
Eosinophils	$\times 10^9/l$	1	$\times 10^3/\mu l$
Hemoglobin	g/l	0.1	g/dl
PCV	l/l	100	%
RBCs	$\times 10^{12}/l$	1	$\times 10^6/\mu l$
WBCs/NCC	$\times 10^9/l$	1	$\times 10^3/\mu l$
Biochemistry			
ACTH	ng/ml	1	pg/ml
Albumin	g/l	0.1	g/dl
ALT	u/l	1	u/l
AST	u/l	1	u/l
Bilirubin	µmol/l	0.059	mg/dl
Calcium	mmol/l	4	mg/dl
Cholesterol	mmol/l	38.61	mg/dl
CK	u/l	1	u/l
Cortisol	nmol/l	0.036	µg/dl
Creatinine	µmol/l	0.0113	mg/dl
GGT	u/l	1	u/l
Globulin	g/l	0.1	g/dl
Glucose	mmol/l	18	mg/dl
Lead	µmol/l	20.7	µg/l
Phosphorus	mmol/l	3.1	mg/dl
Potassium	mmol/l	1	mEq/l
Sodium	mmol/l	1	mEq/l
Total protein	g/l	0.1	g/dl
Total thyroxine (T4)	nmol/l	0.0777	µg/dl
Triglyceride	mmol/l	88.6	mg/dl
Urea nitrogen	mmol/l	2.8	mg/dl
Uric acid	mmol/l	16.9	mg/dl
Zinc	µmol/l	6.54	µg/dl

Normal values: small mammals

	Male adult weight (grams)	Female adult weight (grams)	Birth weight (grams)	Body temperature (°C)	Lifespan (years)	Area of origin
Golden hamster	85–130	95–150	2–3	37–38	18–24	Syria
Rat	450–520	250–300	5–6	35.9–37.5	2.5–3.5	Europe
Rabbit	1,000–6,000	1,000–6,000	30–80	38.5–40.0	5–12	Europe
Guinea pig	900–1,200	700–900	70–100	37.2–39.5	4–5	South America
Gerbil	65–100	55–85	2.5–3.0	37.0–38.5	3–4	Mongolia
Hedgehog	270–700	270–700	10–18	36–37	10	Africa/Europe
Ferret	1,000–2,000	600–1,000	6–12	37.8–40.0	5–12	Europe
Chinchilla	400–500	400–600	35–60	37–38	15–20	South America
Mouse	20–40	20–40	0.75–2.0	36.5–38.0	1–3	Europe

	Heart rate (per minute)	Resp rate (per minute)	Litter number	Gestation (days)	Breeding onset	Weaning age
Golden hamster	250–500	35–135	5–10	15–18	6–8 weeks	20–25 days
Rat	250–450	70–115	6–14	21–23	65–110 days	21–23 days
Rabbit	130–325	30–60	4–10	29–35	4–9 months	4–6 weeks
Guinea pig	230–380	42–104	2–5	59–72	2–3 months	14–21days
Gerbil	360	90	3–7	25–30	70–85 days	20–26 days
Hedgehog	180–300	25–50	1–9	34–37	3–12 months	5–6 weeks
Ferret	180–400	33–40	4–10	42–44	1 year	6–8 weeks
Chinchilla	160	100	1–4	109–120	6–8 months	8–10 weeks
Mouse	300–800	60–220	4–12	19–21	30–60 days	21–28 days

Normal values: birds

	Normal weight (grams)	Life span (years)	Fledging age (days)	Weaning age (days)	Origin
Canary	15–35	6–12	14	21	Europe
Budgerigar	35–70	8–12	22–26	30–40	Australia
Lovebird	46–63	6–8	30–35	40–55	Africa
Cockateil	80–110	10–12	32–38	47–52	Australia
Small conure (Jenday)	80–105	10–12	35–40	45–70	S America
Blue-headed pionus	230	10–15	40–55	45–70	S America
Blue-fronted Amazon	350	>50	45–60	80–100	S America
Eclectus parrot	347–512	35–45	72–80	100–140	Australia
African grey parrot	395–585	45–55	55–65	80–110	Africa
Umbrella cockatoo	850	50–60	45–60	80–110	Australia
Blue and gold macaw	950–1175	75	70–80	120–150	S America
Mallard	M: 1260 F: 1100	10–15	45	1	Widespread
Swan	M: 12200 F: 8900	25–30	70	5	Widespread
Pigeon	240–300	4–9	28–35	35–40	Widespread
Peregrine falcon	M: 550–760 F: 780–1200	15	35–42	50–60	Europe
Barn owl	M: 231–381 F: 295–395	15	50	70–85	Widespread
Harris' hawk	M: 725 F: 834–1047	18	40	90–120	California to Central S America
Red-tailed hawk	M: 690–1300 F: 900–1460	21	42–48	70	N America

Continued overleaf

Normal values: birds (*continued*)

	Heart rate (per minute)	Resp rate (per minute)	Gavage volumes (ml)	Gavage frequency	Blood collection volumes assuming maximum required is 2 ml	Bolus i/v fluid volume (ml)
Canary	235–265	60–80	0.25–0.75	5–6x	0.15	0.5
Budgerigar	260–270	60–75	0.5–3	4–5x	0.3–0.6	1–2
Lovebird	240–250	50–60	1–3	4–5x	0.4–0.6	2–3
Cockateil	210–250	40–50	2–6	4–5x	0.8–1.0	3–4
Small conure (Jenday)	205–220	40–50	2–6	4–5x	0.8–1.0	4–7
Blue-headed pionus	205–220	40–50	5–8	4–5x	1.5–2.0	4–5
Blue-fronted Amazon	125–160	20–45	6–12	4x	2	8–12
Eclectus parrot	115–160	15–40	6–12	4x	2	8–12
African grey parrot	110–155	15–40	8–15	3–4x	2	8–12
Umbrella cockatoo	125–170	15–40	12–16	3–4x	2	10–15
Blue and gold macaw	115–135	20–25	20–40	3–4x	2	15–25
Mallard	180–230	30–95	20–30	3x	2	20–25
Swan	80–150	13–40	100–200	3x	2	150–200
Pigeon	244	35–45	10–12	4–5x	2	4–7
Peregrine falcon	250–320	20–30	15–30	3–4x	2	8–12
Barn owl	205–230	30–45	6–10	4–5x	2	4–6
Harris' hawk	150–180	15–30	15–25	4x	2	10–15
Red-tailed hawk	140–185	15–20	20–30	3–4x	2	10–20

INDEX

For Product Safety Concerns and Information please contact
our EU representative GPSR@taylorandfrancis.com Taylor & Francis
Verlag GmbH, Kaufingerstraße 24, 80331 München, Germany

T - #0307 - 160425 - C320 - 261/194/14 - PB - 9781840760552 - Gloss Lamination